Human Genome Editing

SCIENCE, ETHICS, AND GOVERNANCE

Committee on Human Gene Editing:
Scientific, Medical, and Ethical Considerations

A Report of

The National Academies of
SCIENCES · ENGINEERING · MEDICINE

THE NATIONAL ACADEMIES PRESS
Washington, DC
www.nap.edu

THE NATIONAL ACADEMIES PRESS 500 Fifth Street, NW Washington, DC 20001

This activity was supported by Contract No. HHSP233201400020B/HHSP23337045 with the Defense Advanced Research Projects Agency, the Greenwall Foundation, Grant No. 15-108819-000-DIS with the John D. and Catherine T. MacArthur Foundation, Contract No. HHSP233201400020B/HHSP23337035 with the U.S. Food and Drug Administration of the U.S. Department of Health and Human Services, and the Wellcome Trust, with additional support from the National Academies of Sciences, Engineering, and Medicine's Presidents' Circle Fund and the National Academy of Sciences W.K. Kellogg Foundation Fund. Any opinions, findings, conclusions, or recommendations expressed in this publication do not necessarily reflect the views of any organization or agency that provided support for the project.

International Standard Book Number-13: 978-0-309-45288-5
International Standard Book Number-10: 0-309-45288-0
Digital Object Identifier: https://doi.org/10.17226/24623
Library of Congress Control Number: 2017938606

Additional copies of this publication are available for sale from the National Academies Press, 500 Fifth Street, NW, Keck 360, Washington, DC 20001; (800) 624-6242 or (202) 334-3313; http://www.nap.edu.

Printed in the United States of America

Suggested citation: National Academies of Sciences, Engineering, and Medicine. 2017. *Human Genome Editing: Science, Ethics, and Governance*. Washington, DC: The National Academies Press. doi: https://doi.org/10.17226/24623.

The National Academies of
SCIENCES · ENGINEERING · MEDICINE

The **National Academy of Sciences** was established in 1863 by an Act of Congress, signed by President Lincoln, as a private, nongovernmental institution to advise the nation on issues related to science and technology. Members are elected by their peers for outstanding contributions to research. Dr. Marcia McNutt is president.

The **National Academy of Engineering** was established in 1964 under the charter of the National Academy of Sciences to bring the practices of engineering to advising the nation. Members are elected by their peers for extraordinary contributions to engineering. Dr. C. D. Mote, Jr., is president.

The **National Academy of Medicine** (formerly the Institute of Medicine) was established in 1970 under the charter of the National Academy of Sciences to advise the nation on medical and health issues. Members are elected by their peers for distinguished contributions to medicine and health. Dr. Victor J. Dzau is president.

The three Academies work together as the **National Academies of Sciences, Engineering, and Medicine** to provide independent, objective analysis and advice to the nation and conduct other activities to solve complex problems and inform public policy decisions. The National Academies also encourage education and research, recognize outstanding contributions to knowledge, and increase public understanding in matters of science, engineering, and medicine.

Learn more about the National Academies of Sciences, Engineering, and Medicine at **www.national-academies.org**.

The National Academies of
SCIENCES · ENGINEERING · MEDICINE

Reports document the evidence-based consensus of an authoring committee of experts. Reports typically include findings, conclusions, and recommendations based on information gathered by the committee and committee deliberations. Reports are peer reviewed and are approved by the National Academies of Sciences, Engineering, and Medicine.

Proceedings chronicle the presentations and discussions at a workshop, symposium, or other convening event. The statements and opinions contained in proceedings are those of the participants and have not been endorsed by other participants, the planning committee, or the National Academies of Sciences, Engineering, and Medicine.

For information about other products and activities of the National Academies, please visit nationalacademies.org/whatwedo.

COMMITTEE ON HUMAN GENE EDITING: SCIENTIFIC, MEDICAL, AND ETHICAL CONSIDERATIONS

DIETRAM A. SCHEUFELE, John E. Ross Professor in Science
Communication and Vilas Distinguished Achievement Professor,
University of Wisconsin–Madison
ISMAIL SERAGELDIN, Founding Director, Bibliotheca Alexandrina
SHARON TERRY, President and CEO, Genetic Alliance
JONATHAN WEISSMAN, Professor, Department of Cellular and
Molecular Pharmacology, University of California, San Francisco;
Investigator, Howard Hughes Medical Institute
KEITH R. YAMAMOTO, Vice Chancellor for Science Policy and
Strategy, Vice Dean for Research for the School of Medicine,
Professor, University of California, San Francisco

Study Staff

KATHERINE W. BOWMAN, Study Director
MONICA L. GONZALEZ, Associate Program Officer
JOANNA R. ROBERTS, Senior Program Assistant
ANDREW M. POPE, Director, Board on Health Sciences Policy
FRANCES E. SHARPLES, Director, Board on Life Sciences

Consultants

RONA BRIERE, Editor
HELAINE RESNICK, Editor

Dedication

Dr. Ralph Cicerone (1943-2016) was President of the National Academy of Sciences in 2015 when, in partnership with the President of the National Academy of Medicine, he announced a human genome-editing initiative that would encompass science, ethics, and regulation. He noted that the National Academies of Sciences, Engineering, and Medicine have led the effort to develop responsible, comprehensive policies for many emerging and controversial areas of genetics and cell biology, such as human embryonic stem cell research, human cloning, and "gain-of-function" research. Most notable was its involvement in key events leading up to the 1975 Asilomar conference. But there are important differences between the Asilomar era and today, Dr. Cicerone said in an interview with *Nature*, because few researchers were pursuing recombinant DNA research in 1975. Modern genome-editing techniques are easy to use and widely accessible, leading him to conclude that the situation requires an approach that is "really more international than Asilomar ever had to be."

Dr. Cicerone was as good as his word. In collaboration with science and medicine academies from China and the United Kingdom, an initiative was launched with an international summit. From this came a commitment to future summits and the formation of a study committee, with members hailing from or working in Canada, China, Egypt, France, Germany, Israel, Italy, Spain, the United Kingdom, and the United States. This report is the culmination of the work by that committee and is dedicated to this great leader of the National Academy of Sciences.

Reviewers

This report was reviewed in draft form by individuals chosen for their diverse perspectives and technical expertise. The purpose of this independent review is to provide candid and critical comments that will assist the institution in making its published report as sound as possible and to ensure that the report meets institutional standards for objectivity, evidence, and responsiveness to the study charge. The review comments and draft manuscript remain confidential to protect the integrity of the deliberative process. We wish to thank the following individuals for their review of this report:

Eli Adashi, Brown University
George Annas, Boston University
Dana Carroll, University of Utah
Michael Dahlstrom, Iowa State University
Hank Greely, Stanford University
J. Benjamin Hurlbut, Arizona State University
Maria Jasin, Memorial Sloan Kettering Cancer Center
James Lawford-Davies, Hempsons Law Firm, United Kingdom
Andrew Maynard, Arizona State University
Krishanu Saha, University of Wisconsin–Madison
Fyodor Urnov, Altius Institute
Keith Wailoo, Princeton University

Although the reviewers listed above provided many constructive comments and suggestions, they were not asked to endorse the conclusions or recommendations, nor did they see the final draft of the report before its release. The review of this report was overseen by **Harvey Fineberg** (Moore Foundation) and **Jonathan Moreno** (University of Pennsylvania). They were responsible for making certain that an independent examination of this report was carried out in accordance with institutional procedures and that all review comments were carefully considered. Responsibility for the final content of this report rests entirely with the authoring committee and the institution.

Preface

Genome editing—a suite of methods for creating changes in DNA more accurately and flexibly than previous approaches—was hailed as the 2011 Method of the Year by *Nature Methods*, and the CRISPR/Cas9 system of genome editing was named the 2015 Breakthrough of the Year by *Science*. The technology has excited interest across the globe because of the insights it may offer into fundamental biological processes and the advances it may bring to human health. But with these advances come many questions, about the technical aspects of achieving desired results while avoiding unwanted effects, and about a range of uses that may include not only healing the sick, but also preventing disease in this and future generations, or even altering traits unrelated to health needs. Now is the time to consider these questions. Clinical trials using edited human somatic cells are already underway, and more are anticipated. To help direct the use of genome editing toward broadly promoting human well being, it is important to examine the scientific, ethical, and social issues it raises, and assess the capacity of governance systems to ensure the technologies' responsible development and use. Doing so also entails articulating the larger principles that should underlie such systems.

These were not easy tasks, but we are profoundly grateful to the committee members who joined us in tackling our charge. They willingly and thoughtfully brought their diverse perspectives to bear on our discussions, and we thank them for their commitment to this study and for devoting so much of their time and energy over the past year. It has been a pleasure and a privilege to work with them. The report was also informed by many presentations and discussions with speakers whose contributions provided a wealth of information and insight. We thank them for sharing their research and viewpoints with us. Finally, on behalf of the committee, we would like to thank the staff of the National Academies of Sciences, Engineering, and Medicine for working alongside us throughout the study—their ideas and support were crucial to bringing the project to fruition—and thank the sponsors of the study, who had an expansive vision for its potential.

R. Alta Charo and Richard O. Hynes, *Co-Chairs*
Committee on Human Gene Editing: Scientific,
Medical, and Ethical Considerations

Contents

Boxes, Figures, and Tables

BOXES

FIGURES

TABLES

Summary[1]

Genome editing[2] is a powerful new tool for making precise additions, deletions, and alterations to the genome—an organism's complete set of genetic material. The development of new approaches—involving the use of meganucleases; zinc finger nucleases (ZFNs); transcription activator-like effector nucleases (TALENS); and, most recently, the CRISPR/Cas9 system—has made editing of the genome much more precise, efficient, flexible, and less expensive relative to previous strategies. With these advances has come an explosion of interest in the possible applications of genome editing, both in conducting fundamental research and potentially in promoting human health through the treatment or prevention of disease and disability. The latter possibilities range from restoring normal function in diseased organs by editing somatic cells to preventing genetic diseases in future children and their descendants by editing the human germline.

As with other medical advances, each such application comes with its own set of benefits, risks, regulatory frameworks, ethical issues, and societal implications. Important questions raised with respect to genome editing include how to balance potential benefits against the risk of unintended

---

[1]This summary does not include references. Citations for the discussion presented in the summary appear in the subsequent report chapters.

[2]The term "genome editing" is used throughout this report to refer to the processes by which the genome sequence is changed by adding, replacing, or removing DNA base pairs. This term is used in lieu of "gene editing" because it is more accurate, as the editing could be targeted to sequences that are not part of genes themselves, such as areas that regulate gene expression.

1

harms; how to govern the use of these technologies; how to incorporate societal values into salient clinical and policy considerations; and how to respect the inevitable differences, rooted in national cultures, that will shape perspectives on whether and how to use these technologies.

Recognizing both the promise and concerns related to human genome editing, the National Academy of Sciences and the National Academy of Medicine convened the Committee on Human Gene Editing: Scientific, Medical, and Ethical Considerations to carry out the study that is documented in this report. While genome editing has potential applications in agriculture and nonhuman animals, this committee's task was focused on human applications. The charge to the committee included elements pertaining to the state of the science in genome editing, possible clinical applications of these technologies, potential risks and benefits, whether standards can be established for quantifying unintended effects, whether current regulatory frameworks provide adequate oversight, and what overarching principles should guide the regulation of genome editing in humans.

OVERVIEW OF GENOME-EDITING APPLICATIONS AND POLICY ISSUES

Genome-editing methods based on protein recognition of specific DNA sequences, such as those involving the use of meganucleases, ZFNs, and TALENs, are already being tested in several clinical trials for application in human gene therapy, and recent years have seen the development of a system based on RNA recognition of such DNA sequences. CRISPR (which stands for clustered regularly interspaced short palindromic repeats) refers to short, repeated segments of DNA originally discovered in bacteria. These segments provided the foundation for the development of a system that combines short RNA sequences paired with Cas9 (CRISPR associated protein 9, an RNA-directed nuclease), or with similar nucleases, and can readily be programmed to edit specific segments of DNA. The CRISPR/Cas9 genome-editing system offers several advantages over previous strategies for making changes to the genome and has been at the center of much discussion concerning how genome editing could be applied to promote human health. Like the use of meganucleases, ZFNs, and TALENs, CRISPR/Cas9 genome-editing technology exploits the ability to create double-stranded breaks in DNA and the cells' own DNA repair mechanisms to make precise changes to the genome. CRISPR/Cas9, however, can be engineered more easily and cheaply than these other methods to generate intended edits in the genome.

The fact that these new genome-editing technologies can be used to make precise changes in the genome at a high frequency and with considerable accuracy is driving intense interest in research to develop safe and effective therapies that use these approaches and that offer options beyond simply replacing an entire gene. It is now possible to insert or delete single nucleotides, interrupt a gene or genetic element, make a single-stranded break in DNA, modify a nucleotide, or make epigenetic changes to gene expression. In the realm of biomedicine, genome editing could be used for three broad purposes: for basic research, for somatic interventions, and for germline interventions.

Basic research can focus on cellular, molecular, biochemical, genetic, or immunological mechanisms, including those that affect reproduction and the development and progression of disease, as well as responses to treatment. Such research can involve work on human cells or tissues, but unless it has the incidental effect of revealing information about an identifiable, living individual, it does not involve human subjects as defined by federal regulation in the United States. Most basic research on human cells uses somatic cells—nonreproductive cell types such as skin, liver, lung, and heart cells—although some basic research uses germline (i.e., reproductive) cells, including early-stage human embryos, eggs, sperm, and the cells that give rise to eggs and sperm. These latter cases entail ethical and regulatory considerations regarding how the cells are collected and the purposes for which they are used, even though the research involves no pregnancy and no transmission of changes to another generation.

Unlike basic research, clinical research involves interventions with human subjects. In the United States and most other countries with robust regulatory systems, proposed clinical applications must undergo a supervised research phase before becoming generally available to patients. Clinical applications of genome editing that target somatic cells affect only the patient, and are akin to existing efforts to use gene therapy for disease treatment and prevention; they do not affect offspring. By contrast, germline interventions would be aimed at altering a genome in a way that would affect not only the resulting child but potentially some of the child's descendants as well.

A number of the ethical, legal, and social questions surrounding gene therapy and human reproductive medicine provide a backdrop for consideration of key issues related to genome editing. When conducted carefully and with proper oversight, gene therapy research has enjoyed support from many stakeholder groups. But because such technologies as CRISPR/Cas9 have made genome editing so efficient and precise, they have opened up possible applications that have until now been viewed as largely theoretical. Germline editing to prevent genetically inherited disease is one example. Potential applications of editing for "enhancement"—for changes that go beyond mere restoration or protection of health—are another.

Because genome editing is only beginning to transition from basic research to clinical research applications, now is the time to evaluate the full range of its possible uses in humans and to consider how to advance and govern these scientific developments. The speed at which the science is developing has generated considerable enthusiasm among scientists, industry, health-related advocacy organizations, and patient populations that perceive benefit from these advances. It is also raising concerns, such as those cited earlier, among policy makers and other interested parties to voice concerns about whether appropriate systems are in place to govern the technologies and whether societal values will be reflected in how genome editing is eventually applied in practice.

Public input and engagement are important elements of many scientific and medical advances. This is particularly true with respect to genome editing for potential applications that would be heritable—those involving germline cells—as well as those focused on goals other than disease treatment and prevention. Meaningful engagement with decision makers and stakeholders promotes transparency, confers legitimacy, and improves policy making. There are many ways to engage the public in these debates, ranging from public information campaigns to formal calls for public comment and incorporation of public opinion into policy.

APPLICATIONS OF HUMAN GENOME EDITING

Genome editing is already being widely used for basic science research in laboratories; is in the early stages of development of clinical applications that involve somatic (i.e., nonreproductive) cells; and in the future might be usable for clinical applications involving reproductive cells, which would produce heritable changes.

Basic Science Laboratory Research

Basic laboratory research involving genome editing of human cells and tissues is critical to advancing biomedical science. Genome-editing research using somatic cells can advance understanding of molecular processes that control disease development and progression, potentially facilitating the ability to develop better interventions for affected people. Laboratory research involving genome editing of germline cells can help in understanding human development and fertility, thereby supporting advances in such areas as regenerative medicine and fertility treatment.

The ethical issues associated with basic science research involving genome editing are the same as those that arise with any basic research involving human cells or tissues, and these issues are already addressed by extensive regulatory infrastructures. There are, of course, enduring debates about limitations of the current system, particularly with respect to how it addresses the use of gametes, embryos, and fetal tissue, but the regulations are considered adequate for oversight of basic science research, as evidenced by their longevity. Special considerations may come into play for research involving human gametes and embryos in jurisdictions where such research is permitted; in those cases, the current regulations governing such work will apply to genome-editing research as well. Overall, then, basic laboratory research in human genome editing is already manageable under existing ethical norms and regulatory frameworks at the local, state, and federal levels.

Clinical Uses of Somatic Cell Editing for Treatment and Prevention of Disease and Disability

An example of the application of genome editing to alter somatic (nonreproductive) cells for purposes of treating or preventing disease is a recently authorized clinical trial involving patients whose advanced cancer has failed to respond to such conventional treatments as chemotherapy and radiation. In this study, genome editing is being used to program patients' immune cells to target the cancer.

Somatic cells are all those present in the tissues of the body except for sperm and egg cells and their precursors. This means that the effects of genome editing of somatic cells are limited to treated individuals and are not inherited by their offspring. The idea of making genetic changes to somatic cells—referred to as "gene therapy"—is not new, and genome editing for somatic applications would be similar. Gene therapy has been governed by ethical norms and subject to regulatory oversight for some time, and this experience offers guidance for establishing similar norms and oversight mechanisms for genome editing of somatic cells.

Somatic genome-editing therapies could be used in clinical practice in a number of ways. Some applications could involve removing relevant cells—such as blood or bone marrow cells—from a person's body, making specific genetic changes, and then returning the cells to that same individual. Because the edited cells would be outside the body (ex vivo), the success of the editing could be verified before the cells were replaced in the patient. Somatic genome editing also could be performed directly in the body (in vivo) by injecting a genome-editing tool into the bloodstream or target organ. Technical challenges remain, however, to the effective delivery of in vivo genome editing. Gene-editing tools introduced into the body might not find their target gene within the intended cell type efficiently. The result could be little or no health benefit to the patient, or even unintended harm, such as inadvertent effects on germline cells, for which screening would be necessary. Despite these challenges, however, clinical trials of in vivo editing strategies are already under way for hemophilia B and mucopolysaccharidosis I.

The primary scientific and technical, ethical, and regulatory issues associated with the use of somatic gene therapies to treat or prevent disease or disability concern only the individual. The scientific and technical issues of genome editing, such as the as-yet incompletely developed standards for measuring and evaluating off-target events, can be resolved through ongoing improvements in efficiency and accuracy, while the ethical and regulatory issues would be taken into account as part of existing regulatory frameworks that involve assessing the balance of anticipated risks and benefits to a patient.

Overall, the committee concluded that the ethical norms and regulatory regimes developed for human clinical research, gene transfer research, and existing somatic cell therapy are appropriate for the management of new somatic genome-editing applications aimed at treating or preventing disease and disability. However, off-target effects will vary with the platform technology, cell type, target gene, and other factors. As a result, no single standard for somatic genome-editing efficiency or specificity—and no single acceptable off-target rate—can be defined at this time. For this reason, and because, as noted above, somatic genome editing can be carried out in a number of different ways, regulators will need to consider the technical context of the genome-editing system as well as the proposed clinical application in weighing anticipated risks and benefits.

Germline Editing and Heritable Changes

Although editing of an individual's germline (reproductive) cells has been achieved in animals, there are major technical challenges to be addressed in developing this technology for safe and predictable use in humans. Nonetheless, the technology is of interest because thousands of inherited diseases are caused by mutations in single genes.[3] Thus, editing the germline cells of individuals who carry these mutations could allow them to have genetically related children without the risk of passing on these conditions. Germline genome editing is unlikely to be used often enough in the foreseeable future to have a significant effect on the prevalence of these diseases but could provide some families with their best or most acceptable option for averting disease transmission, either because existing technologies, such as prenatal or preimplantation genetic diagnosis, will not work in some cases or because the existing technologies involve discarding affected embryos or using selective abortion following prenatal diagnosis.

At the same time, however, germline editing is highly contentious precisely because the resulting genetic changes could be inherited by the next

---

[3]OMIM, https://www.omim.org (accessed January 5, 2017); Genetic Alliance, http://www.diseaseinfosearch.org (accessed January 5, 2017).

generation, and the technology therefore would cross a line many have viewed as ethically inviolable. The possibility of making heritable changes through the use of germline genome editing moves the conversation away from individual-level concerns and toward significantly more complex technical, social, and religious concerns regarding the appropriateness of this degree of intervention in nature and the potential effects of such changes on acceptance of children born with disabilities. Policy in this area will require a careful balancing of cultural norms, the physical and emotional well-being of children, parental autonomy, and the ability of regulatory systems to prevent inappropriate or abusive applications.

In light of the technical and social concerns involved, the committee concluded that heritable genome-editing research trials might be permitted, but only following much more research aimed at meeting existing risk/benefit standards for authorizing clinical trials and even then, only for compelling reasons and under strict oversight. It would be essential for this research to be approached with caution, and for it to proceed with broad public input.

In the United States, authorities currently are unable to consider proposals for this research because of an ongoing prohibition on the U.S. Food and Drug Administration's (FDA's) use of federal funds to review "research in which a human embryo is intentionally created or modified to include a heritable genetic modification."[4] In a number of other countries, germline genome-editing trials would be prohibited entirely. If U.S. restrictions on such trials were allowed to expire or if countries without legal prohibitions were to proceed with them, it would be essential to limit these trials only to the most compelling circumstances, to subject them to a comprehensive oversight framework that would protect the research subjects and their descendants, and to institute safeguards against inappropriate expansion into uses that are less compelling or well understood. In particular, clinical trials using heritable genome editing should be permitted only if done within a regulatory framework that includes the following criteria and structures:

- absence of reasonable alternatives;
- restriction to preventing a serious disease or condition;
- restriction to editing genes that have been convincingly demonstrated to cause or to strongly predispose to the disease or condition;
- restriction to converting such genes to versions that are prevalent in the population and are known to be associated with ordinary health with little or no evidence of adverse effects;

---

[4]Consolidated Appropriations Act of 2016, Public Law 114-113 (adopted December 18, 2015).

- availability of credible preclinical and/or clinical data on risks and potential health benefits of the procedures;
- ongoing, rigorous oversight during clinical trials of the effects of the procedure on the health and safety of the research participants;
- comprehensive plans for long-term, multigenerational follow-up that still respect personal autonomy;
- maximum transparency consistent with patient privacy;
- continued reassessment of both health and societal benefits and risks, with broad ongoing participation and input by the public; and
- reliable oversight mechanisms to prevent extension to uses other than preventing a serious disease or condition.

Even those who will support this recommendation are unlikely to arrive at it by the same reasoning. For those who find the benefits sufficiently compelling, the above criteria represent a commitment to promoting well-being within a framework of due care and responsible science. Those not completely persuaded that the benefits outweigh the social concerns may nonetheless conclude that these criteria, if properly implemented, are strict enough to prevent the harms they fear. It is important to note that such concepts as "reasonable alternatives" and "serious disease or condition" embedded in these criteria are necessarily vague. Different societies will interpret these concepts in the context of their diverse historical, cultural, and social characteristics, taking into account input from their publics and their relevant regulatory authorities. Likewise, physicians and patients will interpret them in light of the specifics of individual cases for which germline genome editing may be considered as a possible option. Starting points for defining some of these concepts exist, such as the definition of "serious disease or condition" used by the FDA.[5] Finally, those opposed to heritable editing may even conclude that, properly implemented, the above criteria are so strict that they would have the effect of preventing all clinical trials involving germline genome editing.

Use of Genome Editing for "Enhancement"

Although much of the current discussion around genome editing focuses on how these technologies can be used to treat or prevent disease and

---

[5]While not drafted with the above criteria in mind, the FDA definition of "serious disease or condition" is "a disease or condition associated with morbidity that has substantial impact on day-to-day functioning. Short-lived and self-limiting morbidity will usually not be sufficient, but the morbidity need not be irreversible if it is persistent or recurrent. Whether a disease or condition is serious is a matter of clinical judgment, based on its impact on such factors as survival, day-to-day functioning, or the likelihood that the disease, if left untreated, will progress from a less severe condition to a more serious one" (21 CFR 312.300(b)(1)).

disability, some aspects of the public debate concern other purposes, such as the possibility of enhancing traits and capacities beyond levels considered typical of adequate health. In theory, genome editing for such enhancement purposes could involve both somatic and germline cells. Such uses of the technologies raise questions of fairness, social norms, personal autonomy, and the role of government.

To begin, it is necessary to define what is meant by "enhancement." Formulating this definition requires a careful examination of how various stakeholders conceptualize "normal." For example, using genome editing to lower the cholesterol level of someone with abnormally high cholesterol might be considered prevention of heart disease, but using it to lower cholesterol that is in the desirable range is less easily characterized, and would either intervention differ from the current use of statins? Likewise, using genome editing to improve musculature for patients with muscular dystrophy would be considered a restorative treatment, whereas doing so for individuals with no known pathology and average capabilities just to make them stronger but still within the "normal" range might be considered enhancement. And using the technology to increase someone's muscle strength to the extreme end of human capacity (or beyond) would almost certainly be considered enhancement.

Regardless of the specific definition, there is some indication of public discomfort with using genome editing for what is deemed to be enhancement, whether for fear of exacerbating social inequities or of creating social pressure for people to use technologies they would not otherwise choose. Precisely because of the difficulty of evaluating the benefit of an enhancement to an individual given the large role of subjective factors, public discussion is needed to inform the regulatory risk/benefit analyses that underlie decisions to permit research or approve marketing. Public discussion also is needed to explore social impacts, both real and anticipated, as governance policy for such applications is developed. The committee recommends that genome editing for purposes other than treatment or prevention of disease and disability should not proceed at this time, and that it is essential for these public discussions to precede any decisions about whether or how to pursue clinical trials of such applications.

Public Engagement

Public engagement is always an important part of regulation and oversight for new technologies. As noted above, for somatic genome editing, it is essential that transparent and inclusive public policy debates precede any consideration of whether to authorize clinical trials for indications that go beyond treatment or prevention of disease or disability (e.g., for enhancement). With respect to heritable germline editing, broad participation and input by the public and ongoing reassessment of both health and societal benefits and risks are particularly critical conditions for approval of clinical trials.

At present, a number of mechanisms for public communication and consultation are built into the U.S. regulatory system, including some designed specifically for gene therapy, whose purview would include human genome editing. In some cases, regulatory rules and guidance documents are issued only after extensive public comment and agency response. Discussion is fostered by the various state and federal bioethics commissions, which typically bring together technical experts and social scientists in meetings that are open to the public. And the National Institutes of Health's Recombinant DNA Advisory Committee offers a venue for general public discussion of gene therapy, for review of specific protocols, and for transmission of advice to regulators. Other countries, such as France and the United Kingdom, have mechanisms that involve formal polling or hearings to ensure that diverse and informed viewpoints are heard.

PRINCIPLES TO GUIDE THE GOVERNANCE OF HUMAN GENOME EDITING

One of the charges to the committee was to identify principles that many countries might be able to use to govern human genome editing. The principles identified by the committee are detailed in Box S-1. The committee recommends that any nation considering governance of human genome editing consider incorporating these principles—and the responsibilities that flow therefrom—into its regulatory structures and processes.

RECOMMENDATIONS

In light of the considerations detailed above, the committee made a series of recommendations targeted to basic research and to clinical applications, both somatic and germline. A summary of the key messages in these recommendations is found in Box S-2.

BOX S-1
Principles for the Governance of Human Genome Editing

1. Promoting well-being: *The principle of promoting well-being supports providing benefit and preventing harm to those affected, often referred to in the bioethics literature as the principles of beneficence and nonmaleficence.*

Responsibilities that flow from adherence to this principle include (1) pursuing applications of human genome editing that promote the health and well-being of individuals, such as treating or preventing disease, while minimizing risk to individuals in early applications with a high degree of uncertainty; and (2) ensuring a reasonable balance of risk and benefit for any application of human genome editing.

2. Transparency: *The principle of transparency requires openness and sharing of information in ways that are accessible and understandable to stakeholders.*

Responsibilities that flow from adherence to this principle include (1) a commitment to disclosure of information to the fullest extent possible and in a timely manner, and (2) meaningful public input into the policy-making process related to human genome editing, as well as other novel and disruptive technologies.

3. Due care: *The principle of due care for patients enrolled in research studies or receiving clinical care requires proceeding carefully and deliberately, and only when supported by sufficient and robust evidence.*

Responsibilities that flow from adherence to this principle include proceeding cautiously and incrementally, under appropriate supervision and in ways that allow for frequent reassessment in light of future advances and cultural opinions.

4. Responsible science: *The principle of responsible science underpins adherence to the highest standards of research, from bench to bedside, in accordance with international and professional norms.*

Responsibilities that flow from adherence to this principle include a commitment to (1) high-quality experimental design and analysis, (2) appropriate review and evaluation of protocols and resulting data, (3) transparency, and (4) correction of false or misleading data or analysis.

5. Respect for persons: *The principle of respect for persons requires recognition of the personal dignity of all individuals, acknowledgment of the centrality of personal choice, and respect for individual decisions. All people have equal moral value, regardless of their genetic qualities.*

Responsibilities that flow from adherence to this principle include (1) a commitment to the equal value of all individuals, (2) respect for and promotion of individual decision making, (3) a commitment to preventing recurrence of the abusive

continued

BOX S-1 Continued

forms of eugenics practiced in the past, and (4) a commitment to destigmatizing disability.

6. Fairness: *The principle of fairness requires that like cases be treated alike, and that risks and benefits be equitably distributed (distributive justice).*

Responsibilities that flow from adherence to this principle include (1) equitable distribution of the burdens and benefits of research and (2) broad and equitable access to the benefits of resulting clinical applications of human genome editing.

7. Transnational cooperation: *The principle of transnational cooperation supports a commitment to collaborative approaches to research and governance while respecting different cultural contexts.*

Responsibilities that flow from adherence to this principle include (1) respect for differing national policies, (2) coordination of regulatory standards and procedures whenever possible, and (3) transnational collaboration and data sharing among different scientific communities and responsible regulatory authorities.

BOX S-2
Oversight and Use of Human Gene Editing:
Summary of Recommendations

Global Principles for Research and Clinical Use
Consider and apply the global principles in governance of human genome editing *(2.1)*

Promoting well-being
Transparency
Due care
Responsible science
Respect for persons
Fairness
Transnational cooperation

continued

BOX S-2 Continued

Basic Laboratory Research
Use existing regulatory processes to oversee human genome-editing laboratory research *(3.1)*

Somatic Genome Editing
Use existing regulatory processes for human gene therapy to oversee somatic human genome-editing research and uses *(4.1)*

Limit clinical trials or therapies to treatment and prevention of disease or disability at this time *(4.2)*

Evaluate safety and efficacy in the context of risks and benefits of intended use *(4.3)*

Require broad public input prior to extending uses *(4.4)*

Germline (Heritable) Genome Editing
Permit clinical research trials only for compelling purposes of treating or preventing serious disease or disability, and only if there is a stringent oversight system able to limit uses to specified criteria *(5.1)*

Enhancement
Do not proceed at this time with human genome editing for purposes other than treatment or prevention of disease and disability *(6.1)*

Encourage public discussion and policy debate with respect to somatic human genome editing for uses other than treatment or prevention of disease and disability *(6.2)*

Public Engagement
Public input should precede any clinical trials for an extension of human genome editing beyond disease treatment and prevention *(7.1)*

Ongoing reassessment and public participation should precede any clinical trials of heritable germline editing *(7.2)*

Incorporate public participation into the human genome editing policy process concerning "enhancement" *(7.3)*

When funding genome-editing research, consider including research on strategies to improve public engagement *(7.4)* and for long-term assessment of the ethical, legal, and social implications of human genome editing *(7.5)*

1

Introduction

enome editing[1] is a powerful new tool for making precise additions, deletions, and alterations to the genome—an organism's complete set of genetic material. The development of new approaches—involving the use of meganucleases; zinc finger nucleases (ZFNs); transcription activator-like effector nucleases (TALENs); and, most recently, the CRISPR/Cas9 system—has made editing of the genome much more precise, efficient, flexible, and less expensive relative to previous strategies. With these advances has come an explosion of interest in the possible applications of genome editing, both in conducting fundamental research and potentially in promoting human health through the treatment or prevention of disease and disability. The latter possibilities range from editing somatic cells to restore normal function in diseased organs to editing the human germline to prevent genetic diseases in future children and their descendants.

As with other medical advances, each application comes with its own set of benefits, risks, regulatory questions, ethical issues, and societal implications. Important questions raised with respect to genome editing include how to balance potential benefits against the risk of unintended harms; how to govern the use of these technologies; how to incorporate societal values into salient clinical and policy considerations; and how to respect the in-

---

[1]The term "genome editing" is used throughout this report to refer to the processes by which the genome sequence is changed by adding, replacing, or removing DNA base pairs. This term is used in lieu of "gene editing" because it is more accurate, as the editing could be targeted to sequences that are not part of genes themselves, such as areas that regulate gene expression.

evitable differences, rooted in national cultures, that will shape perspectives on whether and how to use these technologies.

Recognizing both the promise and concerns related to human genome editing, the National Academy of Sciences (NAS) and the National Academy of Medicine (NAM)[2] convened the Committee on Human Gene Editing: Scientific, Medical, and Ethical Considerations to carry out the study that is documented in this report. While genome editing has potential applications for use in agriculture and nonhuman animals,[3] this committee's task (see Box 1-1) was focused on human applications.[4] The charge to the committee included elements pertaining to the state of the science in genome editing, possible clinical applications of these technologies, potential risks and benefits, whether standards can be established for quantifying unintended effects, whether current regulatory frameworks provide adequate oversight, and what overarching principles should guide the regulation of genome editing in humans.

STUDY CONTEXT

The NAS and the NAM Human Gene-Editing Initiative

In light of the promise of genome editing and the associated regulatory and ethical issues, the NAS and the NAM established an initiative to explore these issues in greater depth and facilitate U.S. and international dialogue on how to address them. The first activity of this Human Gene-Editing Initiative was the convening of the International Summit on Human

---

[2]The NAS and the NAM are referred to throughout this report simply as the National Academies, or the U.S. National Academies when discussed in relation to the academies of other nations. Until 2016, the NAM was known as the Institute of Medicine (IOM).

[3]In January 2017, the U.S. Food and Drug Administration (FDA) issued revised draft guidance addressing the regulatory pathway for intentionally altered genomic DNA in plants and nonhuman animals. This would include DNA intentionally altered through genome editing. The guidance does not affect the regulatory pathway for human applications that are regulated as human drugs, devices, and biologics. See FDA "Regulation of Intentionally Altered Genomic DNA in Animals—Draft Guidance" (January 2017) at http://www.fda.gov/downloads/AnimalVeterinary/GuidanceComplianceEnforcement/GuidanceforIndustry/ucm113903.pdf (accessed January 30, 2017) and "Genome Editing in New Plant Varieties Used for Foods; Request for Comments" at https://www.regulations.gov/document?D=FDA-2016-N-4389-0001 (accessed January 30, 2017).

[4]The regulatory roles of the federal departments and agencies and the overall framework for regulation of applications of biotechnology are outlined in "Modernizing the Regulatory System for Biotechnology Products: Final Version of the 2017 Update to the Coordinated Framework for the Regulation of Biotechnology" (January 4, 2017) and "National Strategy for Modernizing the Regulatory System for Biotechnology Products" (September 2016) (https://obamawhitehouse.archives.gov/blog/2017/01/04/increasing-transparency-coordination-and-predictability-biotechnology-regulatory [accessed January 30, 2017]).

BOX 1-1
Statement of Task

The study will examine the scientific underpinnings as well as the clinical, ethical, legal, and social implications of the use of human genome-editing technologies in biomedical research and medicine. It will address the following issues related to human gene editing, including editing of the human germline:

1. What is the current state of the science of human gene editing, as well as possible future directions and challenges to further advances in this research?
2. What are the potential clinical applications that may hold promise for the treatment of human diseases? What alternative approaches exist?
3. What is known about the efficacy and risks of gene editing in humans, and what research might increase the specificity and efficacy of human gene editing while reducing risks? Will further advances in gene editing introduce additional potential clinical applications while reducing concerns about patient safety?
4. Can or should explicit scientific standards be established for quantifying off-target genome alterations and, if so, how should such standards be applied for use in the treatment of human diseases?
5. Do current ethical and legal standards for human subjects research adequately address human gene editing, including germline editing? What are the ethical, legal, and social implications of the use of current and projected gene-editing technologies in humans?
6. What principles or frameworks might provide appropriate oversight for somatic and germline editing in humans? How might they help determine whether, and which applications of, gene editing in humans should or should not go forward? What safeguards should be in place to ensure proper conduct of gene-editing research and use of gene-editing techniques?
7. Provide examples of how these issues are being addressed in the international context. What are the prospects for harmonizing policies? What can be learned from the approaches being applied in different jurisdictions?

The committee will address these questions and prepare a report that contains its findings and recommendations. The report will provide a framework based on fundamental, underlying principles that may be adapted and adopted by any nation that is considering the development of guidelines. The report will also include a focus on advice for the United States.

Gene Editing: A Global Discussion jointly with the Chinese Academy of Sciences and The Royal Society of the United Kingdom. This 3-day event addressed a number of scientific advances in the development of modern genome-editing tools, potential medical uses of these tools in human patients, and ethical and social issues their uses might pose. The organizing committee released a statement that summarized its conclusions from the meeting (NASEM, 2016d). Panel chair David Baltimore also noted "we hope that our discussion here will serve as a foundation for a meaningful and ongoing global dialogue" (NASEM, 2016d, p. 6). All three nations embraced the statement's call for continued research on gene editing, further deliberation with regard to heritable changes, and a continued public discourse on the topic.[5] The summit provided important input to the present study, as did other studies by the NAS and the NAM on related topics (see Box 1-2).

This committee was convened to continue the dialogue initiated by the International Summit and to undertake a year-long, in-depth consensus study. As specified in its statement of task (see Box 1-1), the committee examined the state of the science in human genome editing, its potential applications, and the ethical issues that need to be considered in deciding how to govern the use of these powerful new tools. This report is the product of that study and, as with all other National Academies consensus studies, underwent peer review by an independent panel of experts. Additional activities of the Chinese Academy of Sciences and The Royal Society of the United Kingdom are anticipated, including another international summit to take place in China in 2018.

BACKGROUND

U.S. and International Policy Discussions

Among the earliest calls for a detailed examination of the implications of genome-editing technologies were those made by members of the scientific community engaged in developing these tools and advancing their clinical applications. In 2015 a group of investigators and ethicists, including CRISPR/Cas9 developers, met in Napa, California, and subsequently published a request for the community to explore the nature of human genome editing and provide guidance on its acceptable uses (Baltimore et al., 2015). That same year, a number of articles and commentaries appearing in scientific journals and the popular press called attention to scientific and ethical challenges that would be posed by CRISPR/Cas9 and similar

---

[5]Statement by Ralph J. Cicerone, President, U.S. National Academy of Sciences; Victor J. Dzau, President, U.S. National Academy of Medicine; Chunli Bai, President, Chinese Academy of Sciences; and Venki Ramakrishnan, President, The Royal Society (http://www8. nationalacademies.org/onpinews/newsitem.aspx?RecordID=12032015b [accessed January 24, 2017]).

genetic tools (Bosley et al., 2015; Editing Humanity, 2015; Lanphier et al., 2015; Maxmen, 2015; Specter, 2015).

Professional bodies, international organizations, and national academies of sciences and medicine further raised the profile of genome editing by issuing statements on its appropriate uses, particularly in reference to the potential for creating heritable genetic modifications. Among others, they included the U.K. Academy of Medical Sciences and a number of collaborative partners; the European Group on Ethics in Science and New Technologies, an advisory body to the president of the European Commission; the Council of Europe; and the International Society for Stem Cell Research (AMS et al., 2015; Council of Europe, 2015; EGE, 2016; Friedmann et al., 2015; Hinxton Group, 2015; ISSCR, 2015). The United Nations Educational, Scientific, and Cultural Organization (UNESCO) (2015) issued updated guidance to reflect genome-editing advances. Others launched activities to examine the implications of genome editing in greater detail, including the Académie Nationale de Médecine (France) (ANM, 2016); Institut Nationale de la Santé et de la Récherche Médicale (France) (INSERM; Hirsch et al., 2017); Berlin-Brandenburg Academy of Sciences and Humanities (BBAW, 2015); National Academy of Sciences Leopoldina, in partnership with the Deutsche Akademie der Technikwissenshaften (National Academy of Science and Engineering: "acatech"), Deutsche Forschungsgemeinschaft (German Research Foundation: DFG), and Union der deutschen Akademien der Wissenschaften (Union of German Academies of Sciences and Humanities: Academien Union) (National Academy of Sciences Leopoldina et al., 2015); Federation of European Academies of Medicine (FEAM, UKAMS, and ANM, 2017); Royal Netherlands Academy of Arts and Sciences (KNAW, 2016); Nuffield Council on Bioethics (Nuffield Council, 2016b); and others (see Box 1-3).

The Technologies

New or improved tools facilitate scientific progress by making it possible to investigate new kinds of questions and to generate new solutions. In the area of health and medicine, scientists and clinicians have long sought to apply the techniques of molecular biology to understand basic biology—including embryonic development, physiology, and the immune and nervous systems—and to treat or prevent disease. Much progress has been made in elucidating the role of genetics in diseases, ranging from sickle-cell anemia, muscular dystrophy, and cystic fibrosis, to such conditions as deafness, short stature, and blindness. The development of many such diseases and conditions has a genetic component. Some result from straightforward single-gene changes, but most involve a complex interplay of genetic, environmental, and other factors that remain only imperfectly

BOX 1-2
Related Studies of the NAS and the NAM

Genome Editing in Nonhuman Organisms

Because genome-editing methods such as the CRISPR/Cas9 system are simply tools, they can be applied in myriad ways to achieve genetic changes in cells in the laboratory, in microbes, in nonhuman organisms, or in human subjects. The present study, which focuses on the use of genome editing in humans, is part of a broader examination by the U.S. National Academies of the implications of genome editing across a number of applications that also includes projects addressing the following:

- *Genetically Engineered Crops: Experiences and Prospects*—This report addresses safety, environmental, regulatory, and other aspects of food crops developed through the use of genetic engineering technology. Such crops can be produced using a number of methods, and new genome-editing tools are among them (NASEM, 2016c).
- *Gene Drives on the Horizon: Advancing Science, Navigating Uncertainty, and Aligning Research with Public Values*—This report focuses on a specific application enabled by CRISPR/Cas9 technology that allows genetic changes to spread in a population in the absence of selective advantage. This technology is not applicable to every species and is most commonly proposed for such uses as insect vector control. The ability of heritable genetic changes to spread through an ecosystem raises its own complex set of scientific, ethical, and governance challenges (NASEM, 2016b).
- *Workshop on Gene Editing to Modify Animal Genomes for Research: Scientific and Ethical Considerations (Institute for Animal Laboratory Research [ILAR] Roundtable)*—Genome-editing tools can be used to produce laboratory animal models enabling better study of diseases, as well as to produce livestock with desired traits. The workshop explored animal uses of genome editing, along with associated ethical and regulatory considerations (ILAR Roundtable, 2015).
- *Future Biotechnology Products and Opportunities to Enhance Capabilities of the Biotechnology Regulatory System*—As the types of products that can be created through biotechnology expand, these products are evaluated in regulatory frameworks initially created decades ago. This ongoing study is examining capabilities and expertise that may be needed by U.S. regulatory systems to assess and regulate future products that could be created through a number of technologies, including genome editing. The study is not addressing the development and regulation of human drugs or medical devices (NASEM, 2017).

Other Studies on Clinical Research and Applications

Not specific to genome editing but pertinent to discussions about all of its clinical applications are several other recent National Academies reports:

- *Oversight and Review of Clinical Gene Transfer Protocols: Assessing the Role of the Recombinant DNA Advisory Committee* is a report on the role of the U.S. Recombinant DNA Advisory Committee (RAC), recommending that it move toward more judicious use of its advisory power to review specific protocols, and that it focus primarily on novel applications of gene therapy or on providing a venue for broad public debate about the therapy (IOM, 2014).
- *Mitochondrial Replacement Techniques: Ethical, Social, and Policy Considerations* presents an analysis of the special opportunities and concerns associated with making changes in mitochondrial DNA in gametes or embryos (NASEM, 2016e).
- *Guidelines for Embryonic Stem Cell Research* (IOM, 2005; NRC and IOM, 2007, 2008, 2010) outlines the regulatory landscape and provides a roadmap for professional self-regulation for emerging technologies that generate considerable public interest and controversy.

Studies on Public Engagement and Science Communication

- *Communicating Science Effectively: A Research Agenda* finds that people rarely make decisions based only on scientific information; they also consider their own goals and values, and a focus on knowledge alone is not enough to achieve communication goals (NASEM, 2016a).
- *Public Participation in Environmental Assessment and Decision Making* (NRC, 2008) describes how public participation can improve the quality and legitimacy of policy decisions, and enhance trust and understanding among all parties.
- *Understanding Risk: Informing Decisions in a Democratic Society* describes how risk characterization must be responsive to the problem to be solved and to the interests of the parties affected (NRC, 1996).

In concert with the National Academies' Human Gene-Editing Initiative, these studies represent a series of efforts exploring scientific, ethical, and governance issues raised by potential uses of genome editing.

BOX 1-3
Excerpts from Selected Calls Around the World
for Continued Study and Public Discussion

China, the United Kingdom, and the United States
"This is an important moment in human history and we have a responsibility to provide all sections of society with an informed basis for making decisions about this technology, especially for uses that would affect generations to come" (NASEM, 2016d, p. 8).

France
"Our recommendations include setting up a European committee of experts from different disciplines to assess the scope, efficacy and safety of CRISPR–Cas9, and reviewing the ban on all genetic modifications to the germline" (Hirsch et al., 2017, p. 30).

"[We recommend the] establishment of multidisciplinary discussions on the questions posed by the techniques for the germline and embryonic genome editing . . . considered as part of a wider debate on all the medical technologies . . . with potential effects on the genome of unborn children and, possibly, that of subsequent generations" (ANM, 2016, p. 15).

Germany
"It is important to have an objective debate that informs all stakeholders in a clear and transparent manner about the status of research and development into the techniques, and to ensure that any decisions taken are based on sound scientific evidence" (Leopoldina, 2015, p. 27).

The Netherlands
"Public debate would give patients, care providers and society an opportunity to discuss controversial issues, to assess the risks, advantages and conditions of potential germline applications based on growing scientific insight, and to develop good practices and further regulation" (KNAW, 2016, p. 3).

United Kingdom
"Active early engagement with a wide range of global stakeholders will therefore be needed, which should include, but not be limited to, biomedical and social scientists, ethicists, healthcare professionals, research funders, regulators, affected patients and their families, and the wider public" (AMS et al., 2015).

understood. Furthermore, genetic sequences themselves paint only part of the biological picture. Regulation of how and when genes are turned on and off, including the role of the epigenome,[6] continues to be actively explored. Controlled gene expression and epigenetic alterations influence how tissues develop and differentiate and have clinical ramifications in such areas as cancer and embryonic development.

Tools that enable investigators to alter DNA sequences in order to understand or improve their function are not new. Recent years, however, have seen the development of a suite of genome-editing tools that allow for easier, better controlled, and more accurate changes to DNA inside cells. These tools are based on exogenous enzymes that cut DNA at specific locations, combined with endogenous processes that repair the broken DNA, thereby enabling letters of the genetic code to be added, modified, or deleted. The speed with which this technology has been adopted in research laboratories and further adapted to tackle additional scientific challenges is a reflection of how powerful a technique the editing of genes and genomes will be for the scientific and clinical communities.

The earliest applications of nuclease-based genome-editing methods employed targeted recognition of specific DNA sequences by proteins: homing nucleases (also known as meganucleases), ZFNs, and TALENs. However, the recent development of RNA-based targeting has greatly simplified the process of genome editing. The first publications on the subject, in 2012-2013, explained how the CRISPR/Cas9 system, derived from a natural bacterial defense mechanism against infecting viruses, can be harnessed to make controlled genetic changes in any DNA, including that of human cells (Cho et al., 2013; Cong et al., 2013; Jinek et al., 2012, 2013; Mali et al., 2013). This was a game-changing advance. These methods have rapidly been adopted by scientists worldwide and have greatly accelerated fundamental research that has included altering cells in the laboratory to study the functions of particular genes, developing models for studies of human diseases using stem cells or laboratory animals, creating modified plants and animals to improve food production, and developing therapeutic uses in humans. Genome editing has rapidly become an invaluable core technology in research laboratories and biotechnology companies, and is already moving into clinical trials (e.g., Cyranoski, 2016; Reardon, 2016; Urnov et al., 2010).

---

[6]The term "epigenome" refers to a set of chemical modifications to the DNA of the genome and to proteins and RNAs that bind to DNA in the chromosomes to affect whether and how genes are expressed.

The Issues

Individual-Level Concerns

As with other types of medical interventions, whether genome editing can be used in patients will depend largely on understanding the safety and efficacy of the treatment and evaluating whether the anticipated benefits are reasonable with respect to the risk of adverse effects. Treatments based on genome editing are intended to make controlled modifications to specific portions of the DNA that affect the functions of their target(s) while avoiding changes to other portions whose alteration is not desired. The latter alterations, referred to as off-target events, could have consequences, many unnoticeable but others damaging, depending on their location and their effects. In general, human genome editing raises questions common to the process of researching and developing new treatments: which conditions or diseases are most suitable to address with these technologies, how to identify and evaluate off-target events and other potential side effects, and which patients are most appropriate for studies. As described in this report, regulatory systems for addressing the individual-level concerns associated with genome editing already exist in the United States and many other countries, but can be improved.

Societal-Level Concerns

The use of genome editing also has significant social dimensions that vary depending on the proposed application. The use of a genome-editing treatment whose effects are nonheritable and are restricted to an individual patient may not differ greatly from the use of a traditional drug or medical device. By contrast, making changes that may be inherited by future generations raises questions about the extent to which the long-term effects of proposed edits can be predicted and whether it is appropriate for humans to purposely alter any aspect of their genetic future (Frankel and Chapman, 2000; Juengst, 1991; Parens, 1995). In addition, identifying the increased range of applications made possible by genome editing may be yet another challenge to conventional conceptions of what constitutes a disease or disability. Societal-level concerns are particularly acute with respect to genome-editing interventions aimed at enhancing human capabilities. Such applications also raise questions about how to define and promote fairness and equity (President's Council on Bioethics, 2003). Moreover, as with other genetic technologies, such genome-editing applications may raise concerns about coercive and abusive eugenics programs of the past, which were based on faulty science and served discriminatory political goals (Wailoo et al., 2012).

Looking Beyond Safety and Efficacy

Although the nature of the debate surrounding genome editing is not new, the tools available in the past for making genetic modifications in human cells were time-consuming, difficult, and expensive, and were unlikely to be used outside of specialized medical applications. Recent genome-editing technologies, particularly the CRISPR/Cas9 system, have greatly expanded the landscape of potential applications and potential users. Their rapid development and adoption also have shortened the timeline for discussion of what appropriate governance structures need to be identified or developed. As the safety and efficacy of these technologies continue to improve, the critical question will become not whether scientists and clinicians can use genome editing to make a certain change, but whether they should. There is already discussion of do-it-yourself (DIY) editing and the use of genome-editing tools by the biohacker and DIY biology communities, albeit in nonhuman organisms (Brown, 2016; Ledford, 2015). Thorny issues around acceptable uses of the technology in humans will depend on more than scientific considerations, and may increasingly involve weighing factors beyond individual-level risks and benefits (NRC, 1996).

Layered on the scientific and ethical issues associated with human genome editing is the question of how to govern its application so as to facilitate its appropriate use and avoid its misuse. Determining the limits of the technologies' uses and the regulatory mechanisms needed to enforce these limits will vary according to each nation's cultural, political, and legal context. But whether and how best to move human genome editing forward has implications for transnational scientific cooperation that require ongoing public discussion and input into policy making. There is ample precedent for scientists and other stakeholders to engage in just such activities, and this report is intended to build on points raised by a number of international conventions and declarations, such as the Oviedo Convention (1997), the International Declaration on Human Genetic Data (2003), and the Universal Declaration on Bioethics and Human Rights (2005) (Andorno, 2005a,b; UNESCO, 2004a, 2005).

STUDY APPROACH

To address its complex task (see Box 1-1), the committee included members with expertise in basic and clinical research, in the development of human genetic therapies, and in U.S. and international legal and regulatory frameworks. It included biologists, bioethicists, and social scientists, and incorporated perspectives from potentially affected patient and stakeholder communities. Because the ethical and social issues posed by human genome editing transcend national boundaries, the committee included not only

U.S. members but also those who are citizens of or are currently working in Canada, China, Egypt, France, Germany, Israel, Italy, Spain, and the United Kingdom. Brief biographies of the committee members are found in Appendix D.

This study was informed not only by the International Summit described earlier, which immediately preceded the committee's first meeting, but also by review of the salient literature, additional meetings, and speakers who generously shared their knowledge with the committee. Further information on the process by which the committee conducted this study is provided in Appendix C.

In evaluating the implications of new genome-editing tools, the committee also reviewed scientific progress, ethical debates, and regulatory structures related to the use in humans of medical developments such as assisted reproductive technologies, stem cell therapies, gene transfer, and mitochondrial replacement techniques. These developments interface with those of genome editing because editing of stem cells has potential clinical applications for treating or preventing disease, and reproductive technologies would have to be used in combination with genome editing for any heritable application of the latter technologies. As these other technologies have advanced, legal and regulatory frameworks and ethical norms of conduct have been developed to provide guidance on their appropriate human uses and oversight (Health Canada, 2016; HFEA, 2014; IOM, 2005; NASEM, 2016e; NRC and IOM, 2007, 2008; Nuffield Council, 2016a; Präg and Mills, 2015; Qiao and Feng, 2014). The reports cited here helped provide a basis for the committee's assessment of the use of genome-editing tools in humans and are referenced in subsequent chapters where relevant.

ORGANIZATION OF THE REPORT

The report begins by reviewing international norms that are embodied in the set of overarching principles adopted by the committee for governance of human genome editing (Chapter 2). The chapter continues with an overview of the U.S. regulation of research and clinical application of genome editing, drawing comparisons where appropriate to other national systems of oversight.

With this grounding in principles and regulation, Chapters 3-6 delve into human genome-editing technology and the scientific issues, regulatory context, and ethical implications of four specific applications. Laboratory research conducted in somatic cells and nonheritable laboratory research in human germ cells, gametes, or early-stage embryos is covered in Chapter 3. Chapter 4 examines the uses of genome editing for somatic interventions focused on therapy, including fetal therapy. Chapter 5 addresses the use of genome-editing technology in germline cells for potential research and clinical therapeutic applications in human patients. Chapter 6 considers the potential use of human genome editing to enhance human functions rather than to treat or prevent disease or disability.

The subsequent chapter (Chapter 7) turns from analysis of these categories of application to the role of public input in determining how genome-editing technology should be governed in the future, both in the United States and in other countries. The chapter considers public engagement for different categories of genome-editing applications and explores strengths and limitations of potential models for undertaking such public engagement.

Finally, Chapter 8 returns to the set of overarching principles and the responsibilities that flow from them in the context of human genome editing. The chapter pulls together the report's conclusions and recommendations in light of these fundamental concepts.

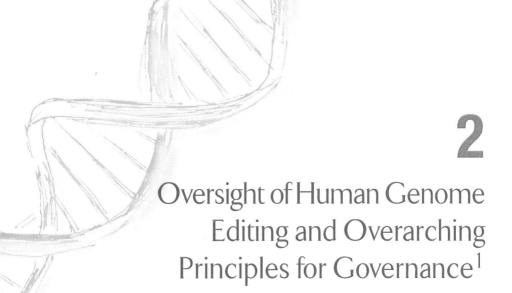

2

Oversight of Human Genome Editing and Overarching Principles for Governance[1]

Oversight of human genome editing fits within the overarching framework of oversight of gene therapy. That framework is embedded within the larger context of international conventions and norms for protection of human rights and, more specifically, for research involving human subjects and clinical care. From these international instruments, one can derive principles for governance of genome editing that have general application within the United States and across the globe, and are reflected in the specific statutory and regulatory rules that are adopted by various nations.

This chapter begins by describing the overarching principles for human genome editing adopted by the committee for this study, which are informed by those international instruments and national rules, and which in turn inform the conclusions and recommendations presented in this report. It then provides an in-depth look at U.S. governance of gene transfer research and therapy, and a brief review of alternative governance approaches used in other countries (some of which are explored in greater depth in Appendix B). Conclusions regarding the adequacy of U.S. oversight systems to deal with the specific technical and ethical issues raised by genome editing appear in Chapters 3 through 6.

---

[1]Portions of this chapter were adapted and updated from the Institute of Medicine (IOM, 2014) and the National Academies of Sciences, Engineering, and Medicine (NASEM, 2016e).

PRINCIPLES FOR GOVERNANCE OF HUMAN GENOME EDITING

Louis Pasteur once said: "La science n'a pas de patrie, parce que le savoir est le patrimoine de l'humanité" (Science has no homeland, because knowledge is the heritage of humanity). But while science is global, it proceeds within a variety of political systems and cultural norms. It is important to identify principles that can transcend these differences and divisions while accommodating cultural diversity. This is no easy task. Achieving consensus around overarching ethical principles to undergird specific recommendations for action can be difficult, whether because no one theory of ethics has been accepted by philosophers and theologians or because no one algorithm for deriving principles from those theories has been found. Utilitarians may agree on the need to evaluate overall beneficial consequences, but may disagree on whether to evaluate the consequences of a rule or of a specific act. Deontologists not only will struggle to derive a defensible list of fundamental rules of behavior, but also will be confronted with specific cases in which adherence leads to results that are intuitively unacceptable or even destructive. Other theories suffer from similar complications.

Bioethics, as a form of applied ethics, has suffered from all these complexities. It has also been dogged by long-standing debates about whether the best approach is high theory, from which all principles and specific actions flow, or anti-theory, in which deductive reasoning from specific cases leads to generalizable principles. And when bioethics is incorporated into public policy making, as opposed to individual clinical ethics analyses, it is necessary to incorporate a wider range of concerns about multicultural civil society, theories of democracy, and just distribution of burdens and benefits.[2]

Regardless of whether reasoning begins with theories grounded in utilitarian consequentialism or deontology or virtue ethics, there has emerged over time what some deem "reflective equilibrium." This concept encompasses the use of both inductive and deductive reasoning, incorporating both theory and case-based casuistry, and accepting the need for reasoning that is understandable to the public, regardless of individual spiritual or religious orientation (Arras, 2016). It has helped shape influential statements and guidance documents across the globe.

The Universal Declaration of Human Rights (UN, 1948), adopted shortly after World War II, became the foundational document for many of the more particularized declarations, conventions, and treaties that followed. In its preamble, it states that "recognition of the inherent dignity and of the equal and inalienable rights of all members of the human family is the foundation of freedom, justice and peace in the world," and its very

---

[2]Further discussion of these issues can be found in Arras (2016).

first provision reads, "All human beings are born free and equal in dignity and rights" (Article 1). Other international documents build on this core principle. The Convention on Rights of the Child, for example, calls for providing conditions for optimal development, such as health care and sanitation (UNICEF, 1990). And the Convention on the Rights of Persons with Disabilities emphasizes "respect for inherent dignity"(Article 3(1)), "respect for difference and acceptance of persons with disabilities as part of human diversity and humanity" (Article 3(4)), and "respect for the evolving capacities of children with disabilities and respect for the right of children with disabilities to preserve their identities" (Article 3(8)) (UN, 2006). Not every convention is legally binding in whole or in part on every country, but even where not incorporated into domestic statutes or applied in domestic court cases, the principles underlying these conventions have become important elements of global norms and aspirations.

Other international activities are focused more closely on biomedical research. The Council for International Organizations of Medical Sciences (CIOMS) is an international, nongovernmental, nonprofit entity, established in 1949 jointly by the World Health Organization (WHO) and the United Nations Educational, Scientific and Cultural Organization (UNESCO), whose members include nearly 50 organizations—professional societies, national academies, research councils—from across the globe. Among other things, it issues international guidelines for health research[3] based on such guidance documents as the World Medical Association's Declaration of Helsinki (WMA, 2013) and UNESCO's (2005) Universal Declaration on Bioethics and Human Rights. The 2016 version of the guidelines (van Delden and van der Graaf, 2016) stresses "the need for research having scientific and social value, by providing special guidelines for health-related research in low-resource settings, by detailing the provisions for involving vulnerable groups in research and for describing under what conditions biological samples and health-related data can be used for research" (CIOMS, 2017, Summary). Of particular relevance to genome-editing policy questions are Guideline 1, emphasizing the need to generate knowledge to protect and promote health, and its relationship to Guidelines 2, 3, and 4, which focus on fairness in the balance and distribution of risks and benefits to individuals and groups (including distribution among populations of high- and low-resource countries). Also of particular relevance is Guideline 7 on public engagement, needed not only to develop and legitimize good policy but also to help translate research into clinical benefit.

In the United States, the landmark 1979 *Belmont Report* of the National Commission for the Protection of Human Subjects in Biomedical and Behavioral Research (HHS, 1979) focused on avoiding infliction of harm,

---

[3]See http://www.cioms.ch (accessed January 5, 2017).

accepting a duty of beneficence, and maintaining a commitment to justice. These pillars of research ethics have been interpreted, expanded, deepened, and applied over the years and incorporated into the U.S. system for governing research with human participants (21 CFR Part 50 and 45 CFR Part 46). In practice, they have resulted in a focus on ensuring a reasonable balance between risk and hoped-for benefits, to the individual and to society, and on ensuring that both risks and benefits are equitably shared. These principles also have come to incorporate particular attention to the need for respect for individual autonomy in the form of generally requiring informed and voluntary participation, and the need to provide special protection against coercion or abuse of those who are vulnerable because of incapacity or circumstances.

Because both the science and the applications of human genome editing will transcend national boundaries, the core principles for governance of these technologies detailed below build on the foundations of these international and national norms. Some of these principles are generally relevant to biomedical research and care, while others are of particular importance in the context of an emerging technology, but all are foundational for the governance of human genome editing.

In this context, the committee focused on principles that are aimed at protecting and promoting the health and well-being of individuals; approaching novel technologies with careful attention to constantly evolving information; respecting individual rights; guarding against unwanted societal effects; and equitably distributing information, burdens, and benefits. Differences in social and legal culture inevitably will lead to different domestic policies governing specific applications of genome editing. Nonetheless, some principles can be shared across national borders. Thus, while the overarching principles presented here are aimed primarily at the U.S. government, they and the responsibilities that underlie them are universal in nature. The principles are listed in Box 2-1 and elaborated below.

   1. **Promoting well-being:** *The principle of promoting well-being supports providing benefit and preventing harm to those affected, often referred to in the bioethics literature as the principles of beneficence and nonmaleficence.*

Responsibilities that flow from adherence to this principle include (1) pursuing applications of human genome editing that promote the health and well-being of individuals, such as treating or preventing disease, while minimizing risk to individuals in early applications with a high degree of uncertainty; and (2) ensuring a reasonable balance of risk and benefit for any application of human genome editing.

BOX 2-1
Overarching Principles for Research on and
Clinical Applications of Human Gene Editing

Genome editing holds great promise for deepening understanding of biology
and for preventing, ameliorating, or eliminating many human diseases and conditions. Along with this promise comes the need for responsible and ethically appropriate approaches to research and clinical use. The following general principles
are essential foundations for those approaches:

1. Promoting well-being
2. Transparency
3. Due care
4. Responsible science
5. Respect for persons
6. Fairness
7. Transnational cooperation

---

2. Transparency: *The principle of transparency requires openness and
sharing of information in ways that are accessible and understandable to stakeholders.*

Responsibilities that flow from adherence to this principle include (1)
a commitment to disclosure of information to the fullest extent possible
and in a timely manner, and (2) meaningful public input into the policy-
making process related to human genome editing, as well as other novel
and disruptive technologies.

3. Due care: *The principle of due care for patients enrolled in research studies or receiving clinical care requires proceeding carefully
and deliberately, and only when supported by sufficient and robust
evidence.*

Responsibilities that flow from adherence to this principle include proceeding cautiously and incrementally, under appropriate supervision and in
ways that allow for frequent reassessment in light of future advances and
cultural opinions.

4. Responsible science: *The principle of responsible science underpins
adherence to the highest standards of research, from bench to bedside, in accordance with international and professional norms.*

Responsibilities that flow from adherence to this principle include a
commitment to (1) high-quality experimental design and analysis, (2) ap-

propriate review and evaluation of protocols and resulting data, (3) transparency, and (4) correction of false or misleading data or analysis.

5. **Respect for persons:** *The principle of respect for persons requires recognition of the personal dignity of all individuals, acknowledgment of the centrality of personal choice, and respect for individual decisions. All people have equal moral value, regardless of their genetic qualities.*

Responsibilities that flow from adherence to this principle include (1) a commitment to the equal value of all individuals, (2) respect for and promotion of individual decision making, (3) a commitment to preventing recurrence of the abusive forms of eugenics practiced in the past, and (4) a commitment to destigmatizing disability.

6. **Fairness:** *The principle of fairness requires that like cases be treated alike, and that risks and benefits be equitably distributed (distributive justice).*

Responsibilities that flow from adherence to this principle include (1) equitable distribution of the burdens and benefits of research and (2) broad and equitable access to the benefits of resulting clinical applications of human genome editing.

7. **Transnational cooperation:** *The principle of transnational cooperation supports a commitment to collaborative approaches to research and governance while respecting different cultural contexts.*

Responsibilities that flow from adherence to this principle include (1) respect for differing national policies, (2) coordination of regulatory standards and procedures whenever possible, and (3) transnational collaboration and data sharing among different scientific communities and responsible regulatory authorities.

In U.S. regulation, these principles underlie the insistence on voluntary, informed consent from competent persons; special protections for those lacking competence; a reasonable balance between the risks of harm and potential benefits; attention to minimizing risks whenever possible; and equitable selection of research participants.

REGULATION OF GENE THERAPY IN THE UNITED STATES

Both somatic and germline human genome editing would be regulated in the United States within the framework for gene-transfer research and, once approved, for gene therapy, which applies to work with human tissues and cells from the early stages of laboratory research through preclinical testing, human clinical trials, approval for introduction into medical therapy, and postapproval surveillance. At the national level, regulation may be mandatory in all cases—for example, when the work is to be submitted to the U.S. Food and Drug Administration (FDA) for approval—or it may be mandatory only for those who are using federal funds. Oversight also can proceed according to voluntary self-regulation pursuant to professional guidelines. In addition to national rules, individual states have at times issued rules on specific topics, such as embryo research, or attached restrictions to the use of state funds, such as for embryonic stem cell work. As a result, unlike some jurisdictions, such as the United Kingdom, in which work with embryos generally falls under a single statutory framework or regulatory body, the United States has individual rules related to stage of work and source of funding that overlap and interact in a manner that, in the end, provides fairly comprehensive coverage.

In general, laboratory work is subject to local oversight by institutional biosafety committees (IBCs), whose focus is on safety, and in many cases to federal oversight for quality assurance under the Clinical Laboratory Improvement Amendments as well.[4] In some cases, laboratory work using cells from identifiable living donors also is subject to review by institutional review boards (IRBs), whose focus is on protecting donors from the effects of being identified and on ensuring appropriate informed consent. Laboratory work using human embryos does not fall within IRB jurisdiction unless the progenitor-donors are identifiable, but this work may be overseen by voluntary oversight bodies, such as embryonic stem cell research oversight committees (ESCROs) created pursuant to NAS/IOM recommendations (IOM, 2005) or the embryo research oversight committees (EMROs) recently proposed by the International Society for Stem Cell Research (ISSCR, 2016a). Preclinical animal work is subject to regulation and oversight by institutional animal care and use committees pursuant to the Animal Welfare Act. Clinical trials may be the subject of discussion and advisory protocol review by the National Institutes of Health (NIH) Recombinant DNA Advisory Committee (RAC), but will nonetheless require approval by an IRB and permission from the FDA.

Human genome-editing technologies are considered to be gene therapies with regard to FDA oversight, and the agency regulates human genome editing under the existing framework for biological products, which includes gene therapy products. The FDA has authorized a number of gene therapy trials but has not yet approved a gene therapy for market. If one is approved, it will still be subject to the FDA's ongoing monitoring and, if necessary, restrictions on its use. This FDA oversight entails review under rules governing biologics and, in many cases, under rules governing drugs.

Once gene therapies have been introduced into clinical care, not only will the FDA maintain surveillance to detect safety concerns, but also formal studies of the labeled uses may be conducted to take a fresh look at

---

[4]See https://www.cms.gov/Regulations-and-Guidance/Legislation/CLIA/index.html?redirect=/clia (accessed January 5, 2017).

the safety and efficacy of the therapy. Postmarket use may also encompass uses that go beyond the indications for which a therapy was approved. Formal studies of an approved biologic for a use other than specified in the labeling would generally not be considered "off-label" use and would require FDA oversight. But outside of a study, off-label use in clinical care is entirely legal and has become a common practice among physicians with respect to drugs, and might be available for a gene-transfer product using genome editing once it is approved. Physicians use their own expertise and sources of information, as well as the advice of professional societies. They are regulated at the state level by their licensing and disciplinary bodies, may be limited by availability of patients' insurance coverage for novel interventions, and are constrained by the prospect of tort liability for medical malpractice should they be deemed negligent or reckless.

Table 2-1 provides a summary of the major steps in the anticipated regulatory pathway for the development of a new medical product created

TABLE 2-1 Summary of U.S. Regulatory Pathway for a Medical Product Created Using Genome Editing

Step	Primary Regulatory Authorities (U.S. System)	Examples of Considerations
Laboratory research in cells and tissues (nonembryonic), including human induced pluripotent stem cells (iPSCs)	• Institutional biosafety committee • Institutional review board (certain uses of human tissue) • National Institutes of Health (NIH)-funded researchers must comply with NIH Guidelines for Human Stem Cell Research (certain uses of iPSC lines are prohibited) • NIH-funded researchers must comply with NIH Guidelines for Human Stem Cell Research (only human embryonic stem cell [hESC] lines approved by NIH may be used; certain uses of hESC lines are prohibited)	Laboratory worker safety Tissue donor safety, privacy, and rights (human cells and tissue); adequacy of consent process

TABLE 2-1 Continued

Step	Primary Regulatory Authorities (U.S. System)	Examples of Considerations
Laboratory research in human embryonic stem cells or embryos	• Institutional embryonic stem cell research oversight committees (ESCROs) or embryo research oversight (EMRO) committees (voluntary but widespread) • Prohibition on use of federal funds for research in which human embryos are created for research purposes, destroyed, or subject to a certain level of risk of harm Additional state laws as applicable	Special ethical concerns and regulations (federal and state) associated with research using human embryo and hESC lines
Preclinical animal studies	• U.S. Department of Agriculture • Public Health Service Policy on Humane Care and Use of Laboratory Animals • Institutional animal care and use committee	Humane care, study design, and pain minimization
Clinical trials (Investigational New Drug [IND] application)	• Institutional review board • Institutional biosafety committee • NIH Recombinant DNA Advisory Committee (RAC) (advisory) • U.S. Food and Drug Administration (FDA), Office of Tissues and Advanced Therapies, Center for Biologics Evaluation and Research (CBER)	Balance of anticipated risks and benefits to human subjects Appropriate protocol design and informed consent
New medical product application (Biologic Licensing Application)	• FDA CBER	Evaluation of safety and efficacy data
Licensed medical product (postmarket measures)	• FDA CBER	Long-term patient safety

using genome editing. The individual steps and considerations listed in this table are discussed in greater detail in the remainder of the chapter.

Oversight of Laboratory-Based Research

Rules governing research with human cells and tissues, including somatic cells, gametes, embryos, and fetal tissue tend to focus on several key issues. For most cells and tissues, an initial question is whether the donor can receive any kind of payment, in cash or kind. This has been a particularly sensitive issue with respect to gametes used in research, with debate being focused less on the ethics of research using gametes and more on the ethics of how they are obtained and whether it involves anything that resembles undue inducement. For embryos and fetal tissue, rules are influenced by broader legal regimes governing human reproduction and products of conception, to the extent such regimes exist in a given country. And for all tissues, attention is given to whether the tissue is obtained with required permissions from the donor and whether its use poses any risk to the donor's privacy. These rules can change, of course, when tissue is obtained from cadavers rather than live donors.

In the United States, human tissue is donated for research in various ways. Rules governing that donation depend on several factors, the most important of which are whether the tissue is left over from a clinical procedure or is being obtained through a new intervention specifically for research, and whether the resulting tissue specimen has information attached to it that makes the donor's identity readily ascertainable. When tissue is collected through a physical intervention (such as a blood draw) specifically for research, the donor is a human subject, and an IRB oversees the recruitment of donors, the procedures used for collection, and the information provided to obtain consent.[5] However, as discussed below, merely giving consent to use of already excised tissue does not render the donor a human subject, unless the tissue has information that makes the donor's identity readily ascertainable.

Once the tissue has been obtained, it is available for laboratory research, subject to the usual rules for oversight of recombinant DNA research by IBCs. This pattern of regulation is the same regardless of whether genome editing will be carried out on the tissues.

---

[5]Donating embryos or fetal tissue remaining after miscarriage or abortion does not render the donor a human subject unless identifying information about the donor is retained and insufficiently obscured.

Recombinant DNA Research and Institutional Biosafety Committees

Research with human tissues and cells that takes place entirely within a laboratory and does not involve either preclinical testing on nonhuman animals or clinical testing on humans is subject to regulations and requirements, many focused primarily on ensuring the safety of the laboratory environment for workers. For experiments subject to the *NIH Guidelines for Research Involving Recombinant or Synthetic Nucleic Acid Molecules* (*NIH Guidelines*), there is a requirement that the research be reviewed and approved by an IBC. The *NIH Guidelines* are applicable to all research that is conducted at or sponsored by an institution that receives NIH funding for such research; however, many institutions follow requirements of the *NIH Guidelines* even when they are not required. IBCs review nearly all forms of research utilizing recombinant (or synthetic) nucleic acid molecules at the local institutional level (e.g., university or research center). The IBCs ensure research is conducted in conformity with the biosafety provisions of the *NIH Guidelines* and assess the research for potential risks to human health and the environment. This biosafety review is accomplished by assessing the appropriate physical and biological containment for the research and ensuring the researchers are adequately trained to conduct the work they are proposing safely.

An IBC is required to have at least five members with expertise in recombinant or synthetic nucleic acid molecule technology, at least two of whom are independent of the institution at which the research is being conducted. The *NIH Guidelines* encourage institutions to open IBC meetings to the public when possible and when consistent with the protection of privacy and proprietary interests (NIH, 2013c). The *NIH Guidelines* also require institutions to make IBC meeting minutes available to the public upon request.

Human Tissue Use and Institutional Review Boards

Laboratory-based research using human tissue may also trigger certain human subjects protections, even though all the work is done in vitro. Two situations trigger this additional level of regulation.

First, as noted above, if the tissue is being collected from a living individual, specifically for research, this interaction generally will be subject to oversight by an IRB. Although IRBs are designed primarily to protect the rights and welfare of research subjects in clinical investigations, the act of collecting tissue for research is considered to render the donor a research subject, even if subsequent work with the tissue will yield no information that could be traced to or in any way affect the donor.

The second situation may occur when tissue is collected without interaction with the person from whom it is derived, such as when surgical tissue that would otherwise be discarded is collected for use in research. If the tissue is sufficiently anonymized, the use of the tissue in research will not trigger IRB review. But if the donor's identity can be readily ascertained, the donor is considered a research subject, and IRB review is triggered unless the work is eligible for exemption or waiver of some or all elements of informed consent.

The rules will change with respect to research using stored human specimens upon the effective date of the January 2017 revisions to the "Common Rule" that sets out the framework and requirements for human subjects research that is funded by most federal agencies and departments or is otherwise subject to its jurisdiction.[6] Effective as of January 2018, the revised rule covering use of identifiable tissue

> Allows the use of broad consent (i.e., seeking prospective consent to unspecified future research) from a subject for storage, maintenance, and secondary research use of identifiable private information and identifiable biospecimens. Broad consent will be an optional alternative that an investigator may choose instead of, for example, conducting the research on nonidentified information and nonidentified biospecimens, having an institutional review board (IRB) waive the requirement for informed consent, or obtaining consent for a specific study.

> Establishes new exempt categories of research based on their risk profile. Under some of the new categories, exempt research would be required to undergo limited IRB review to ensure that there are adequate privacy safeguards for identifiable private information and identifiable biospecimens.[7]

---

[6]The FDA has its own set of regulations governing human subjects research, which can differ in some details (e.g., regarding waivers of consent in minimal-risk research). Those regulations can be found at 21 Code of Federal Regulations (CFR) Part 50. The Common Rule applies to research funded by the following departments and agencies: Agency for International Development, Environmental Protection Agency, National Aeronautics and Space Administration, National Science Foundation (NSF), Social Security Administration, U.S. Department of Agriculture, U.S. Department of Commerce, U.S. Department of Defense, U.S. Department of Education, U.S. Department of Energy (DOE), U.S. Department of Health and Human Services (HHS), U.S. Department of Homeland Security, U.S. Department of Housing and Urban Development, U.S. Department of Labor, U.S. Department of Transportation, and U.S. Department of Veterans Affairs. Historically, genetics research funding has come from NSF, DOE, and HHS, in particular (Rine and Fagen, 2015). The Common Rule also applies to research conducted at institutions that have voluntarily extended the rule's application to research funded by sources other than those listed above.

[7]Federal Policy for the Protection of Human Subjects; Final Rule Federal Register, Vol. 82, no. 12 (January 19, 2017), 7149-7274.

The rules governing use of anonymous, de-identified, or coded materials[8] will allow for even broader use. Research will be exempted from all or most IRB oversight if it is for secondary research use[9] of identifiable private information and identifiable biospecimens for which consent is not required, and when

- The identifiable private information or identifiable biospecimens are publicly available;

- The information is recorded by the investigator in such a way that the identity of subjects cannot readily be ascertained, and the investigator does not contact subjects or try to re-identify subjects;

- The secondary research activity is regulated under HIPAA [Health Insurance Portability and Accountability Act] or

- The secondary research activity is conducted by or on behalf of a federal entity and involves the use of federally generated nonresearch information provided that the original collection was subject to specific federal privacy protections and continues to be protected.

With IRB review comes a set of protections focused on ensuring that the risks (physical, psychological, and socioeconomic) and possible benefits to the research subject and society are in reasonable balance. Furthermore, except when eligible for waiver, informed and voluntary consent is required from the research subject (in the present context, the person whose tissue is being used) or from a legally authorized representative.

Additional Rules Governing Laboratory Research on Human Gametes and Embryos

Basic science research on genome editing may entail experimentation on human gametes and embryos, with no intention of performing intrauterine transfer to establish a pregnancy in a woman (see Chapter 3). Indeed, such in vitro research on embryos has already proceeded in China (using nonviable embryos) and has been approved (with viable embryos) by the

---

[8]Anonymous tissue is collected and stored without any personal identifiers at any time; de-identified tissue has earlier identifiers removed; and coded tissue has identifiers that are obscured by virtue of coding. Where the investigators lack easy access to a key with which to break the code, the tissue will no longer have a personal identity that is "readily ascertainable."

[9]"By "secondary research," this exemption is referring to reusing identifiable information and identifiable biospecimens that are collected for some other "primary" or "initial" activity. The information or biospecimens covered by this exemption would generally be found by the investigator in some type of records (in the case of information) or some type of tissue repository (such as a hospital's department for storing clinical pathology specimens). Federal Policy for the Protection of Human Subjects; Final Rule Federal Register, Vol. 82, no. 12 (January 19, 2017), 7149-7274 at 7191.

relevant regulatory bodies in Sweden and the United Kingdom. Work also is proceeding on understanding human germ cell development, research in which genome editing is one of many tools that can be used to explore the roles of specific genes (Irie et al., 2015).

This laboratory research might take a number of forms, each raising slightly different ethical and legal issues. First, it might involve editing somatic tissue in such a way that gametes would or might also be affected. Second, it might involve editing an existing gamete or gamete progenitor, such as a spermatogonial stem cell, in vitro or in vivo. Third, it might involve editing an egg in the process of fertilization (e.g., during intracytoplasmic sperm injection), or editing an already fertilized egg (zygote) or embryo.

As long as the work on gametes and embryos remains preclinical—that is, there is no transfer for gestation—the regulatory oversight and limits in the United States derive from state embryo research laws or limitations imposed by federal or other funders. Should there be a clinical trial involving efforts to gestate the edited reproductive materials, the research would come under FDA jurisdiction, and approval of an Investigational New Drug (IND) application would be required prior to beginning each such trial (see Chapter 5 for discussion of such potential future applications).

In the United States, the public policy issues surrounding laboratory research with human embryos were debated extensively by the 1994 NIH Human Embryo Research Panel, which was convened to provide recommendations to the Advisory Committee to the NIH Director. Its conclusions reflect the view that embryos should be regarded as different from ordinary human tissue but nonetheless be used for some areas of research if in the service of important scientific knowledge that cannot be obtained with less controversial methods. In addition, the panel's report called for the use of human embryos at the earliest stages and in the smallest numbers consistent with needs of the research. Except in very limited circumstances, the panel called for use of only those embryos that, although originally created in the course of a reproductive effort, now would otherwise be discarded. Donation to research would require the informed consent of those who had created the embryos for reproductive purposes (NIH, 1994). While technically the panel's report addressed conditions for federal funding of research that uses human embryos (which was subsequently prohibited by congressional action[10]), its recommendations came to be recognized within

---

[10]The Dickey-Wicker Amendment prohibits the use of most federal funds for research that involves creating or destroying embryos, and for research that puts embryos at risk of injury or destruction except when necessary to increase their chance for healthy development. The amendment has been attached to the annual appropriations bills for the Departments of Health and Human Services, Labor, and Education since 1996.

the scientific community as a more general evaluation of the ethics and acceptability of such research.

Regulatory protections for human research subjects do not apply to the ex vivo embryo.[11] Nonetheless, many (if not most) institutions housing embryonic stem cell research have put voluntary oversight measures in place (Devereaux and Kalichman, 2013), and the International Society for Stem Cell Research recently adopted guidelines calling for expanding these oversight committees to almost all research involving human embryos, regardless of whether stem cells will be derived and regardless of funding source (ISSCR, 2016b).

Some preclinical research on germline genome editing would likely take advantage of embryos left over from reproductive attempts using in vitro fertilization (IVF). Although no official numbers are available, a conservative estimate indicates that more than one million embryos, most of them produced but ultimately not used for IVF, remain in storage across the United States (Lomax and Trounson, 2013), with many more being stored around the world. As noted earlier, U.S. federal funding for research on embryos generally is prohibited. The work can, however, be supported with funds from individual states and private sources, often with policies similar to those proposed by the 1994 embryo research panel. California, for example, has been funding embryo research and embryonic stem cell research for a decade using funds from a state bond issued during the years when federal funding was limited to a small number of older embryonic stem cell lines. Connecticut, Maryland, New Jersey, and New York also created funds for research that could not be federally funded (NIH, 2016c).

Genome-editing research that generates human gametes from pluripotent stem cells would not be governed by the laws or funding policies governing embryo research unless a fertilized egg would be made in order to test the gametes. A single-cell fertilized egg is treated as if it were an embryo for most relevant state and federal laws, and restrictions on the work or on the funding would apply. In addition, such a step would constitute making an embryo solely for research purposes (i.e., without any intent to gestate the embryo and bring a fetus to term), and this has remained the most controversial form of embryo research in the United States. Some of those opposed to making embryos in research argue that fertilization brings a new, morally significant human being into existence, and that making embryos for research purposes is inherently disrespectful of human life and potentially open to significant abuses (NIH, 1994, p. 42). In some cases, this reasoning is extended to encompass totipotent cells made with somatic cell nuclear transfer ("cloning"). Even those who do not accord full moral

---

[11]Other rules, particularly state laws governing research using embryos, may apply (see Chapter 5).

status to an embryo might be wary of creating embryos for research (Green, 1994; *The Washington Post*, 1994).

On the other hand, the panel concluded that making embryos is justified when "the research by its very nature cannot otherwise be validly conducted" or when it is necessary for a study that is "potentially of outstanding scientific and therapeutic value" (NIH, 1994, p. 45). This would appear to include research on in vitro-derived gametes and on techniques for avoiding mitochondrial disease, neither of which were on the immediate horizon for human application at the time of the embryo research panel's report. The genome-editing research necessary to test edited gametes would seem to fall within this exception, as would the introduction of genome-editing components along with sperm during IVF procedures such as intracytoplasmic sperm injection. Among those countries that permit research on human embryos, rules differ on whether this exception also would permit making embryos specifically for research (UNESCO, 2004b).

Oversight in Other Nations for Research Using Human Embryos

As noted earlier, in the United States, a handful of states have laws governing or forbidding research using human embryos (NCSL, 2016). At the federal level, there is no prohibition on such research, although there are limits on the use of federal funds to perform the research.

By contrast, much of what is permitted in the United States would be more tightly regulated in the United Kingdom, where research on human gametes and embryos is subject to review by the Human Fertilisation and Embryology Authority, and a license is required for each specific set of experiments. (See Chapter 5 for discussion of clinical use of germline editing.) In other countries, such as Chile,[12] Germany (DRZE, 2016), Italy (Boggio, 2005), Lithuania,[13] and Slovakia,[14] the research would not be legal under any regulatory regime.

This variation in governance approaches reflects the fact that research with gametes, and in particular with embryos, has been controversial in many countries. Views on the legal and moral status of the human embryo range from treating it the same as any other human tissue, to considering

---

[12]Chile, Congreso Nacional, Sobre la investigacion científica en el ser humano, su genoma, y prohibe la clonacion humana, September 22, 2006, no. 20.120, art. 1, Witherspoon Council staff translation, http://www.leychile.cl/Navegar?idNorma=253478 (accessed April 25, 2017) (Spanish).

[13]Lithuania, Seimas, Law on Ethics of Biomedical Research, no. VIII-1679, May 11, 2000, last amended June 26, 2014, no. XII-981, art. 3, § 2, http://e-seimas.lrs.lt/rs/legalact/TAD/d7231dc0489411e4ba2fc5e712e90cd4 (accessed April 25, 2017).

[14]Slovakia, Health Care Act No. 277/1994, art. 42, 3(c), as quoted in UNESCO (2004b); Slovakia, Slovak Penal Code, art. 246a added in 2003, as quoted in UNESCO (2004b, p. 14).

it a tissue deserving of some extra degree of respect, to viewing it as tissue that should be accorded the same respect or even the same legal rights as a live-born child. These views vary both among and within countries and reflect both religious and secular influences. The result has been public policies ranging from permissive, to regulated, to prohibitionist.

While genome editing is a powerful new technology for making genetic modifications in cells, its use in the context of research on human embryos raises issues essentially the same as those discussed in the past: the moral status of the embryo, the acceptability of making embryos for research or using embryos that would otherwise be discarded, and the legal or voluntary limits that apply to the use of embryos in research (CIRM, 2015; ISSCR, 2016b; NIH, 1994, 2015b). This report does not address those ethical arguments, and accepts as given the current legal and regulatory policies that apply in each country. If any of those general policies were to change in the future, genome-editing research would be affected as well.

Research Using Nonhuman Animals

The 1966 Animal Welfare Act (7 U.S.C. § 2131), the federal law covering the use of animals in research, regulates testing and maintenance of a number of species, although notably not some of those which are most commonly used, such as rats and mice. It is enforced by the U.S. Department of Agriculture's (USDA's) Animal and Plant Health Inspection Service, and at the local level requires that research institutions establish an institutional animal care and use committee "to oversee and evaluate all aspects of the institution's animal care and use program," such as ensuring that the standards for physical containment and pain minimization are met.

If genome-editing research at any point were to require the creation of chimeric organisms, funding from NIH would come with rules limiting certain combinations (NIH, 2015a). NIH has recently requested public comment on proposed changes to provisions relevant to chimeras in its guidelines for human stem cell research, including work that involves chimeras (NIH, 2016b).

Clinical Trials of Human Genome Editing—The Role of IRBs

Clinical genome-editing trials—that is, studies involving human subjects—cannot commence without permission from the FDA, the details of which are discussed below. Along with FDA review, three other bodies—IRBs, IBCs, and the RAC—have clinical trial oversight responsibilities for genome editing.

IRB review and approval focuses on the risks and benefits of a clinical study and on the manner in which people are recruited for the study. It is required for any research involving human subjects that is supported by the U.S. Department of Health and Human Services (HHS) or regulated by the FDA. It is also required for research conducted or supported by any of the other federal agencies subscribing to the Common Rule, for research on products regulated by the FDA, and for research conducted by investigators at any institution that has voluntarily extended these protections to research that is otherwise not subject to these rules. The Common Rule addresses research with living individuals, and some federal funding agencies have adopted additional rules specifically with respect to research with fetuses. Research on embryos, as noted earlier, is regulated separately by some states and through federal funding restrictions.

IRBs have the authority to approve or deny approval for research protocols, human subject recruitment plans, and informed consent documents. They also may require modifications to a protocol as a condition of approval. IRBs also oversee amendments to ongoing studies and can suspend studies proving to be problematic—for example, due to the rate or severity of adverse events. In this task, IRBs may be assisted by data and safety monitoring boards, designed to track interim data while a study is ongoing. They provide additional expert and independent review to help ensure that a study continues to meet the standard for a reasonable balance of risks and potential benefits and that the information provided during initial recruitment of subjects remains a fair reflection of their risks and benefits as additional information is obtained during the study.

Federal regulations do not specify whether an IRB must hold open meetings or make its minutes and other documents available to the public; these are matters for individual institutional policies or state law. But an IRB, in addition to including experts with appropriate technical training, must include at least one member whose primary concern is in a nonscientific area and one lay member who is not otherwise affiliated with the institution. In addition, an IRB has the discretion to invite individuals with competence in special areas to assist in the review of complex issues.

Federal regulations require an IRB to determine that risks to research subjects are minimized and are reasonable in relation to the potential benefits to the subjects and the importance of the knowledge that may be expected to result from the research. They are also required to ensure that selection of subjects is equitable and that subjects are freely volunteering for the research with sufficient information. In pediatric protocols, risk tolerance is lower. If benefit to the child is possible, the research may proceed with the consent of one parent and risk tolerance will be geared to the potential benefits. But if the research offers no prospect of medical benefit, the child may not be exposed to more than a "minor increment over minimal risk" absent special intervention by the secretary of HHS.

When research is done on fetuses, certain federal funders insist on special provisions related to the degree of risk that is permitted and to how (and from whom) consent must be sought (Subpart B 45 CFR 46); while not required, these same provisions may be adopted by investigators who use other funds. These provisions state that risk to the fetus is tolerated when it has been minimized to the extent possible and when it is balanced by the prospect of direct benefit for the pregnant woman or the fetus. If there is no such prospect of benefit, the risk to the fetus may not be greater than minimal, and the purpose of the research must be the development of important biomedical knowledge that cannot be obtained by any other means. Consent by the pregnant woman is sufficient when the research holds the prospect of benefit to her as well as the fetus. If the research holds the prospect of benefit only to the fetus and not to the pregnant woman herself, then paternal consent is also required, if feasible.

Requiring voluntary and informed consent is one of the key protections for human subjects. The elements, as listed in HHS regulations, include among other items

- an explanation of the purposes of the research, the procedures that will be used, and whether any procedures are experimental;
- a description of any reasonably foreseeable risks or benefits to the subject or to others;
- a disclosure of appropriate alternative procedures;
- a statement describing the extent, if any, to which confidentiality will be maintained;
- for research involving more than minimal risk, an explanation as to whether any compensation and medical treatments are available in case of injury; and
- a statement that participation is voluntary, refusal to participate will involve no penalty, and that the subject may discontinue participation at any time.[15]

First-in-human trials make compliance with these provisions difficult, given that by definition, it is very difficult to assess the degree of uncertainty that pertains when research is moving from preclinical models to human interventions. Nonetheless, such trials must take place, and IRBs work to ensure that subjects not only understand what is known from preclinical work but also appreciate the existence of knowledge gaps that will affect the extent to which the outcome of the trials can be predicted.

The federal rules include a provision stating that an "IRB should not consider possible long-range effects of applying knowledge gained in the

---

[15]Federal Policy for the Protection of Human Subjects; Final Rule Federal Register, Vol. 82, no. 12 (January 19, 2017), 7149-7274 at 7266.

research (for example, the possible effects of the research on public policy) as among those research risks that fall within the purview of its responsibility" (21 CFR 56.111(a)(2)). This provision therefore excludes from IRBs the power to withhold approval of a study solely because the knowledge it produces or the policies it affects may be socially controversial or because of fears that the study will represent the beginning of a slippery slope to future applications that are controversial. The provision does, however, allow IRBs to withhold approval of a study because it may cause physical, psychological, or emotional harm to the subjects.

Clinical Trials of Human Genome Editing: The Role of the Recombinant DNA Advisory Committee

The late 1960s and early 1970s saw the rapid progression of the concepts and technology that led to the first intentional creation of recombinant DNA molecules (Berg and Mertz, 2010). The RAC was established by then–NIH Director Donald Frederickson in 1974 in response to scientific, public, and political concerns about the potential use and misuse of recombinant DNA technologies, as well as the associated known and unknown risks. The proposed RAC membership included requirements designed to ensure broader public perspective, such as a diverse membership that included scientists, clinicians, ethicists, biosafety experts, theologians, and public representatives, among others. Over time, the RAC's membership and responsibilities have evolved in response to scientific developments and shifting public concerns.

Early actions by the RAC included requiring that every research institution create a biohazard review committee (later renamed an IBC) to review risks and certify the presence of adequate safety measures. The major initial task of the RAC was the drafting of guidelines for recombinant DNA research discussed that, while lacking the legal force of regulations, have had an enormous influence on practices for preventing the unintended release of or human exposure to genetically modified organisms and material (Rainsbury, 2000). The NIH Guidelines are a term and condition of NIH funding, and are applicable to all recombinant DNA research that is conducted or sponsored by a public or private institution that receives NIH funding for any such research (NIH, 2013a). Many other U.S. government agencies and private institutions require that their funded research be conducted in accordance with the NIH Guidelines (Corrigan-Curay, 2013).

Initially, the RAC reviewed and approved all proposals for gene-transfer research protocols to be performed at institutions receiving NIH funds for recombinant DNA research and advised the NIH director on the issuing of official approvals, as technically, official approvals came from the NIH director, based on the RAC's decision (Freidmann et al., 2001). Over time, the interplay between RAC review and FDA review has evolved. The RAC's initial focus on safety broadened over time to include providing a venue for discussion of social and ethical issues. And in the mid-1990s, the FDA assumed sole authority to approve gene transfer research protocols, with some protocols selected for in-depth review and public discussion after an initial review by RAC members. Provision was also made for a compassionate use exemption process (Rainsbury, 2000; Wolf et al., 2009).

Appendix M of the *NIH Guidelines* is a "Points to Consider" document that details the requirements for human gene-transfer protocol submission and reporting and review by the RAC (NIH, 2013c). The *NIH Guidelines* state that "NIH will not at present entertain proposals for germline alteration" (p. 100). With regard to in utero gene transfer, the *NIH Guidelines* state that NIH may be willing to consider such research, but only after significant additional preclinical and clinical studies satisfy criteria developed at a RAC conference. In April 2015, the NIH director issued a statement that "NIH will not fund any use of gene editing technologies in human embryos" (Collins, 2015).

Within the entire system of oversight for gene-transfer research, the RAC provides a forum for the in-depth review and public discussion of a protocol. The IRBs convene in private, although, as noted earlier, they do include nonscientists as members. The public nature of the RAC is due to its status as a public advisory committee under the Federal Advisory Committee Act (FACA) of 1972. To comply with FACA regulations, the RAC must hold open meetings, giving advance notice of the time and place; provide minutes; and allow for public participation (Steinbrook, 2004).

The RAC also sponsors public symposia on important scientific and policy issues related to recombinant DNA research (Friedmann et al., 2001), providing a public forum for scientific, clinical, ethics, and safety experts along with the public to discuss emerging issues in the field of gene transfer. Along with the RAC's protocol review and mechanisms for informing institutional oversight bodies, this transparent system is intended to optimize the conduct of individual research protocols and to advance gene-transfer research generally (O'Reilly et al., 2012). In this way, the RAC serves as an important channel for scientific debate, informing institution-level oversight, increasing transparency, and promoting public trust and confidence in the field of gene transfer.

In April 2016, amendments to the *NIH Guidelines* (NIH, 2016a) went into effect. Under the revised guidelines, which reflected many of the recommendations of an earlier National Academies study (IOM, 2014), individual human gene-transfer trials are limited to cases in which NIH concurs with a request from an oversight body (such as an IRB or an IBC) that has determined that a protocol would significantly benefit from RAC review and has met one or more of the following criteria:

- The protocol uses a new vector, genetic material, or delivery methodology that represents a first-in-human experience, thus presenting an unknown risk.
- The protocol relies on preclinical safety data that were obtained using a new preclinical model system of unknown and unconfirmed value.
- The proposed vector, gene construct, or method of delivery is associated with possible toxicities that are not widely known and that may render it difficult for oversight bodies involved to evaluate the protocol rigorously. (IOM, 2014, p. 4)

Human gene-transfer protocols may also be reviewed by the RAC if the NIH director determines that the research presents significant scientific, societal, or ethical concerns. The RAC has reviewed several protocols involving the three major genome-editing technologies, and certain human genome-editing protocols, at this early stage of development, would be expected to meet these criteria.

Public Engagement Under the Auspices of the Recombinant DNA Advisory Committee

Public review of protocols for gene-transfer research is intended (1) to disseminate information so that other scientists can incorporate new scientific findings and ethical considerations into their research, and (2) to enhance public awareness of and build public trust in such research, allowing for a public voice in the review of the research (Scharschmidt and Lo, 2006). According to NIH's Office of Science Policy (OSP), protocol review by the RAC serves many functions (Corrigan-Curay, 2013), including

- optimizing clinical trial design and increasing safety for research subjects, and in some instances strengthening biosafety protections necessary for researchers, health care workers, and close contacts of research subjects;
- improving the efficiency of gene therapy research by allowing scientists to build on a common foundation of new knowledge emanating from a timely, transparent analytic process; and
- informing the deliberations of the FDA, the NIH Office of Human Research Protections (OHRP), IRBs, IBCs, and other oversight bodies whose approval is necessary for gene therapy research projects to be undertaken.

The current process aims to be highly transparent. The OSP website provides information about protocols and the public discussions at the

RAC meetings, and the protocols themselves are made available to members of the public upon request (OBA, 2013). All correspondence between the RAC and investigators also is part of the public record for the protocol and is available to the investigators, sponsor(s), IRB(s), IBC(s), the FDA, and OHRP (NIH, 2013a). For protocols selected for in-depth review and public discussion, the protocol registration process is defined as complete when, following the review, the investigator receives a letter based on the recommendations discussed at the RAC meeting. The letter is also sent to the relevant IRB(s) and IBC(s) (NIH, 2013b). Minutes and webcasts of the RAC meetings are made available on the RAC's public website. Neither investigators nor IRBs or IBCs are required to follow any of the RAC's recommendations. Rather, a protocol's approval comes from a collection of other regulatory bodies. A protocol must be approved by the relevant IBC(s) and IRB(s) before research participants can be enrolled in a clinical trial. These bodies often rely on the RAC's recommendations in making their decisions, but the RAC's approval per se is not required for the research to move forward (Wolf et al., 2009). The FDA, the agency responsible for regulatory approval, also takes into account the views of the RAC when reviewing IND applications (Takefman, 2013).

U.S. Food and Drug Administration Review of Investigational New Drug Applications

Regardless of the funding source, the FDA is the agency ultimately responsible for the regulation and approval of genome-editing products. Most of these products will be viewed as biologic drugs rather than devices. Thus, before being used in human trials, they will need to have FDA review and approval of their IND application. INDs for gene therapy are regulated by the Office of Tissues and Advanced Therapies (previously the Office of Cellular, Tissue and Gene Therapies) within the Center for Biologics Evaluation and Research (CBER). The review follows a regulatory framework in which the FDA and the sponsor interact throughout the product's life cycle, from pre-IND to postmarketing surveillance.

CBER regulates a range of biologics, including human gene therapy products, and certain devices related to gene transfer. The FDA defines gene therapy products as products that "mediat[e] their effects by transcription and/or translation of transferred genetic material and/or by integrating into the host genome . . . and [that] are administered as nucleic acids, viruses, or genetically engineered microorganisms" (FDA, 2006, p. 4). The general types of gene therapy products reviewed by the FDA to date, pursuant to its authority under the Federal Food, Drug, and Cosmetic Act (Public Law 75-717) and the Public Health Service Act (Public Law 78-410) as amended, are nonviral vectors (plasmids), replication-deficient viral vectors (e.g.,

adenovirus, adeno-associated virus), replication-competent oncolytic vectors (e.g., measles, reovirus), replication-deficient retroviral and lentiviral
vectors, cytolytic herpes viral vectors, genetically modified microorganisms
(e.g., *Listeria, Salmonella, E. coli*), and ex vivo genetically modified cells.

The FDA also maintains a federal advisory committee—the Cellular,
Tissue and Gene Therapies Advisory Committee—that reviews and evalu-
ates available data related to the safety, effectiveness, and appropriate use
of human cells, human tissues, gene-transfer therapies, and xenotransplantation products that are intended for transplantation, implantation, infusion, and transfer in the treatment and prevention of a broad spectrum of
human diseases and in the reconstruction, repair, or replacement of tissues
for various conditions.[16]

The FDA process applies to all gene-therapy clinical research, regardless of funding source. During the FDA's review of INDs and its subsequent
review of major steps in the research process (e.g., movement from phase
I to phase II studies), any RAC preliminary scientific and ethical review of
human gene transfer, as well as its public discussion of novel applications, is
taken into account (Takefman, 2013). Unlike RAC review, the FDA's review
process for granting an IND to begin a gene-therapy clinical trial is closed
to the public. To go on the market, products must have received approval
of their Biologic Licensing Application (BLA) (21 CFR 600-680), which
focuses on manufacturing information, labeling, and preclinical and clinical
studies. The process for approving the BLA may include some public participation. Many first-in-class products are taken to an advisory committee,
which typically includes members with medical and scientific expertise, as
well as ethicists, industry representatives, and patient representatives. These
meetings often represent the FDA's first public discussion of a new medical
product, providing access to information for patients, physicians, and other
stakeholders who observe the meeting, and to those who use the meeting
transcripts made available on the agency website. Meetings are publicly
announced in advance, and include public comment periods.

The FDA offers assistance to the research community in the form of
"Points to Consider" documents that present the current thinking of FDA/
CBER staff about important issues in gene transfer and gene therapy (FDA,
1991). These documents are intended to guide investigators in understanding FDA perspectives and requirements for development and testing as they
prepare their IND applications. In 2015 the FDA released "Considerations
for the Design of Early-Phase Clinical Trials of Cellular and Gene Therapy
Products" (FDA, 2015b).

To ensure that all regulatory requirements are met, the FDA encourages a "pre-IND" meeting between investigators and agency officials early

---

[16]51 *Federal Register* 23309 (1986).

in the protocol development process at which specific questions related to the planned clinical trial design are discussed. The meeting also provides an opportunity for the discussion of various scientific and regulatory aspects of the medical product as they relate to safety and/or potential clinical hold issues,[17] such as plans for studying the gene-transfer product in pediatric populations (FDA, 2001). For the meeting, the investigator must submit an information package that describes the structure of the gene-transfer product, its proposed clinical indication, dosage, and administration; provides preclinical and clinical study descriptions and a data summary; includes chemistry, manufacturing, and controls (CMC) information; and specifies objectives expected from the meeting (FDA, 2000).

For certain types of protocols—including those involving gene-transfer products—it is sometimes necessary to discuss special issues regarding recombinant DNA proteins from cell-line sources, such as the adequacy of characterization of cells, potential contamination of cell lines, removal or inactivation of adventitious agents, or potential antigenicity of the product (FDA, 2015b). An investigator is expected to consider and address FDA guidance resulting from the pre-IND meeting before submitting an application for an IND.

As a general rule, when reviewing IND submissions, the FDA balances potential benefits and risks to participants in the clinical trials (Au et al., 2012; Takefman and Bryan, 2012). Once the investigator has submitted the IND, the FDA has 30 days either to allow it to proceed or to put it on clinical hold while more data are obtained from the sponsor. The application includes details on product manufacturing, safety and quality testing, and purity and potency, as well as preclinical, pharmacological, and toxicological testing. Safety testing required specifically of gene-therapy products includes (1) potential adverse immune responses to the ex vivo transduced cells, the vector, or the transgene; (2) vector and transgene toxicities, including distribution of the vector to germ cells in testicular and ovarian tissues; and (3) potential risks of the delivery procedure (FDA, 2012b).

The clinical protocol section of the application includes information about phase I, II, and/or III studies, including starting dose, dose escalation, route of administration, dosing schedules, definition of patient population (detailed entry and exclusion criteria), and safety monitoring plans. It also includes information regarding study design, including description of clinical procedures, laboratory tests, or other measures to be used to monitor the effects of the product. Because vectors and transgenes of gene-therapy

---

[17]A clinical hold is an order to delay a proposed clinical investigation or suspend an ongoing investigation. Conditions for issuing a clinical hold include unreasonable risk to research subjects or discovery of information that undermines confidence in the investigators or the study protocol (*Clinical Holds and Requests for Modification*, 21 CFR, Sec. 312.42 [April 1, 2016]).

products may persist for the lifetime of the research subject, the FDA has issued guidance on observation of subjects for delayed adverse events (FDA, 2006).

Federal regulations require that information about many clinical trials be posted at ClinicalTrials.gov, the government's database for information about a large proportion of clinical trials, or a similar site. This applies to many clinical trials of drug products (including biological products) and device products that are regulated by the FDA. Effective as of January 2017, there is an expanded registry with additional results data to help patients find trials.[18] The goals are to enhance trial design, to prevent duplication of unsuccessful trials, to improve the evidence base and efficiency of drug and device development, and to build public trust.

In accordance with statutory mandates, however, there is little or no transparency in FDA reviews during the IND stage, including whether the agency is considering an IND for a specific product. But once the FDA has approved a license for a product, it may post the clinical, pharmacological, and other technical reviews of the product on its website (see, for example, information for Ducord, an umbilical cord–derived, stem cell product for use in certain transplantation procedures, as reported by Zhu and Rees [2012]). Although proprietary information is redacted from these posted reviews, the clinical reviews provide considerable information about the trials.[19] They may summarize early-stage discussions about trial design and assessments of whether sponsors conformed to certain ethical and good trial practice standards. When necessary, the FDA can engage its Cellular, Tissue and Gene Therapies Advisory Committee to receive public input on a pressing issue of broad applicability.

The FDA's Sentinel Initiative—launched in 2008 to establish a national risk identification and analysis system using electronic health care data to monitor the safety of drugs, biologics, and devices after they have reached the market—complements the Adverse Event Reporting System. Through Sentinel, the FDA can access information from electronic health records, insurance claims data and registries, and other sources using a process that also maintains patient privacy. CBER has launched several projects within Sentinel aimed at improving postlicensure safety surveillance of vaccines and other biologics. In addition to monitoring, other postmarket quality control measures include registries, special patient information pamphlets, and requirements for formal phase IV studies. The European Union has its

---

[18]81 *Federal Register* 64981-65157.

[19]Section 916 of the Food and Drug Administration Amendments Act (2007) requires posting of certain information about a BLA approval on the FDA website. See SOPP8401.7 Action Package for Posting, http://www.fda.gov/BiologicsBloodVaccines/GuidanceComplianceRegulatory Information/ProceduresSOPPs/ucm211616.htm (accessed February 2, 2017).

own tools for postmarket monitoring and control, different in detail but similar in purpose (Borg et al., 2011).

Once the FDA has approved a drug, it may be prescribed for uses that differ from those for which it was approved and labeled. As noted earlier, such off-label prescribing is a legal and common practice of health care providers when they deem it medically appropriate. This may mean use of the product for a different medical condition from that for which it was approved (e.g., approved for one kind of cancer and used for another), or its administration at different doses, in different forms, or to different categories of patients. Off-label prescribing allows for physician discretion and the efficient use of information following a drug's initial approval, while still maintaining postmarket surveillance for safety. In the United States, some areas of medicine, such as pediatrics (AAP, 2014) and cancer care (American Cancer Society, 2015), are known to have a high rate of off-label use.

There are a number of mechanisms by which products may follow an accelerated regulatory pathway, including Fast Track, Breakthrough Therapy, Accelerated Approval, and Priority Review (FDA, 2015a). The means used to accelerate the review range from earlier, more frequent, and more intensive consultations with FDA staff; to easing rules for the submission of materials; to changing the endpoints required in the study; to conducting the review before that of other products for which the applications were submitted earlier.

This provision for accelerated review was expanded to include regenerative medicine and other cell therapy products in the 21st Century Cures Act,[20] signed into law in December 2016. The act allows for approval of a "regenerative-medicine therapy" based on surrogate endpoints reasonably expected to predict clinical outcomes and on evidence provided by a wider range of sources, including those outside the realm of controlled clinical trials. Postapproval measures can still include requirements for further trials, as well as surveillance, patient information brochures, registries, and other risk mitigation measures. This process resembles to some extent the "conditional approval" mechanism adopted in Japan for regenerative-medicine products, although it lacks any trigger that automatically withdraws approval if postmarket risk mitigation and clinical trial commitments are not fulfilled.

The therapies being developed with human genome editing were not excluded from this new expanded category, and some might be eligible for a variety of accelerating mechanisms if they meet the definition of

---

[20]21st Century Cures Act, Public Law No. 114-255, HR 34, 114th Cong. (2015-2016) (https://www.congress.gov/bill/114th-congress/house-bill/34/text?format=txt). See also http://www.fda.gov/BiologicsBloodVaccines/CellularGeneTherapyProducts/ucm537670.htm (accessed January 30, 2017).

"regenerative-medicine therapy" (which "includes cell therapy, therapeutic tissue engineering products, human cell and tissue products"), as well as the criterion of having the potential to fulfill an unmet need for a "serious or life-threatening disease or condition." Since passage of the new law, the FDA has been working on implementing these provisions and considering a number of issues, including the scope of the products that meet the definition of regenerative-medicine therapy as specified in the legislation. As written, though, the criterion of fulfilling an unmet need for a serious or life-threatening disease would seem to exclude intended uses for enhancement.[21]

The Interplay Between the FDA and the NIH RAC

Concern about the conduct of gene-transfer trials reached a new level of intensity after the 1999 death of Jesse Gelsinger, a participant in one such trial (Shalala, 2000; Steinbrook, 2002). In response, NIH took steps to coordinate reporting of adverse events and expand public access to information regarding human gene transfer trials, for example, through the creation of the Genetic Modification Clinical Research Information System (GeMCRIS) (NIH, 2004). This database, which became operational in 2004, includes summary information on human gene-transfer trials registered with NIH (2004). Included in the GeMCRIS summaries is information about the medical conditions under study, institutions where trials are being conducted, investigators carrying out these trials, gene products being used, and routes of gene product delivery, as well as summaries of study protocols.

Differences remain between the RAC's and the FDA's approach to oversight of gene-transfer research. The FDA, as the sole federal regulatory agency for biomedical products in the United States, focuses on safety and efficacy when evaluating gene-transfer products, from the first time they are used in humans through their commercial distribution (Kessler et al., 1993) and over the lifetime of their use. FDA regulation includes many steps that, by statutory provision, are confidential because of the presence of proprietary information (Wolf et al., 2009). In contrast, the RAC is able to address broader scientific, social, and ethical issues raised by gene-transfer and gene therapy research, and—unlike IRBs—the RAC is permitted to address these broader issues in its review of individual protocols as well (NIH, 2016b, Sec. IV-C-2-e). In addition, RAC review is conducted publicly by experts who are not employed by the government (Wolf et al., 2009).

---

[21]21st Century Cures Act, Public Law No. 114-255, HR 34, 114th Cong. (2015-2016) (https://www.congress.gov/bill/114th-congress/house-bill/34/text?format=txt [accessed January 30, 2017]).

To encourage communication between the agencies, the RAC charter calls for a member of CBER to be one of the nonvoting federal representatives to the RAC (NIH, 2011). NIH and the FDA also have harmonized reporting of adverse events.

GOVERNANCE IN OTHER NATIONS

As noted by former FDA Commissioner Robert Califf, "[s]cientific advances do not adhere to national boundaries and therefore it is critical that we understand the evolving views of our international counterparts." To that end, the FDA actively participates in the International Pharmaceutical Regulators' Forum and its Gene Therapy working group for the purpose of exchanging technical information and identifying areas for regulatory coordination (Califf and Nalubola, 2017).

The regulatory pathways for gene therapy in other jurisdictions are similar to those in the United States in important ways (see Appendix B), particularly with respect to the centrality of premarket risk and benefit assessment. For example, gene therapy in South Korea has a pathway very similar to that in the United States except that it includes a system of conditional approval that allows for use with less robust evidentiary bases. The United Kingdom has rigorous premarket risk and benefit review, as in the United States, but singles out therapies involving gametes or embryos for more intensive regulation (see Box 2-2). The European Union has additional layers of quality control for "advanced therapy medicinal products," which would include some gene therapy products, although as in the United States, off-label use would be permissible (George, 2011). Japan uses a system for gene therapy products that resembles the U.S. device regulations, in which new products are sorted prospectively by level of anticipated risk and regulated accordingly. Singapore also has adopted a risk-based approach, with such criteria as whether the manipulation is substantial or minimal; whether the intended use is homologous or nonhomologous;[22] and whether it will be combined with a drug, a device, or another biologic. These criteria resemble many of those used by American authorities in determining whether tissues should be subject to rules governing transplant medicine or rules governing the marketing of cell-therapy products (Charo, 2016b). Box 2-2 illustrates the differences between the United States and other regulatory regimes by describing the example of the United Kingdom.

---

[22]The FDA defines homologous use as the repair, reconstruction, replacement, or supplementation of a recipient's cells or tissues with a human cell, tissue, or cellular or tissue-based product (HCT/P) that performs the same basic function or functions in the recipient as in the donor (21 CFR 1271.3(c)), including when such cells or tissues are for autologous use.

BOX 2-2
Example of an Alternative Governance Regime

The United Kingdom serves as an example of an alternative governance regime for gene therapy. For somatic gene therapy, its approach is not unlike that in the United States, but it has more centralized and intensive regulatory control over therapies that involve gametes and embryos.

For somatic gene therapy, the United Kingdom's biotechnology advisory system involves interplay between the Gene Therapy Advisory Committee and the Health and Safety Executive Scientific Advisory Committee on Genetically Modified Organisms (Contained Use). The U.K. Clinical Trials Regulations require that before clinical trials of gene therapy are conducted, approval must be obtained from the Medicines and Healthcare Products Regulatory Agency. Approval from the Gene Therapy Advisory Committee is also required, and additional laws and regulations govern quality control at facilities producing the cell-based therapy products (Bamford et al., 2005). Public input is sought by these regulatory agencies and by professional societies. For example, each year the British Society for Gene and Cell Therapy runs a Public Engagement Day to bring students at all levels, patients, caregivers, and scientists together for discussion and debate. Once available clinically, gene therapies may be used off-label, as in the United States.

With respect to the possibility of germline editing, the United Kingdom has a more focused and vertically integrated regulatory regime, with tighter controls over whether and when a procedure can be carried out and by which professionals and clinics. Unlike the U.S. system, which has a formal "investigational" phase of defined uses for a therapy followed by an approval for commercial marketing (i.e., clinical use in the market), and which then allows professionals wide latitude in how to use the therapy, the U.K. system foregoes these separate categories and limits physician discretion in the area of therapies using embryos or gametes. It is a rigorous system of oversight that can track the fate of every embryo used for research or treatment.

To implement this system, the United Kingdom created the Human Fertilisation and Embryology Authority (HFEA), an independent regulator of treatments using eggs and sperm and of treatments or research involving human embryos. It develops standards, and then issues licenses to specific clinics to proceed with specific interventions. To be licensed, clinics must meet safety and quality assurance standards, offer counseling to patients, monitor birth outcomes and the well-being of children conceived through the new technologies, and generally provide personnel and systems that allow for ongoing compliance monitoring. In addition to the clinic/research center (with named individuals involved), HFEA issues licenses for the specific project or treatment. The latter can be on a broad basis for common, well-established procedures or specific to each individual case. For preimplantation genetic diagnosis, for example, licenses were originally for specific diseases. With experience, this constraint was relaxed. Centers can now obtain licenses for a range of genetic diseases, but these still must be on the HFEA's approved list, so off-label use is not allowed for applications involving gametes and embryos.

CONCLUSIONS AND RECOMMENDATION

Genome editing holds great promise for preventing, ameliorating, or eliminating many human diseases and conditions. Along with this promise, however, comes the need for ethically responsible research and clinical use.

The existing U.S. regulatory structures discussed in this chapter provide a starting framework for governance of laboratory research, preclinical testing, clinical trials, and potential medical uses involving human genome editing in the United States, as well as for an understanding of differences between the U.S. system and the regulatory infrastructures of other nations.

There is considerable similarity in the structures for product regulation among different jurisdictions, with an emphasis on premarket balancing of risk and benefit. Some differences exist in the availability of conditional approval or other accelerated approval mechanisms for cell-therapy products, as well as in the management of embryos and gametes. In clinical care, off-label use is commonly permitted, again with the notable exception of the more comprehensive controls on therapies involving embryos and gametes in the United Kingdom.

Overall, while capable of improvement, the structure of the U.S. regulatory system is adequate for overseeing human genome-editing research and product approval. Specific areas in which additional effort might be made are identified in Chapters 3-7.

> **RECOMMENDATION 2-1. The following principles should undergird the oversight systems, the research on, and the clinical uses of human genome editing:**
> 1. **Promoting well-being**
> 2. **Transparency**
> 3. **Due care**
> 4. **Responsible science**
> 5. **Respect for persons**
> 6. **Fairness**
> 7. **Transnational cooperation**

3

Basic Research Using Genome Editing

The recent remarkable advances in methods for editing the DNA of genes and genomes have engendered much excitement and activity and had a major impact on many areas of both basic and applied research. It has been known for 60 years that all life on Earth is encoded in the sequence of DNA, which is inherited in each succeeding generation, but accelerating advances have greatly enhanced understanding of and the ability to manipulate DNA.

This chapter reviews the various types of and purposes for basic laboratory research involving human genome editing. It begins by describing the basic tools of genome editing and the rapid advances in genome-editing technology. The chapter then details how genome editing can be used in basic laboratory research aimed at advancing understanding of human cells and tissues; of human stem cells, diseases, and regenerative medicine; and of mammalian reproduction and development. Ethical and regulatory issues entailed in this research are then summarized. Throughout the chapter, key terms and concepts germane to basic research involving genome editing are defined; Box 3-1 defines the most foundational of these terms.

THE BASIC TOOLS OF GENOME EDITING

All living organisms, from bacteria to plants to humans, use similar mechanisms to encode and express genes, although the sizes of their genomes and their numbers of genes differ greatly. Hence, understanding of

---

BOX 3-1
Foundational Terms

The following terms are foundational to understanding any research involving DNA.

DNA is a long polymer of similar repeating units of four types (A,T,C,G), where the letters denote distinct units called **nucleotide bases.** The bases pair specifically with each other (A with T and C with G) to form the well-known double helix of DNA with its two complementary strands. Segments of DNA sequence encode **genes** that can be copied (**transcribed**) from the DNA into a second type of nucleotide polymer called **RNA.** Some of these RNAs act by pairing with other RNAs to affect their functions, while others contribute to structures necessary for cellular activities, including the copying of some of the RNA molecules to encode proteins. **Proteins** are polymers of a different type of unit, called amino acids, of 20 different types; hence the copying of RNA to form proteins is known as **translation** since the copying is into a different "language"—"written" in amino acids rather than nucleotides. These protein polymers fold into complex three-dimensional shapes that form the building blocks of the cells that make up the human body and perform the myriad functions of living organisms. The combination of **transcription** from DNA to RNA and **translation** of RNA to protein is known as **gene expression**, and is tightly regulated so that genes are expressed at the appropriate times and places and in the correct amounts. Thus, the functions of individual cells are dependent on the genes they express. The complete set of genes in an organism is called its **genome.** Most human cells contain two complete copies of the human genome, each comprising 3 billion base pairs and encoding approximately 20,000 genes encoding proteins, plus the regulatory elements that control their expression. One can think of the genome as the "code" or "software" and RNA and proteins and the structures they form as the "hardware" of cells and living organisms.

---

any form of life is immensely informative with respect to understanding all other forms, and provides insights and applications that obtain across species—a fact that has been particularly invaluable in the development of methods for editing genes and genomes.

The earliest studies in molecular biology were on bacteria and their viruses. Their relative simplicity and ease of analysis were key in establishing the basis of the genetic code and the expression of genes. Parallel research on more complex organisms built on the advances in these studies of bacteria, and by the mid-1960s, it was clear that bacteria, plants, and animals shared many fundamental molecular mechanisms. Key discoveries in bacteria uncovered some of their mechanisms for protection against viruses, including so-called **restriction endonucleases,** proteins bacteria use to cleave the DNA of infecting viruses and "restrict" their growth. This discovery allowed scientists to cut DNA in predictable and reproducible ways and to reassemble the cut pieces into **recombinant DNA.**

By the mid-1970s, it was evident that recombinant DNA offered a powerful means of combining DNA in productive ways, with promising applications in biotechnology. However, this potential also raised questions about whether the application of these novel methods might entail some risk. In light of those concerns, a group of scientists and others convened a meeting at Asilomar in 1975 to consider what precautions might be needed to oversee this new technology and established a set of guidelines to regulate the containment and conduct of the research. The descendants of those guidelines still regulate recombinant DNA research to this day, some of them incorporated into official regulatory systems. In practice, the most extreme concerns did not eventuate. Today, the use of recombinant DNA methods is widespread worldwide and has yielded enormous benefits to humankind in terms of scientific understanding and medical advances, including many valuable drugs and treatments, and the biotechnology industry is now a thriving part of the world economy.

Among methods developed through the use of recombinant DNA technology is the ability to introduce DNA into cells where it can be expressed—a so-called **transgene.** This method is widely used in fundamental laboratory research (see Appendix A for more detail). When such exogenous DNA is introduced into a cell, it can insert into the DNA of the cell's genome largely at random and, depending on how and where it is inserted, can be expressed as RNA and protein, although this overall process is not very efficient. A key advance was the development of techniques for generating molecular tools that could be used to cut the DNA of genes and genomes in specific places to allow targeted alterations in the DNA sequence. It was found that **double-strand breaks (DSBs)** could be deliberately generated by nucleases that cut DNA at defined sites (**homing nucleases,** sometimes also called **meganucleases,** originally discovered in yeast) (Choulika et al., 1995; Roux et al., 1994a,b). In the succeeding 20 years, based on these groundbreaking discoveries, several additional types of nucleases that can be targeted to specific sites were developed and adapted for use in targeted DNA cleavage (Carroll, 2014).

Such double-strand breaks also occur naturally during DNA replication or through radiation or chemical damage, and cells have evolved mechanisms for repairing them by rejoining the ends (a process known as **nonhomologous end joining [NHEJ]**). However, this rejoining often is not perfect, and small insertions and deletions can be introduced during the repair. Such insertions and deletions (**indels**) can disrupt the sequence of the DNA and often inactivate the gene that was cut. This targeted cleavage and inaccurate repair through NHEJ provide a means of inactivating genes or gene-regulatory elements. Although the resulting indels are usually one or a few nucleotides long, in some cases they can consist of thousands of base pairs. Genome editing through NHEJ can also be harnessed to create defined chromosomal deletions or chromosomal translocations by simultaneously creating two double-strand breaks at different sites, followed by rejoining at those two sites. These sites can be either on the same chromosome (producing a deletion) or on different chromosomes (producing a translocation).

More precise editing can be achieved if, during the breakage-repair process in the cell, an extra piece of DNA is provided that shares sequence (i.e., is homologous) with the cleaved DNA. Such homologous repair also is used by normal cellular repair mechanisms. These mechanisms can be exploited to make precise changes. If homologous DNA slightly different in sequence from the cleaved sequence is introduced into the cell, that difference can be inserted into the sequence of the gene or genome, a process termed **homology-directed repair (HDR)**. HDR can also be used to insert a novel sequence (e.g., one or more genes) of variable length at a precise genomic location. In contrast to NHEJ, HDR-mediated genome editing allows scientists to predict both where the edit will occur and the size and sequence of the resulting change. Thus, HDR-mediated editing is very much like editing a document because precise changes in the characters can be made.

Two types of targeted nucleases that have been widely developed for use in editing genes and genomes are **zinc finger nucleases (ZFNs)** and **transcription activator-like effector nucleases (TALENs)**. Both rely on proteins whose normal function is to bind to specific relatively short DNA sequences. Zinc fingers are segments of proteins used by multicellular organisms to control the expression of their genes by binding to DNA (they also typically bind zinc as part of their structure; hence their name). They can be engineered by molecular biologists to recognize different short DNA sequences and can be joined to nucleases that cleave DNA. Thus, the zinc fingers target specific sequences in genes and genomes, and the attached nucleases cleave the DNA to generate a double-strand break by cleaving both strands of the DNA. ZFNs have been developed for gene editing and are in clinical trials—for example, in attempts to confer resistance to the HIV virus in AIDS patients (Tebas et al., 2014). TALENs work similarly to ZFNs, also using DNA recognition proteins (transcription activator-like effectors or TALEs) originally identified in bacteria that infect plants. The DNA recognition sequences of TALE proteins are made of repeating units, each of which recognizes a single base pair in the DNA. TALEs are simpler and easier to engineer than are zinc fingers and can similarly be joined to DNA-cleaving nucleases to yield TALENs. The preclinical application of TALENs to engineer lymphocytes for the treatment of acute lymphoblastic leukemia was recently reported (Poirot et al., 2015).

Thus, these tools are already well-established approaches to the use of genome editing for applications in gene therapy, and many of the associated safety and regulatory issues have already been addressed (see Chapter 4). However, the protein engineering required to design site-specific versions of TALENs and, even more so, of ZFNs, remains technically challenging, time-consuming, and expensive.

The past 5 years have seen the development of a completely novel system, known as **CRISPR/Cas9** (CRISPR stands for clustered regularly interspaced short palindromic repeats) (Doudna and Charpentier, 2014; Hsu et al., 2014). Short RNA sequences modeled on the CRISPR system, when paired with **Cas9** (CRISPR associated protein 9, an RNA-targeted nuclease), or alternatively with other similar nucleases, can readily be programmed to edit specific segments of DNA. The CRISPR/Cas9 system is simpler, faster, and cheaper relative to earlier methods and can be highly efficient. CRISPR/Cas9, like TALEs, was originally discovered in bacteria, where it functions as part of an immunity system to protect bacteria from invading viruses (Barrangou and Dudley, 2016; Doudna and Charpentier, 2014). The key distinguishing feature of CRISPR/Cas9 is that it uses RNA sequences instead of protein segments to recognize specific sequences in the DNA by complementary base pairing.

As first reengineered in 2012 (Jinek et al., 2012), the bacterial nuclease Cas9 binds a single RNA sequence known as a **guide RNA** tailored to recognize any sequence of choice. This two-component system can bind to the chosen site in DNA via the guide RNA and cleave the DNA using the Cas9 nuclease. Since it is simple to synthesize RNA of any desired sequence, generation of CRISPR/Cas9 targeting nucleases is straightforward—the system is readily programmed to target any sequence in any genome. Programs exist for choosing suitable guide RNAs, and while not all guides work equally well, testing a number of guides to find effective ones is not difficult or expensive. This ease of design, together with the remarkable specificity and efficiency of CRISPR/Cas9 has revolutionized the field of genome editing and has major implications for advances in fundamental research, as well as in such applications as biotechnology, agriculture, insect control, and gene therapy.

Figure 3-1 provides a summary of the ZFN, TALEN, and CRISPR methods of genome editing. As mentioned, these genome-editing methods are being widely applied across a broad range of biological sciences, from fundamental laboratory research on cells and laboratory animals; to applications in agriculture involving improvements in crop plants and farm animals; to applications in human health, both at the research level and, increasingly, in clinical applications. Agricultural applications have been addressed in other studies by the U.S. National Academies of Sciences, Engineering, and Medicine (see Chapter 1) and potential clinical applica-

FIGURE 3-1 Methods of genome editing.
Top: Zinc finger nucleases (ZFNs): The colored modules represent the Zn fingers, each engineered to recognize three adjacent base pairs in the DNA; these modules are coupled to a dimer of the FokI nuclease that makes a double-stranded cut in the DNA.
Middle: Transcription activator-like effector nucleases (TALENs). The colored modules each recognize a single base pair in the DNA; these modules are coupled to a dimer of the FokI nuclease that makes a double-stranded cut in the DNA.
Bottom: CRISPR/Cas9. Two components derived from the clustered regularly interspaced short palindromic repeat (CRISPR) region are needed. A nuclease such as Cas9 (blue) is targeted to a specific site on the DNA by the guide RNA (purple), which binds a 20-base sequence in the genome adjacent to a short protospacer adjacent motif (PAM) sequence (yellow) and targets a double-stranded cut in the DNA. NOTE: In all three cases, the DNA cut can be repaired by nonhomologous end joining of the ends or by repair directed by a stretch of homologous DNA (green), producing alterations in the genome of the target organism, which can be from any species. (For more detail, see Appendix A.)
SOURCES: Top and middle (Beumer and Carroll, 2014); bottom (Charpentier and Doudna, 2013).

tions are the subject of subsequent chapters of this report. The focus in this chapter is on basic laboratory research using genome editing.

This research addresses fundamental questions concerning the use and optimization of genome-editing methods both in cultured cells and in experimental multicellular organisms (e.g., mice, flies, plants). Such basic discovery research is essential for improving any future applications of genome editing. Applications of genome editing in laboratory research also have added powerful new tools that are contributing greatly to understanding of basic cellular functions, metabolic processes, immunity and resistance to pathological infections, and diseases such as cancer and cardiovascular disease. These laboratory studies are overseen by standard laboratory safety mechanisms. In addition to these applications, this chapter reviews the potential for using similar approaches in basic research on human germline cells, not for the purposes of procreation but solely for laboratory research. This work will provide valuable insights into the processes of early human development and reproductive success, and could lead to clinical benefits, directly as a result of work with human embryos and germline cells or through improvements in the derivation and maintenance of stem cells in vitro.

RAPID ADVANCES IN GENOME-EDITING TECHNOLOGY

The development of CRISPR/Cas9 has revolutionized the science of gene and genome editing, and the basic science is advancing extremely rapidly, with additional CRISPR-based systems being developed and deployed for multiple different purposes. Different species of bacteria use somewhat different CRISPR systems, and although the CRISPR/Cas9 system is currently the most widely used because of its simplicity, alternative systems being developed will provide increased flexibility in methodology (Wright et al., 2016; Zetsche et al., 2015).

Among the issues that need to be addressed going forward are the specificity and efficiency of the DNA cleavage mediated by CRISPR-guided nucleases. While the roughly 20-base sequence recognized by the guide RNA provides a great deal of specificity (an exact match should occur by chance in approximately 1×10^{12} base pairs—1 in a trillion—the equivalent of several hundred mammalian genomes), there is some small potential for so-called **off-target events,** in which the nucleases make cuts in unintended places, especially if the guide RNA binds to DNA sequences that are slightly different from the intended target. Some early experiments suggested that off-target events might occur at a significant rate, but as the methods have been improved and as their application has increasingly been in normal cells rather than cultured cell lines, the frequency of off-target cleavages appears to be very low. Advances have been achieved in the specificity of Cas9 cleavage (Kleinstiver et al., 2016; Slaymaker et al., 2016), and methods have been developed for monitoring the frequency of off-target cleavage. (See Appendix A for more detail.)

Another significant advance has occurred in the development of methods for modifying the CRISPR/Cas9 system so that DNA cleavage is avoided. For example, the nuclease function of Cas9 can be inactivated so that a complex of guide RNA and such a "dead" Cas9 (dCas9) will target a specific site via the guide RNA but will not cleave the DNA (Qi et al., 2013). By coupling other proteins with different activities to the dCas9, however, different sorts of modifications can be made to the DNA or its associated proteins. Thus, it is possible to design variants of CRISPR/Cas9, ZFN, or TALE that will turn on or turn off adjacent genes, make single-base changes, or modify the chromatin proteins that associate with DNA in chromosomes and thus modify the epigenetic regulation of genes (Ding et al., 2016; Gaj et al., 2016; Konerman et al., 2015; Sander and Joung, 2014). All of these noncleaving variants fail to cleave DNA, thus reducing the potential for deleterious off-target events, and many other modifications are being introduced to enhance specificity and reduce off-target events (see Appendix A for further detail). Most recently, CRISPR/C2c2, a programmable RNA-guided, RNA-cleaving nuclease, has been described (Abudayyeh et al., 2016; East-Seletsky et al., 2016) that could be used to knock down specific RNA copies of genes without affecting the gene itself. This development raises the future possibility of nonheritable or reversible editing.

As can be seen from this brief survey, the rapidly developing versatility of these RNA-guided genome-editing systems is opening up numerous means of manipulating the expression and function of genes. A recent report of methods for inducibly knocking down or knocking out genes in a multiplex fashion in many cell types, including human pluripotent stem cells, as well as in mice (Bertero et al., 2016) further expands the potential of these methods. These and other advances have rapidly rendered these methods basic tools of molecular biology worldwide, adding to the existing toolkit assembled over the past 40 years. These methods are now being applied to study with unprecedented ease the functions of genes in cells and in experimental animals, such as yeast, fish, mice, and many others, to enhance understanding of life. They also are being used to investigate the derivation and differentiation of stem cells, providing fundamental insights relevant to regenerative medicine, and to develop culture models of human disease both to advance understanding of disease processes and to enable testing of drugs on human cells ex vivo.

BASIC LABORATORY RESEARCH TO ADVANCE
UNDERSTANDING OF HUMAN CELLS AND TISSUES

Basic biomedical research aimed at discovering more about the mechanisms and capabilities of genome editing offers significant opportunities to advance human medicine. Genome-editing research conducted on human cells, tissues, embryos, and gametes in the laboratory offers important avenues for learning more about human gene functions, genomic rearrangements, DNA-repair mechanisms, early human development, the links between genes and disease, and the progression of cancer and other diseases that have a strong genetic basis. Manipulation of genes and gene expression by genome editing allows one to understand the functions of genes in the behavior of human cells, including why they malfunction in disease. For example, editing of cultured human cells to model the changes that arise in cancer or in genetically inherited diseases provides culture models of those diseases with which to understand the molecular basis of the resulting defects. Such laboratory studies also allow the development of means of combating those defects, such as the testing of potential drugs in cell culture. All of those approaches are much easier now than they were just a few years ago.

Certain cells derived from an early embryo, after fertilization but prior to the developmental stage at which it would implant in a woman's uterus, are referred to as **embryonic stem (ES) cells.** These ES cells have scientific advantages because they can reproduce in cell culture and have the potential to form all the different body cell types while lacking the potential themselves to develop into a fetus. It is now also possible to create stem cells by manipulating adult somatic cells to convert them to a state in which they, too, have the ability to form multiple cell types, reducing the need to take stem cells from an early embryo. These are referred to as **induced pluripotent stem (iPS) cells.** Such pluripotent stem cells can be cultured in vitro and induced to develop into many different cell types, such as neurons, muscle or skin cells, and many others. Advances over the past several decades in understanding stem cells and how they can be used form the foundation for the field of **regenerative medicine,** which seeks to repair or replace damaged cells within human tissues or to generate new tissues after disease or injury. Although these are increasingly areas of clinical practice, and the application of genetically altered cells in humans is not covered in this chapter (see Chapter 4), there are nevertheless a number of important reasons why scientists aim to undertake basic investigations in human and animal stem cells in the laboratory.

Genome-editing methods have been extremely useful in generating a variety of genetic modifications in human ES and iPS cells. Before the advent of efficient genome-editing tools, these cells had proven resistant to genetic modification with the standard tools of homologous recombination that had been used effectively in mouse ES cells. Using those tools in human cells resulted in very low frequencies of targeted recombination. Improvements in efficiency resulting from the use of CRISPR/Cas9 have enabled rapid generation of tagged reporter cell lines, making it possible to follow differentiation pathways, look for interacting proteins, sort appropriate cell types, and investigate the functions of individual genes and pathways in cells, among many other applications (Hockemeyer and Jaenisch, 2016). For example, the ability to make precisely targeted mutations or corrections in specific genes has made possible the generation of human ES lines with different specific disease alleles on the same genetic background (Halevy et al., 2016) for use in research on the consequences of such disease genes. Conversely, genome editing also allows the targeted correction of disease mutations in patient-specific iPS cell lines to generate genetically matched control lines. Such modified stem cell lines are used primarily to conduct experimental and preclinical studies, to investigate specific disease processes, and to test drugs that could be used to treat such diseases. In the future, such edited stem cell lines could be used for various forms of somatic cell–based therapies (see Chapter 4).

BASIC LABORATORY RESEARCH TO ADVANCE UNDERSTANDING OF MAMMALIAN REPRODUCTION AND DEVELOPMENT

Germline cells are cells with the capacity to be involved in forming a new individual and to have their genetic material passed on to a new generation. They include precursor cells that form eggs and sperm, as well as the eggs and sperm cells themselves. When fertilization occurs to create an embryo, the earliest stages of this embryo, referred to as the **zygote** (fertilized egg) and **blastocyst,** have the potential to divide and form all the cells that will make up the future individual, including **somatic** (body) cells and new germ cells. As the embryo continues to develop, its cells differentiate into specific cell types that become increasingly restricted in their functions (e.g., to form specialized cells such as those in the nervous system, skin, or gut).

During reproduction and development, genetic changes made directly in **gametes** (egg and sperm), in egg or sperm precursor cells, or in very early embryos would be propagated throughout the future cells of an organism and may therefore be heritable by subsequent generations. As emphasized above, this chapter focuses exclusively on the use of genome-editing technologies in the laboratory, and not on clinical applications in humans or in embryos for the purposes of implantation to initiate pregnancy. Nevertheless, it is important to understand which cell types are involved in human development and their functions, because this information informs researchers' decisions about how to study particular scientific questions and informs ethical, regulatory, and social discussions around when and why it may be useful to use human cells, including embryos, in basic laboratory research.

Genome Editing of Germline Stem Cells and Progenitor Cells

It is already possible in mice to genetically modify the genome in a fertilized egg (the zygote), in individual cells of the early embryo, in pluripotent ES cells, or in spermatogonial stem cells, just as in somatic cells. In all these cases, the effects of the genetic modifications can be studied directly in the embryo or in cells in culture. There are a number of ways to undertake these genetic manipulations and a number of cell types in which they can be conducted. The cell types below are all considered part of the germline or have the capacity to contribute to the germline:

- embryonic stem cells derived from normal early embryos (blastocyst stages)
- cells from early embryos produced after somatic cell nuclear transfer (SCNT)[1]
- iPS cells obtained by reprogramming somatic cells into an ES cell-like state

In mice, these cell types can all be manipulated experimentally through genome editing. Stem cells of the types listed above can contribute to the germline in vivo after they are introduced into mouse embryos at the morula or blastocyst stage. This process generally creates an embryo that is a chimera, in which some cells are derived from the stem cells introduced into the embryo, and some are formed from the initial embryonic cells. Mouse or rat spermatogonial stem cells can be cultured and their genomes edited, and the cells can then be introduced into recipient mouse or rat testes, where they can give rise to sperm able to fertilize oocytes, at least in vitro (see Appendix A and Chapman et al., 2015). In all of these cases, when the resultant embryos are transferred back into the uterus to complete pregnancy, it is possible to establish lines of mice carrying the genetic alterations. These approaches provide unprecedented opportunities to explore the functions of all the genes in the genome and to develop rodent models of human diseases. Proof-of-principle experiments also have been

---

[1] SCNT is a technique in which the original nucleus of an egg cell is removed and replaced with a "donor" nucleus taken from another cell (e.g., from a somatic cell that has undergone genome editing). This is the technique that was used to create Dolly, the first cloned mammal obtained from an adult cell.

reported in which disease-related genetic mutations have been corrected in mouse zygotes (Long et al., 2014; Wu et al., 2013), embryonic stem cells, or spermatogonial stem cells (Wu et al., 2015) and then transmitted though the germline to produce genetically corrected mice.

The application of genome-editing technologies to the equivalent human cell types holds considerable potential value for fundamental research without any intent to use such manipulated cells for human reproductive purposes. Improved knowledge of how an early human embryo develops also is valuable in its own right, and because such knowledge can help answer questions about humans' own early development, as well as facilitate understanding and potential prevention or treatment of a wide range of clinical problems. A number of these applications are described below.

Improvements in Assisted Reproductive Technology

The success of human reproductive technologies and **preimplantation genetic diagnosis (PGD)** of inherited diseases has been, and continues to be, dependent on **in vitro fertilization (IVF)** and on culturing of human embryos from the zygote to the blastocyst stage. However, tools for ensuring that an individual embryo in culture is normal and capable of completing pregnancy remain limited. Most embryo research has been conducted on mouse embryos, which are similar to human embryos in certain respects but significantly different in others (see Box 3-2). Even the conditions in which human embryos are kept in culture are based largely on those established for mouse embryos. High rates of aneuploidy[2] are found in cultured human embryos relative to other species. This aneuploidy is often mosaic—that is, it varies among cells in the embryo (Taylor et al., 2014)—but how it arises and how it relates to in vitro culture conditions are not well understood. There is also concern that epigenetic[3] abnormalities might occur in human embryos in vitro (Lazaraviciute et al., 2014), which might compromise development or health, even later in life. Research on early-stage human embryos in culture should enable scientists to better understand the cellular and molecular pathways that control early human embryo development and the conditions under which human embryos in culture can develop successfully. This knowledge could in turn help improve IVF outcomes.

All of the differences between humans and mice discussed above mean that it is not possible to accurately infer developmental events in human embryos from studying mice. This limitation has practical consequences for

---

[2]Having a chromosome number that is not an exact multiple of the usual haploid number.

[3]The term "epigenome" refers to a set of chemical modifications to the DNA of the genome and to proteins and RNAs that bind to DNA in the chromosomes to affect whether and how genes are expressed.

the development of improved IVF technologies, as well as for the ability to derive the best pluripotent or other stem cells for modeling of human disease and for future regenerative therapies. Thus, there is considerable interest in experimental investigation of preimplantation human development in culture, in jurisdictions where such research on human embryos is permitted. The goals of this work are to understand the fundamental events of fertilization, activation of the embryonic genome, cell lineage development, epigenetic events such as X-inactivation, and others, and how these events compare and contrast with what is understood from studying mice.

Similar research also could provide insights into the reasons for the high rates of early pregnancy loss in natural human pregnancies (10 to 45 percent, depending on the age of the mother), as well as the causes of infertility. Better understanding of sperm development would be crucial in addressing issues of male infertility. Pluripotent stem cells arise from the early embryo, and these cells can generate ES cells in culture. Better understanding of human embryonic development would provide insights into the origins and regulation of pluripotency and how to translate that knowledge into improved stem cells for regenerative medicine. The potential benefits of such research are not limited to embryonic stem cells. Cell types that give rise to the yolk sac and the placenta also are determined in the early embryo prior to implantation. The yolk sac and placenta establish the crucial links with the mother during pregnancy and provide nutrients and other factors that enable the embryo to survive. Defects in these tissues can compromise a pregnancy, leading to miscarriage, premature birth, or postnatal abnormalities. Better understanding of how the yolk sac and placenta originate would help in improving techniques for overcoming infertility and preventing early miscarriage, as well as understanding and preventing congenital malformations. These extraembryonic cell types also provide cues that pattern the early postimplantation embryo, although almost nothing is known about these processes in humans. These possibilities and others discussed in this chapter are summarized in Table 3-1.

Understanding of Human Development

Genome editing by CRISPR/Cas9 and similar techniques has a key place in the tool set needed to undertake such experiments. CRISPR/Cas9-guided activation or inactivation of specific target pathways could be used to understand overall gene regulation in development. Indeed, as the efficiency of CRISPR/Cas9 continues to increase, it should be possible to use genome editing to knock out[4] genes in zygotes and study the effects directly

---

[4]A gene is said to be "knocked out" when it is inactivated because the original DNA sequence has either been replaced or disrupted.

BOX 3-2
Differences Between Mouse and Human Development

In the past few years, considerable progress has been made in understanding the events that allow the zygote to develop into the blastocyst, the earliest stage of embryonic development in which different cell types are formed. Much of this research has been conducted on mouse embryos. However, it is clear that a number of important differences exist between the development of mouse and rodent embryos and those of humans and most other mammals (see the figure below). Significant research remains necessary to understand what these differences are, how they arise, and why they are significant. Genome editing in human cells and early embryos in the laboratory provides an important tool to help address these questions.

A mouse blastocyst takes 3-4 days to develop, whereas a human blastocyst takes 5-6 days. The blastocyst has about 100 cells, is about 1/10th of a millimeter in diameter, and contains only three cell types; there is an outer layer called *trophectoderm* that encloses an inner cell mass consisting of *primitive endoderm* and *epiblast* cells. Mice, humans, and all mammalian embryos spend their first few days of development making mainly the cell types needed to survive in the uterus, the placenta, and the yolk sac, which are derived from trophectoderm and primitive endoderm, respectively (Cockburn and Rossant, 2010). The epiblast cells are the pluripotent cells that give rise to the entire embryo, including its germ cells (Gardner and Rossant, 1979).

In addition to the differences summarized in the figure above, there are clearly other differences in the control of development of the early embryos of the two species. In a mouse embryo, the signaling pathways and downstream gene regulatory pathways that drive the formation of the three cell types of the blastocyst are fairly well understood (Frum and Ralston, 2015). Each cell is restricted to one of these three fates by the blastocyst stage. Information from the molecular analysis of events in the early mouse embryo has helped in understanding the underlying principles of the establishment of cellular pluripotency. Together with knowledge gained from studying embryonic stem (ES) cells, this information aided in the momentous development of induced pluripotent stem (iPS) cells in which adult cells are reprogrammed to pluripotency using factors known to be expressed in the early embryo (Takahashi and Yamanaka, 2006; Takahashi et al., 2007). The ability to create iPS cells represents an example in which basic laboratory research contributed to critical advances in a field—in this case regenerative medicine. Scientists can use these cells to generate cells to study or treat disease, greatly reducing the need to use cells derived from embryos. Because iPS cells can be created from a person's own cells, they also minimize the immune rejection that can occur if cells arising from one individual are used in another.

In contrast to understanding of mouse development, much less is known about the cellular and molecular events of blastocyst formation in human embryos. Some experiments on the timing of cell-lineage restriction have been performed, but not with as much precision as in mice because of the restricted number of embryos that are available for research. Compounding the challenges of studying

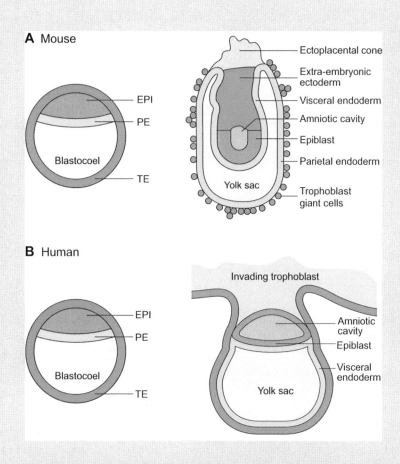

A Mouse

- Ectoplacental cone
- Extra-embryonic ectoderm
- Visceral endoderm
- Amniotic cavity
- Epiblast
- Parietal endoderm
- EPI
- PE
- Blastocoel
- TE
- Yolk sac
- Trophoblast giant cells

B Human

Invading trophoblast

- EPI
- PE
- Blastocoel
- TE
- Amniotic cavity
- Epiblast
- Visceral endoderm
- Yolk sac

Comparison of blastocyst and early postimplantation development between mouse and human. Whereas the blastocysts of the two species (left-hand figures) look very similar, later stages at the time of implantation (right-hand figures) show significant differences, particularly in the extraembryonic tissues.

(A) The trophectoderm of a mouse blastocyst after implantation undergoes a proliferative phase stimulated by FGF4 signals from the epiblast (EPI, blue) to form the extraembryonic ectoderm (green) and ectoplacental cone (light green). There is only limited invasion of the maternal uterus by mouse trophoblast cells until much later in placental development. PE = primitive endoderm; TE = trophectoderm.

(B) The trophectoderm of the human blastocyst does not stay in close contact with the epiblast after implantation but invades into the endometrium, where it will later form the chorionic villi.

SOURCE: Rossant, 2015.

continued

BOX 3-2 Continued

development in human embryos has been the absence of appropriate methods. The development of genome-editing tools can help address this gap.

The early postimplantation stages of mouse and human development differ morphologically and perhaps in other ways not currently understood. Current data suggest that cell-lineage restriction occurs later in a human embryo than in a mouse embryo, probably not until after the blastocyst is fully developed. New technologies for analyzing gene expression in small amounts of tissue, and even from single cells, are helping scientists gain insights into the molecular pathways controlling lineage development. Single-cell RNA sequencing, a method for looking at genome-wide gene expression in single cells, has been applied to early human embryos (Blakeley et al., 2015; Petropoulos et al., 2016). From these data it is already apparent that there are both similarities and significant differences between humans and mice in the developmental profiles of gene expression, including in some of the key genetic drivers known for mouse preimplantation development. It is possible to speculate about which of these genes are required to drive human preimplantation development, but it is not yet known how critical they are. Genome-editing methods such as CRISPR/Cas9 will allow determination of the roles of those genes expressed specifically during human preimplantation development.

Differences between mouse and human blastocyst formation also are thought to underlie the significant differences in the properties of ES cells derived from these two species (Rossant, 2015). Although both mouse and human ES cells are derived from the pluripotent cells of the blastocyst and share expression of some key pluripotency genes, they have many different properties, including

---

in genetically altered embryos. None of these experiments would involve human pregnancies, so none could result in heritable germline modifications. They would all be in vitro experiments, with results being analyzed primarily at the blastocyst stage in the first 1-6 days of development.

In some cases, there could be interest in exploring the effects of altering specific genes at the next stages of human development, notably the early stages after the embryo would implant in a uterus. At present, culture of human embryos up to the stage just prior to germ-layer formation (at 14 days after fertilization or the formation of the "primitive streak") is permitted in many countries. Improved culture systems that allow human embryos to develop in culture during the implantation period are being developed. Recent results suggest that these systems could be used to study the elaboration of extraembryonic structures and of the epiblast into an "embryonic disc"—processes that occur in humans in ways not found in mice (Deglincerti et al., 2016; Shahbazi et al., 2016). These improved cell their dependence on different growth factors for their self-renewal. Many of the properties of human ES cells are more similar to those of epiblast cells found in early postimplantation stages of mouse development, leading to the question of whether human embryos actually go through the same so-called naïve state of pluripotency observed in mouse blastocysts and ES cells (Huang et al., 2014; Pera, 2014).

In addition to ES cells obtained from the pluripotent cell lineage in the blastocyst, it is possible in mice to derive stem cells corresponding to progenitors of both trophectoderm and extraembryonic endoderm, termed TS and XEN cells, respectively (Rossant, 2015). These stem cell types are valuable for understanding molecular mechanisms of differentiation, as well as the properties of these cell lineages, which are relevant to placental and yolk sac biology in health and disease. However, attempts to derive equivalent extraembryonic stem cell types from human blastocysts have not yet been successful (Hayakawa et al., 2014). Such cell lines would be of great value, especially given the considerable evolutionary divergence seen in placental types among mammals. This divergence includes substantial differences in the types of cells making up the human placenta compared with mice and other mammals. For example, syncytiotrophoblast cells that invade and directly interact with the endometrium (the cells lining the uterus/womb) are present in the placenta of great apes and may even have unique properties in humans. As a result, it is not possible to rely on knowledge gained from studying mouse cells to understand normal development of the human placenta. Similarly, it is not possible to understand pathologies in which the placenta or placental interaction with the mother fails, which can cause miscarriage, or the placenta invades too vigorously into the uterus, which can lead to choriocarcinoma.

culture systems, combined with better ways of analyzing gene function using genome editing, can be expected to lead to better understanding of the fundamental processes of early human development. Already at least two research groups (in the United Kingdom and Sweden) have received regulatory permission to carry out CRISPR/Cas9 experiments on human embryos, aimed at addressing these kinds of fundamental biological questions.

Knowledge gained from such studies is expected to inform and improve IVF procedures and embryo implantation rates and reduce rates of miscarriage. Conversely, the same studies may lead to novel methods of contraception. Such research also should lead to better ways of establishing and maintaining stem cells from these early embryonic stages, which could facilitate efforts to derive cell types for studies and treatments of disease and traumatic injury. Knowledge gained from these laboratory studies using genome-editing methods in early human embryos should also provide information about the suitability of these methods for any eventual

TABLE 3-1 Reasons for Laboratory Studies of Human Embryos

In Vitro Studies	Clinical Outcomes
Studies of fertilization in vitro	Improvements in in vitro fertilization (IVF) and preimplantation genetic diagnosis (PGD) Possible improvements in contraception
Improved culture of early human embryos	Improvements in IVF and PGD Insights into reasons for miscarriages and congenital malformations
Development of extraembryonic tissues (yolk sac and placenta)	Insights into reasons for failures in implantation and for miscarriages
Isolation and in vitro differentiation of pluripotent stem cells	In vitro models for human diseases for experimental testing of drugs and other therapies Improved cells for somatic gene/cell therapies and for regenerative medicine
Investigations of sperm and oocyte development	Possible novel approaches to infertility

potential clinical use. That is, basic research can be expected to inform an understanding of the feasibility of making heritable, and preferably non-mosaic, changes in the genome (see Chapter 5). Because human embryos that can be used in research are a valuable and relatively scarce resource, it will be important to ensure that the most efficient methods are used for these laboratory studies of their basic biology. Thus, it is likely that in the course of this research, various technical issues associated with improving the use of genome-editing methods in human embryos will be addressed. Relevant questions include

- the type and form of genome-editing components to be introduced;
- whether to use Cas9 or an alternative nuclease;
- what method to use to introduce the genome-editing components—for example, as DNA, mRNA, protein, or ribonucleoprotein complex;
- whether to use single guide RNAs, pairs, or multiple guide RNAs as part of the editing machinery;
- the size of the DNA template and whether such a template is required;
- the optimal timing for genome editing, that is, whether information can be obtained by using two-cell embryos, whether it is necessary to use one-cell embryos, or whether it is best to introduce the reagents along with the sperm during in vitro fertilization;

- whether mosaicism can be tolerated, keeping in mind that it may be an advantage for certain experiments, as when cell fate is to be followed, but may need to be avoided in other cases, such as when investigating a gene whose product is a secreted protein; and
- how to test and improve modified versions of nucleases such as Cas9 or inhibitors of certain repair mechanisms (e.g., an effective inhibitor of nonhomologous end joining may be needed if the experiment demands homology-directed repair [Howden et al., 2016]).

Understanding of Gametogenesis and Infertility

In mice, the generation of spermatogonial stem cell (SSC) lines from the adult testes has provided a rich source of cells with which to study the process of spermatogenesis in vitro and in vivo, after regrafting to the testes. It is possible to alter these cells genetically and study the impact of the changes on the process of spermatogenesis itself or, in mice, the impact on the offspring. It is also possible to correct genetic mutations in the stem cells in vitro using CRISPR/Cas9. Proof of principle for such an approach has been published (Wu et al., 2015). This work used CRISPR/Cas9 editing in mouse SSCs to correct a gene mutation that causes cataracts in mice. The edited SSCs were transferred back to mouse testes, and round spermatids were collected for intracytoplasmic sperm injection (ICSI), a form of IVF, to create embryos. Resulting offspring were correctly edited at 100 percent efficiency. Similar experiments have been conducted using SSCs from other species, including macaques (Hermann et al., 2012). Stable human SSC lines have not yet been reported, but would clearly be an important tool for understanding male infertility and for exploring such issues as the higher rate of mutations associated with age. This is an active area of research because it may enable restoration of fertility in male cancer patients after radiation or chemotherapy. The ability to grow and manipulate human SSCs would, however, raise the possibility of generating human germline alterations if the cells were grafted back to the testes or used in IVF.

Related issues arise from experiments in which both oocytes and sperm progenitors have been generated from mouse ES cells. ES-derived oocytes can be fertilized by normal sperm, and ES-derived spermatids can fertilize eggs by ICSI (Hayashi et al., 2012; Hikabe et al., 2016; Saitou and Miyauchi, 2016; Zhou et al., 2016). Human gametes have not yet been generated successfully from pluripotent stem cells, although two recent papers report the generation of early germ cell progenitors from human ES cells (Irie et al., 2015; Sasaki et al., 2015). Through the use of genome-editing methods, this work also highlighted significant differences between mice and humans in the genes involved in specification of primordial germ cells. There is evidence as well that knowledge gained from studying later stages of spermatogenesis in mice may not always be applicable to the same process in humans. These findings reflect the role of research on human cells in answering questions about human biology. If human haploid gametes could be generated from human pluripotent cells, as they can be in mice, it would open up new avenues for understanding gametogenesis and the causes of infertility. It would also open up possibilities for using heritable genome modifications to address health problems that originate from genetic causes.

ETHICAL AND REGULATORY ISSUES IN BASIC RESEARCH

As described in more detail in Chapter 2, basic science research performed in the laboratory on somatic cells will be subject to regulation focused on safety for laboratory workers and the environment, including special review by institutional biosafety committees for work involving recombinant DNA. Few new ethical issues are raised, although if the cells and tissues come from identifiable living individuals, donor consent and privacy will be a concern, and in most cases the protocols will be subject to at least some review by institutional review boards.

Research with embryos is more controversial. As noted earlier, research using viable embryos is illegal in a small number of U.S. states (NCSL, 2016), and while permitted in most states, research that exposes embryos to risk generally may not be funded by the U.S. Department of Health and Human Services (HHS); this is due to the Dickey-Wicker Amendment,[5] which has been adopted repeatedly since the 1990s as part of the HHS appropriations process, including in the bills introduced for 2017 funding (see Chapter 2).[6] It states

(a) None of the funds made available in this Act may be used for—

(1) the creation of a human embryo or embryos for research purposes; or

(2) research in which a human embryo or embryos are destroyed, discarded, or knowingly subjected to risk of injury or death greater than that allowed for research on fetuses in utero under 45 CFR 46.204(b) and section 498(b) of the Public Health Service Act (42 U.S.C. 289g(b)).

(b) For purposes of this section, the term "human embryo or embryos" includes any organism, not protected as a human subject under 45 CFR 46 as of the date of the enactment of this Act, that is derived by fertilization, parthenogenesis, cloning, or any other means from one or more human gametes or human diploid cells.

---

[5]Public Law No. 114-113, Division H, Title V, § 508.
[6]§ 508(a) in both S. 3040 and H.R. 5926.

The effect of this combination of state and federal law is to make embryo research legal in most of the United States but generally not eligible for HHS funding.

Additional, extralegal oversight of laboratory research using human embryos comes from the stem cell research oversight committees that were widely adopted pursuant to recommendations of the National Academies regarding embryonic stem cell research (IOM, 2005; NRC and IOM, 2010). Recently, the International Society for Stem Cell Research, whose membership includes investigators from around the world as well as the United States, adopted guidelines calling for the transformation of these voluntary stem cell research oversight committees into human embryo research oversight (EMRO) committees that would oversee "all research that (a) involves preimplantation stages of human development, human embryos, or embryo-derived cells or (b) entails the production of human gametes in vitro when such gametes are tested by fertilization or used for the creation of embryos" (ISSCR, 2016a, p. 5). The review would include details of the proposal and the credentials of the researchers under the auspices of these independent, multidisciplinary committees of scientists, ethicists, and members of the public. The proposed committees would assess research goals "within an ethical framework to ensure that research proceeds in a transparent and responsible manner. The project proposal should include a discussion of alternative methods and provide a rationale for employing the requested human materials, including justification for the numbers of preimplantation embryos to be used, the proposed methodology, and for performing the experiments in a human rather than animal model system" (ISSCR, 2016a, p. 6).

CONCLUSIONS AND RECOMMENDATION

Laboratory research involving human genome editing—that is, research that does not involve contact with patients—follows regulatory pathways that are the same as those for other basic laboratory in vitro research with human tissues, and raises issues already managed under existing ethical norms and regulatory regimes. This includes not only work with somatic cells, but also the donation and use of human gametes and embryos for research purposes, where this research is permitted. While there are those who disagree with the policies embodied in some of those rules, the rules continue to be in effect. Important scientific and clinical issues relevant to human fertility and reproduction require continued laboratory research on human gametes and their progenitors, human embryos, and pluripotent stem cells. This research is necessary for medical and scientific purposes that are not directed at heritable genome editing, though it will also provide valuable information and techniques that could be applied if heritable genome editing were to be attempted in the future.

RECOMMENDATION 3-1. Existing regulatory infrastructure and processes for reviewing and evaluating basic laboratory genome-editing research with human cells and tissues should be used to evaluate future basic laboratory research on human genome editing.

4

Somatic Genome Editing

The use of human genome editing to make edits in somatic cells for purposes of treating genetically inherited diseases is already in clinical trials. Somatic cells contribute to the various tissues of the body but not to the germline, meaning that, in contrast with heritable germline editing (discussed in Chapter 5), the effects of changes made to somatic cells are limited to the treated individual and would not be inherited by future generations. The idea of making genetic changes to somatic cells, referred to as gene therapy, is not new,[1] and considerable progress has been made over the past several decades toward clinical applications of gene therapy to treat disease (Cox et al., 2015; Naldini, 2015). Hundreds of early-stage and a small number of late-stage trials are under way (Mullin, 2016), although only two gene therapies have been approved as of late 2016 (Reeves, 2016). Existing technical approaches to gene therapy are based on the results of extensive laboratory research on individual cells and on nonhuman organisms, establishing the means to add, delete, or modify genes in living cells or organisms. Prospects for future applications of gene therapy have recently been greatly enhanced by improvements in genome-editing methods, particularly the development of nuclease-based editing tools (see Chapter 3).

This chapter begins by providing background information on human somatic cell genome editing, including definitions of key terms. It then summarizes the advantages of genome editing over traditional gene therapy and

---

[1]Gene therapy denotes the replacement of faulty genes or the addition of new genes to cure or improve the ability to fight disease.

earlier approaches, and briefly reviews the repair methods—homologous and nonhomologous—used for nuclease-based genome editing. Next is a discussion of potential human applications of somatic cell genome editing. Scientific and technical considerations and ethical and regulatory issues are then examined in turn. The chapter ends with conclusions and recommendations. Additional scientific and technical detail on methods for genome editing are provided in Appendix A.

BACKGROUND

Genes, Genomes, and Genetic Variants

All humans contain two sets of genes inherited from their parents; each of these sets of genes is called a genome and is packaged into 23 chromosomes. The **haploid** (single) human genome is around 3 billion (3×10^9) base pairs long, and the two inherited genomes in each somatic cell (**diploid**) encode the information required for the assembly and functioning of a person's cells and body throughout life. Although people speak of the human genome, each genome differs from any other at many positions (around 1 in 1,000 base pairs, or about 3 million positions), and these genetic differences contribute to what makes individual humans unique (The 1000 Genomes Project Consortium, 2015). Many of these variations probably have little or no effect, but some affect the expression and/or functions of genes. Within the human genome lie approximately 20,000 genes that encode proteins, the molecules that actually build human cells and bodies, plus many other DNA elements that control when, where, and how much each gene is expressed (Ezkurdia et al., 2014). Some variants in genes can change the properties of the proteins they encode, while other genomic variants can affect the expression of genes. Such variants influence the color of hair or eyes, blood type, height, weight, and many other individual features, although most human traits are affected by interactions among multiple genes. Furthermore, other influences, such as diet, exercise, education, and environment, have major impacts by interacting with a person's genetic makeup.

Many of the variations in genomic sequences arise from alterations in the sequences of base pairs that arise during **replication** (copying) of the DNA during cell division (one can think of them as typographical changes). These alterations occur continually at a certain rate, and although cells have mechanisms for proofreading and correcting (editing) such changes, some escape the proofreading process and persist. Furthermore, the frequency of DNA alterations can be increased by radiation (e.g., by ultraviolet rays in sunlight or by cosmic or X-rays) or by environmental chemicals (e.g., cigarette smoke and other carcinogens). As mentioned, many of these variants have little or no effect, but others have positive or deleterious effects. This process of variation in human genomes has been going on since before humans evolved as a separate species and continues to this day. Evolution relies on this continual generation of variants—those that are advantageous are selected for, whereas those that are deleterious are selected against. Whether a particular variant is advantageous or deleterious, however, can vary with the context and may be a consideration in deciding whether to edit variants for clinical benefit.

Genetically Inherited Diseases

One primary impetus for interest in possible clinical applications of the recent advances in genome editing is the possibility that they provide new avenues for treating and preventing human disease. One such possible use is in the treatment of genetically inherited diseases, thousands of which are known.[2] Certain deleterious variants can be inherited from one or both parents, while others can arise de novo in the embryo rather than being inherited from either parent. The pattern of inheritance varies with the nature of the variant. If a variation that causes loss of function in a gene is inherited from one parent, it often has no evident effect, because the unaltered variant inherited from the other parent is sufficient to provide the function needed. Geneticists refer to this mode of inheritance as **recessive.** Recessive gene variants usually (but not always) have little or no effect in the so-called **heterozygous** state, when two different variants are present in the fertilized egg (zygote) and in the subsequent child and adult. That is, a person generally will not have the disease caused by a recessive deleterious gene variant unless that variant is inherited from both parents. If both parents are heterozygous, each having one copy of a deleterious variant, each of their children will have a 25 percent chance of inheriting two copies of that variant—the so-called **homozygous** state. In that case, there is no functional variant available, and the consequence may be a genetically inherited disease. Many examples of this phenomenon exist (e.g., certain forms of severe combined immunodeficiencies, such as bubble boy disease, as well as sickle-cell anemia and Tay-Sachs disease).

Other variants may actually produce medical problems even when present in a single copy despite the presence of a functional gene variant. Such variants, called **dominant,** produce deleterious effects even in the heterozygous state. A clear example is Huntington's disease, in which a single copy of a dominant disease-causing variant produces late-onset disease.

---

[2]OMIM, https://www.omim.org (accessed January 10, 2017); Genetic Alliance, http://www.diseaseinfosearch.org (accessed January 25, 2017).

Some inherited diseases, such as certain forms of hemophilia, which affect blood clotting, involve genes that are present on the X chromosome (so-called **X-linked**). Because men have only one X chromosome, whereas women have two, a single abnormal X-linked hemophilia gene in a man will lead to the disease being manifest, whereas women with just one deleterious variant will be carriers of the altered gene, usually without having bleeding symptoms (so called silent **carriers**).

Adding to the complexity of understanding genetic disorders is the observation, noted above, that some variants may be either deleterious or advantageous depending on the context. Probably the best known example is sickle-cell disease, which is caused by a variation in one of the genes encoding hemoglobin, the protein that carries oxygen in red blood cells. If the sickle hemoglobin variant is inherited from both parents (homozygous), it causes the hemoglobin protein to aggregate under certain conditions, leading to deformation of the red blood cells into a sickled shape that interferes with blood circulation, causing multiple difficulties and much pain and impairment of normal tissue functions. Heterozygous individuals (heterozygotes) who inherit just one sickle gene variant have few if any signs of disease and are known as carriers since they carry the sickle-cell variant and can pass it on to their children. It turns out that heterozygosity for this variant makes carriers somewhat resistant to malaria parasites that infect their red blood cells. That is, the sickle-cell variant provides a significant survival advantage in areas where malaria is present, and for that reason has been selected for and is relatively prevalent in such areas such as Africa, India, and the Mediterranean, where carriers are more common than in other areas. There are other examples of such balanced selection based on heterozygous advantage, balanced against the disadvantage of inheriting two disease-associated variants.

Finally, it is important to note that most human diseases are thought to be affected by genetic variants in multiple genes, with each variant having only a minor effect on disease progression. Thus, while the prospect of human genome editing to treat genetically inherited diseases has great appeal in some cases—for example, those in which a single gene can be clearly identified as causal—that is not true of the majority of common human diseases.

ADVANTAGES OF GENOME EDITING OVER TRADITIONAL GENE THERAPY AND EARLIER APPROACHES

Gene therapy is the introduction of exogenous genes into cells with the goal of ameliorating a disease condition. This is most efficiently done using viral vectors that take advantage of a virus's natural ability to enter cells. The viral vectors are used to introduce a functional transgene and compensate the malfunction of an inherited mutant gene (gene replacement) or to instruct a novel function in the modified cells (gene addition). The vectors also include exogenous transcriptional regulatory sequences (promoter) to drive transgene expression. Because viral vectors have a limited cargo capacity, both the transgene and the promoter have to be modified from the natural version present in the genome and may thus fail to properly recapitulate physiological expression patterns. According to the choice of vector and type of target cells, the genetic modification may be transient, long-lasting, or permanent. Permanent modification is achieved using lentiviral or gamma-retroviral vectors that physically insert into the genome of the infected cells (integration). However, because insertion is semi-random, it may affect the function and expression of genes at or nearby the insertion site, thus representing a potential risk (insertional mutagenesis). Currently, tremendous progress is being made in gene therapy because of improved viral vectors, particularly lentiviral and recombinant adeno-associated viruses (rAAV), and these strategies are being intensively investigated in the clinic. However, despite the fact that remarkable benefits are being reported in most treated patients (Naldini, 2015), more flexible and precise genetic modifications, such as those made possible by targeted genome editing, are needed to further improve the safety of gene therapy and broaden its application to the treatment of more diseases and conditions.

Until the past decade, attempts to use genome modification in the treatment of genetically inherited disease, also called **gene targeting,** were made by introducing a DNA template carrying the desired sequence into a cell population in culture, and then either allowing insertion at a random location or relying on rare homologous recombination events to incorporate that template sequence at an intended location in the genome. The DNA template generally was introduced into the cell using such systems as recombinant plasmids (small circular pieces of DNA) or viral vectors, which take advantage of a virus's natural ability to enter cells. The rare cells that acquired the desired sequence then had to be genetically selected and clonally expanded. Despite the limitations of this approach, the importance of gene targeting as an experimental tool is reflected in the broad use of homologous recombination to modify yeast, vertebrate cell lines, or even mice to genetically dissect a wide range of biological processes (Mak, 2007; Orr-Weaver et al., 1981).

The frequency of successful gene targeting using these older strategies ranged from 10^{-6} (1 in 1 million cells) for plasmid DNA to 10^{-2}-10^{-3} (1 in 100 to 1 in 1,000 cells) using viral vectors (such as rAAV). When scientists modify DNA with a nuclease that makes a double-strand break (DSB) at a desired location in the genome, however, the frequency of successful genome editing increases dramatically (Carroll, 2014; Jasin, 1996). Nuclease-based systems that make targeted genetic alterations are at the root of the genome-editing technologies discussed in this report. With nuclease-based editing systems, it is now possible to cut and, consequently, modify up to 100 percent of the desired target sequence in the genome, either by small insertions or deletions introduced by the nonhomologous end-joining DSB repair, or by relying on homologous recombination to introduce a new sequence at the target site, albeit with a somewhat lower efficiency. These dramatic improvements in efficiency have enabled scientists and clinicians to consider using genome editing for a greatly expanded range of applications, including application to the treatment of diseases.

Flexibility

Nuclease-based genome editing encompasses various methods for altering the DNA sequence of a cell. This editing can achieve several types of results, depending on where in the DNA the edits are made and for what purpose. Changes that can be made with genome editing include

- targeted disruption (inactivation) of the coding sequence of a gene (gene disruption);
- precise substitution of one or more nucleotides (e.g., in situ conversion of a genetic variant to wild type or to another allelic variant);
- targeted insertion of a transgene into a predetermined site for protein-coding genes;
- targeted alterations made to non–protein coding genetic elements that regulate gene expression levels (e.g., promoters, enhancers, and other types of regulatory elements);[3] and
- creation of large deletions at chosen genome locations.

Safety and Effectiveness

Nuclease-based genome editing may abrogate the risk of insertional mutagenesis inherently associated with prior gene-replacement vectors that integrate quasi-randomly throughout the genome, although late-generation integrating vectors used today may mitigate this risk. In addition, in situ gene correction of inherited mutations using genome editing reconstitutes both the function and the physiological control of expression of the mutant gene. This provides a safer and more effective correction strategy than gene

---

[3]Small insertions or deletions can be created to inactivate an element; larger defined deletions can be created to remove entire elements; specific nucleotide substitutions can be made in the element; or new genetic elements can be inserted into precise locations in the genome.

replacement, in which expression of the therapeutic transgene is driven by a reconstituted artificial promoter. Such randomly inserted transgenes may fail to reproduce the physiological expression pattern faithfully, and they can be strongly influenced by the insertion site, giving rise to substantial variegation of expression among a population of transduced cells. Indeed, one of the first potential applications of ex vivo genome editing may well be stem cell–mediated correction of primary immunodeficiencies—an improvement over prior transgenic approaches in which ectopic or constitutive expression of the therapeutic gene posed a risk of cancerous transformation or malfunction. If on-target editing frequencies of clinically relevant cell types are high enough to be therapeutically useful, genome editing may eventually outperform gene replacement (traditional gene therapy) in terms of safety, provided that off-target changes do not pose similar risks by modifying genes associated with cancer.

Another potential broad application of genome editing is precisely targeted integration of a gene expression cassette into a so-called safe genomic harbor, chosen because it is conducive to robust transgene expression and allows a safe insertion that does not have a detrimental effect on adjacent genes. This approach may ensure predictable and robust expression of a therapeutic gene without the risk of oncogenesis caused by inadvertent insertional activation of an oncogene. Targeted integration into a safe harbor and in situ correction of mutations are both potentially widely applicable to stem cell–based therapies as long as the targeted cells are amenable to extensive in vitro culture selection and expansion prior to clinical use. One can envisage increasing application of these types of genome editing as the ability to grow and differentiate different types of cells in culture improves, particularly in conjunction with differentiation from pluripotent cells (Hockemeyer and Jaenisch, 2016).

Gene Disruption

A unique application of genome editing relative to standard gene therapy strategies is targeted gene disruption. Indeed, clinical testing of gene disruption using zinc finger nucleases (ZFNs) is already under way, with some indication of benefit for T-cells (Tebas et al., 2014), and this approach has recently been extended to hematopoietic stem cells (HSCs). These trials aim to disrupt expression of a cytokine receptor, C-C chemokine receptor type 5 (CCR5), which also functions as a coreceptor for HIV infection and is not essential for T-cell function, thus making the T-cells of an HIV-infected individual resistant to viral infection.[4] Gene disruption could, in principle, also be used to eliminate a dominant disease-causing gene variant.

Accessibility

Multiple nuclease platforms have been developed or improved in the past 5-10 years, making it likely that additional such platforms will be developed in the near future. The CRISPR/Cas9 nuclease platform, developed just since 2012, has generated significant optimism among research, clinical, and patient communities and has democratized genome editing, making it usable by many more laboratories. As a result, CRISPR/Cas9 has raised awareness of genome editing as a therapeutic tool and motivated consideration of the ethical and regulatory issues associated with its use (Baltimore et al., 2015; Corrigan-Curay et al., 2015; Kohn et al., 2016). These issues are not new, however, nor are they specific to the CRISPR-Cas9 system; many of them have already been confronted and addressed in the context of earlier gene therapy and genome-editing applications.

HOMOLOGOUS AND NONHOMOLOGOUS REPAIR METHODS USED FOR NUCLEASE-BASED GENOME EDITING

Nuclease-based genome editing relies on the design of an artificial enzyme—a nuclease—to bind a specific target sequence in the genome where it creates either a DNA double-strand break or a DNA single-strand cut known as a "nick." The cell usually repairs the break through one of two major mechanisms: (1) nonhomologous end joining (NHEJ), which frequently inactivates the gene or genetic element during the repair process; or (2) homology-based mechanisms, generically described as homology directed repair (HDR). (See also Chapter 3.)

Genome editing by NHEJ creates an insertion or deletion ("indel") at the break site that alters the sequence of the edited gene. Importantly, while genome editing by NHEJ is precisely located by where the DNA break or nick is produced, it is not possible to predict the size or sequence of the resulting change in a single cell or the variability of the changes (indels) among a group of cells.

In genome editing by HDR, a DNA template is used either to create one or more nucleotide changes, perhaps to match a known human reference sequence, or to insert a novel sequence (e.g., one or more genes) at a precise

---

[4]There are six clinical trials involving the use of ZFNs to disrupt expression of CCR5. Three of these trials have been completed, one is ongoing, and two are currently recruiting participants. For more information, see https://www.clinicaltrials.gov/ct2/show/NCT02500849?term=zinc+finger+nuclease+CCR5&rank=1 (accessed January 10, 2017).

genomic location. In contrast to NHEJ, HDR-mediated genome editing allows scientists to predict both where the edit will occur and the size and sequence of the resulting change. Thus, HDR-mediated editing is analogous to editing a document because it enables precise changes in DNA sequence.

POTENTIAL HUMAN APPLICATIONS OF
SOMATIC CELL GENOME EDITING

Genome-editing applications can be categorized based on several general features:

- **Which cells or tissue(s) are modified**—in particular, whether the modification is made in somatic cells or tissues, which do not contribute to future generations; in a germ cell or germ cell progenitor, which can result in heritable changes passed to future children; or in a zygote, in which case both somatic and germ cells would be modified. (The focus here is on somatic editing; germline editing is discussed in Chapter 5).
- **Where the editing takes place**—in the test tube, followed by return of the cells or tissues to the individual (ex vivo), or directly in the person's body (in vivo).
- **The specific goal(s) of the modification**—for example, to treat or prevent disease or to introduce additional or new traits. These goals may be achieved by modifying a pathogenic DNA variant to a known nonpathogenic variant present in human reference sequences, or by modifying a gene to a sequence other than one that is a known existing human sequence.
- **The precise nature of the modification**—simple modification of a disease-causing mutation or risk-associated allelic variant, or more a complex change, such as disruption or ectopic/overexpression of an endogenous gene or addition of a novel function that augments a biological response or establishes resistance to a disease or pathogen.

The intent of each of these modifications could be to treat or prevent a disease but could also be to modify (or, in principle, even create novel) phenotypic traits in the treated cells or tissues. It is important to note, for example, that one can use genome editing to achieve enhancement of a cellular property (e.g., secreting supranormal amounts of protein or resisting a viral infection) with the intent of curing a disease. Such cellular enhancement with intent to modify disease course needs to be distinguished from the concept of enhancement aimed at creating a desired or novel organismal feature in humans (a topic discussed in detail in Chapter 6).

Table 4-1 provides examples of the types of human diseases that might

TABLE 4-1 Examples of Potential Therapeutic Applications of Somatic Cell Genome Editing*

Disease	Inheritance/ Transmission Pattern	Ex vivo or In vivo	NHEJ or HDR Mediated Editing	Stage of Development	General Strategy
Sickle-Cell Disease	Autosomal recessive	Ex vivo (HSPC)	HDR	Clinical development	Edit to non-disease-causing variant
Sickle-Cell Disease/β-Thalassemia	Autosomal recessive	Ex vivo (HSPC)	NHEJ	Preclinical	Induction of fetal hemoglobin
Severe Combined Immunodeficiency X-linked (SCID-X1)	X-linked recessive	Ex vivo (HSPC)	HDR	Clinical development	Knock-in of full or partial complementary DNA (cDNA) to correct downstream disease-causing variants
X-Linked Hyper IgM Syndrome	X-linked recessive	Ex vivo (T-cells)	HDR	Preclinical–clinical development	Knock-in of full cDNA to correct downstream disease-causing variants
Hemophilia B	X-linked recessive	In vivo (liver)	HDR	Clinical trial*	Express clotting factor from a strong promoter
Cystic Fibrosis	Autosomal recessive	In vivo (lung)	HDR	Discovery	Edit to non-disease-causing variant

HIV	Viral infection	Ex vivo (T-cells and HSPC)	NHEJ	Clinical trial	Engineer resistance to HIV
HIV	Viral infection	Ex vivo	HDR	Discovery	Engineer constitutive secretion of anti-HIV factors
Cancer Immunotherapy	NR	Ex vivo (T-cells)	NHEJ or HDR	Conceptual through clinical trial	Engineer more potent cancer-specific T-cells by genome editing
Duchenne's Muscular Dystrophy (DMD)	X-linked recessive	In vivo	NHEJ	Preclinical	Deletion of pathologic variant to convert Duchenne muscular dystrophy (DMD) to milder Becker's muscular dystrophy
Huntington's Disease	Autosomal dominant	In vivo	NHEJ	Discovery	Delete disease-causing expanded triplet repeat
Neurodegenerative Diseases	Various	Ex vivo or in vivo	HDR	Conceptual	Engineer cells to secrete neuroprotective factors

*Current information on clinical trials is available at ClinicalTrials.gov.
NOTE: HDR = homology-directed repair; HSPC = hematopoietic (blood) stem and progenitor cells; NHEJ = nonhomologous end joining; NR = not relevant (the edits are to lymphocytes designed to kill the cancer).

be treated using somatic cell genome editing. Even though this list is not comprehensive, it highlights the broad range of potential applications.

Clear examples of how genome editing might be applied to cure disease are to use homologous recombination to change the variant that causes sickle-cell disease back to the sequence that encodes wild-type β hemoglobin (Dever et al., 2016; DeWitt et al., 2016) or correct the deficits in severe combined immune deficiencies (Booth et al., 2016). A more subtle use of genome editing to correct a disease-causing variant is to insert the wild-type DNA copy of the mRNA (complementary or cDNA) into an endogenous locus to correct downstream mutations (Genovese et al., 2014; Hubbard et al., 2016; Porteus, 2016). Concerning the liver as a target organ, it has been shown that targeted insertion of a clotting factor transgene downstream of the promoter of the albumin gene in a fraction of hepatocytes may rescue the hemophilia bleeding phenotype in mouse models (Anguela et al., 2013; Sharma et al., 2015).

Several potential applications of genome editing entail causing gene disruption, provided that the delivery of the nuclease does not lead to loss of the treated cells because of toxicity or immune rejection. Among these applications are the disruption of dominant mutations and expanded triplet repeats in some neurodegenerative diseases, such as Huntington's disease (Malkki, 2016), and the reconstitution of a functional dystrophin in Duchenne's muscular dystrophy by deletion or forced skipping of the exon carrying the disease-causing mutation (Long et al., 2016; Nelson et al., 2016; Tabebordbar et al., 2016). Other examples include disruption of an endogenous gene repressor to rescue expression of a fetal gene compensating for a defective adult form, as is currently being attempted by disrupting expression of BCL11A in the erythroid lineage; to rescue fetal globin expression to compensate for the lack of expression of adult β globin in thalassemia major; or to counteract the sickling β globin mutant in sickle-cell anemia (Hoban et al., 2016). In T-cell immunotherapy, a promising application of genome editing is single or multiplex disruption of genes that may antagonize, counteract, or inhibit the activity of exogenous cell-surface receptors introduced into T-cells to direct them against tumor-associated antigens (Qasim et al., 2017). These strategies can strongly potentiate current cell-based immunotherapy strategies, possibly overcoming current barriers that limit efficacy in most solid tumors.

SCIENTIFIC AND TECHNICAL CONSIDERATIONS ASSOCIATED WITH THE DESIGN AND APPLICATION OF GENOME-EDITING STRATEGIES

All types of genome editing involve consideration of certain parameters that together determine the efficacy and potential toxicity of a genome-editing tool. These scientific and technical considerations inform how and why a particular approach is chosen to meet a research or therapeutic goal; they also impact the nature of the data that will be available for the regulatory evaluations that will be required for potential preclinical testing, clinical trials, review, and ongoing oversight of these methods.

Choice of Engineered Nuclease Platform

The choice of nuclease includes the platform type, which can be based on protein-DNA recognition (e.g., meganucleases, ZFNs, or transcription activator-like effector nucleases [TALENs]) or on nucleic acid base-pairing recognition (e.g., CRISPR/Cas9), and the design and generation of the components that target the intended genomic sequence. When developing protein-based DNA-binding domains that are made using zinc fingers and TAL effectors, extensive engineering and improvement are possible for each specific sequence-binding domain, such that it is difficult to make a general prediction on the performance and specificity of the overall platform. That is, for ZFNs and TALENs, optimization of performance (activity and specificity) often requires work for each nuclease that may or may not translate to another nuclease.

In contrast, when RNA-based nucleases such as Cas9 are developed, general improvements are made to the platform itself and should translate to each specific target sequence. Because the only major difference among CRISPR-Cas9 systems is the targeting guide RNA, optimization of one Cas9 nuclease often will generalize to improved performance of other nucleases. This fact has implications for the ease or speed with which genome-editing systems designed for one clinical application could be adapted to target others.

Delivery Strategy: Ex Vivo and In Vivo Genome Editing

Genome editing can be carried out **ex vivo** or **in vivo**. In ex vivo editing, it is possible to conduct a number of checks on the edited cells before they are administered to a patient because the cells are first manipulated in the laboratory. Ex vivo editing, which occurs outside the body, is suitable only for certain cell types, however. By contrast, in vivo editing allows other types of cells and tissues to be edited, but poses additional safety and technical challenges because it involves administering the genome-editing tool directly into a patient's body fluids (e.g., blood), body cavities, or organs in order to modify targeted cells in situ.

Ex vivo genome editing can be performed by isolating and manipulating a population of the intended target cells outside the body and then transplanting those cells into an individual. The source of cells can be autologous or allogeneic: autologous cells are derived from the same individual, while allogeneic cells are derived from an immunologically matched donor. Whether the cells are sourced from the same patient or a matched donor, the administered cells often have stem cell–like properties, which may allow their self-renewal and long-term maintenance in vivo, as well as repopulation of the treated tissue with their genetically modified progeny. In some approaches, the cells can be treated in culture to induce commitment or differentiation toward a desired cell type or lineage before being administered to the patient. Otherwise, the edited cells can be differentiated somatic cells, such as short-lived or long-lived immune effector cells that are expanded and genetically modified ex vivo to enhance their activity against a tumor or infectious agent. Several somatic cell types have been isolated, genetically modified, and transplanted, including blood-forming hematopoietic (blood) stem and progenitor cells, fibroblasts, keratinocytes (skin stem cells), neural stem cells, and mesenchymal stromal/stem cells. This list likely will grow as scientific knowledge and techniques improve. An expanded repertoire of cell types has the potential to increase the range of possible ex vivo genome-editing applications.

In in vivo genome editing, the editing machinery that needs to be delivered to the cells includes the nuclease that cuts the DNA and, in the case of CRISPR/Cas9, the guide RNA that targets the editing to a specific genomic location. If HDR is intended, a homologous template is also required. Targets of in vivo genome editing may include long-lived tissue-specific cells, such as muscle fibers, liver hepatocytes, neurons of the central nervous system, or photoreceptors in the retina, but may also include rare, tissue-specific stem cells and other types of cells that cannot easily be harvested and transplanted. Relative to ex vivo approaches, however, in vivo approaches pose greater challenges with respect to efficient delivery of the genome-editing machinery to the right cells in the body, ensuring that the correct location in the genome has been successfully edited, and minimizing errors resulting from off-target editing.

Additional Considerations

A number of additional scientific and technical considerations related to both ex vivo and in vivo genome editing inform the development of human genome-editing systems.

Ability to Isolate the Relevant Cell Types

To carry out ex vivo genome editing, it is necessary first to isolate the relevant cell types from an appropriate tissue source or to generate them from pluripotent stem cells, and then to grow and modify them ex vivo and finally administer them to the patient so that they can engraft and/or deliver the intended biological activity. There are several advantages to the ex vivo strategy: only the intended cells are exposed to the editing reagents, there is a wide choice of delivery platforms that can best be fitted to each cell type and application, and it is possible to characterize and even purify and expand the edited cells before administration. Currently this process has been established for only a few cell types, including cells that will eventually give rise to skin, bone, muscle, blood, and neurons. The range of possible ex vivo genome-editing applications will expand with the development of scientific knowledge about how to isolate additional primary cell types and derive other cell types from pluripotent cells, grow the cells ex vivo, and ultimately transplant them back into patients successfully and safely.

Ex vivo genome-editing strategies have a number of expected limitations, which are common to all attempts at culturing cells ex vivo. These limitations include the need for prolonged culture and expansion from a few cells or even a single founder cell, both of which entail the risk of accumulating mutations, as well as incurring replicative exhaustion. This issue is particularly relevant for genome editing because inducing double stranded breaks in DNA, as is required to initiate the process, may itself trigger such cellular responses as apoptosis (cell death), differentiation (changing cell type), cell senescence (aging), and replicative arrest (cells stop dividing). All of these cellular responses are detrimental to cell expansion and maintenance of pluripotency.

These limitations represent significant hurdles to ex vivo genome editing because most therapeutic applications require substantial numbers of cells for infusion. Overcoming these hurdles will require better ways to culture cells, better understanding of the safety risks associated with genomic accrual of random mutations in these settings, and reliable assays for assessing such events. Additional hurdles are the ability to fully control the commitment and differentiation of cells in culture and their purification from the source pluripotent cells. This is an important consideration because administration of immature cells may be associated with a risk of tumorigenesis or failure to integrate functionally within the tissue. Despite these limitations, ex vivo genome editing has the advantage that cells with the desired alteration can be selected and the accuracy of the alterations validated before transplantation to the patient.

Ability to Control Biodistribution of the Genome-Editing Tool

Additional considerations for in vivo genome editing are linked to the choice of the delivery platform for the editing machinery because this choice impacts the extent, time course, and in vivo biodistribution of the genome-editing tool. This consideration has major implications for potential efficacy, acute and long-term toxicity, and immunogenicity and even the risk of unintentional editing of germ cells. Efficient editing of the intended genomic site usually requires a high level of intracellular nuclease expression, even though this often can be for only a short time to prevent excess toxicity and off-target activity. Whereas short-term, high expression of the genome-editing nuclease can be obtained relatively easily for cells cultured in vitro, it is more challenging in vivo. Finally, in an in vivo setting there could be unintentional (inadvertent) modification of the germ cells or primordial germ cells; therefore, preclinical development of in vivo editing should address the risk of modification of germ cells resulting in heritable changes that could be passed on to future generations and minimize this potential risk in humans enrolled in clinical trials.

In general, the risk of germline transmission associated with the administration of ex vivo genome-edited cells is likely to be low if one can show that the editing reagents do not remain associated with the treated cells and are not shed in active form at the time of administration. In these conditions, nonclinical studies of germline transmission may not be necessary. On the other hand, in vivo administration of editing reagents would require assessment of their potential biodistribution to the gonads and activity on germ cell genomes. These parameters will be strongly influenced by the delivery platforms used and the timing and route of delivery. When viral vectors are used to deliver the nuclease, the preclinical studies might take into consideration accumulating knowledge from animal and human studies concerning the potential of these vectors to reach germline cells. Preclinical studies in animal models such as nonhuman primates could be designed to monitor both the biodistribution of the vector/vehicle as well as the activity of the nuclease in cells from off-target tissues, including the gonads.

A suggested approach to studying the potential of germline transmission in such nonclinical models would be to follow a decision tree, in which a positive finding triggers the next level of investigation. One could first investigate the presence of the reagent and/or genomic signs (indels) of its activity in the gonads; next identify their actual occurrence in germ cells isolated from the positive gonads; and then determine the transient or sustained occurrence of this finding and, eventually, the transmission of the genetic modification to the viable progeny of the treated animals. Molecular assays could be designed to track the occurrence of indels at the intended or surrogate nuclease target sites, provided that such sites exist in the genome of the species used for the study with sufficient affinity for the nuclease to support the sensitivity of the assay. Many limitations exist when conducting such studies in surrogate animal species, as already discovered for several gene therapy products, including the low sensitivity of the available assays, species-specific differences in vehicle biodistribution and access to the gonadal cells, and the general difficulties of testing transmission to the female versus male germline. Because of these limitations, regardless of the outcome of nonclinical biodistribution data, contraceptive measures are usually recommended (if meaningful or applicable) for patients undergoing in vivo gene therapy in clinical trials, at least for the expected time of clearance of the administered vector/vehicle from the body fluids, and usually extended to encompass at least one cycle of spermatogenesis (approximately 64-74 days in men). Testing of semen can be done at various points during this time interval; if samples are positive, the testing should continue, and the respective regulatory authorities should be notified. On the other hand, there are currently no noninvasive means of monitoring women for germline transmission.

Ability to Limit Immune Response to Delivery Vectors or Genome-Editing Proteins

In vivo delivery of proteins and nucleic acids is currently done with either of two types of platforms. The first is based on chemical conjugates (lipo- and/or glyco-complexes) that provide short-lived but relatively inefficient expression across multiple different tissue types, although advances have been achieved in targeting specific cell types, such as liver (Yin et al., 2014). This approach can expose therapeutically irrelevant cell types in the patient to the potential toxicity of the nuclease. The second type of platform relies on viral vectors that can provide robust and tissue-specific expression, but they also are frequently long-lived and more likely to provoke an immune response. Self-complementary rAAV8 vectors (scAAV), for example, have been shown to mediate continued expression of the engineered nuclease. Sustained nuclease expression increases the risk of DNA damage and genotoxicity, with subsequent potential risk of widespread (albeit possibly slow) cell death or malignant transformation of the patient's cells. Moreover, all current formulations of editing machinery contain elements that are derived from proteins of common microbial pathogens, which could trigger primary or secondary immune responses in treated individuals. As has been well documented in viral gene therapy studies, immune recognition of viral vector proteins may lead to rapid and complete clearance of cells that have received the editing machinery, which eliminates the benefit of the treatment. The risk of clearance of the edited cells is exacerbated by preexisting immunity and by the extent and duration of expression of the antigen.

Ability to Make Genome Edits in Nondividing Cells

Another major hurdle for both ex vivo and in vivo editing is that targeted insertion of a DNA sequence into postmitotic cells, such as neurons, is not feasible because of their low or absent homologous recombination activity. In contrast, NHEJ, which is active in nondividing cells, has been harnessed mainly for the generation of indels to inactivate a gene. However, NHEJ can, with modifications to the methods, be used to generate site-specific gene insertions (e.g., Maresca et al., 2013; Suzuki et al., 2016). Most recently, it was reported that one of these methods, homology-independent targeted gene integration, or HITI, allows targeted knock-in of DNA sequences in dividing cells (e.g., stem cells) and most importantly, in nondividing cells (e.g., neurons) both in vitro and in vivo (Suzuki et al., 2016).

In vivo genome editing is a highly sought-after application that has been shown to be feasible and potentially therapeutic in some mouse models. Substantial challenges to its translation to the clinic remain, however, at least in the current modalities of administration. Also considering the well-known difficulties of predicting immune response in animal models, stable expression of nucleases, despite being apparently well tolerated in some animal models, may not be the preferred route to clinical development.

Assessment of the Activity and Specificity of Genome Editing

Each targeting nuclease can be characterized by the *efficiency* and *specificity* of DNA cleavage. Efficiency can be relatively easily measured (by sequencing the targeted site). Specificity reflects on-target versus off-target site activity, which also can be measured by various assays, each with advantages and disadvantages (see Appendix A for details). While whole-genome sequencing could be the gold standard for analyzing single cells or clones, the depth of this sequencing is not sufficient to assess the off-target spectrum in populations of cells.

Comparing Off-Target Editing Rate with the Natural Mutation Rate of the Human Genome

It is important to note that accurate assessment of the specificity of a genome-editing approach requires that mutations created by the genome-editing process be distinguished from those that occur spontaneously throughout a life span. The natural error frequency of normal genome replication varies among sites in the genome but is approximately 10^{-10} per base per round of DNA replication. Because each human cell contains approximately 6 billion DNA base pairs, even the naturally low error rate means that DNA replication can be expected to generate, on average, approximately one or a few de novo mutations in each round of cellular replication. Thus, as cells proliferate, they naturally accumulate mutations at this rate. In addition to this background mutation frequency, a significant amount of DNA damage results from normal environmental exposures such as radiation, oxidative stress, and DNA-damaging agents in the environment. A direct comparison between the mutation frequency generated by a genome-editing nuclease and the spontaneous mutation frequency has not yet been conducted, but results from this type of analysis are likely to depend on the specific nuclease in question and on which cell type is examined. The error rate of nuclease technologies continues to improve and may at some point, if it is not already, be less than the spontaneous mutation frequency.

Measuring Efficiency and Specificity for Each Delivery Platform

For genome-editing applications, the system (nuclease and targeting sequences) must be delivered inside cells. Because the choice of delivery platform determines the extent, level, and time course of expression of the genome-editing machinery, it affects the efficiency and specificity displayed in a given set of experimental conditions and furthermore determines the toxicity and immunogenicity profile. In addition, several intrinsic features of the chosen delivery platform (DNA, RNA, or protein; delivery mechanism) also influence its potential toxicity (see Table A-1 in Appendix A). These effects usually are due to normal innate target-cell responses to exogenous molecules, and they often are stronger for DNA—especially DNA plasmids—than for RNA or proteins. The innate responses to viruses may vary with virus and cell type: usually they are very low for AAV or lentivirus in human somatic cells (Kajaste-Rudnitski and Naldini, 2015), with the exception of some immune cell types, such as dendritic cells and macrophages, which have a large complement of built-in viral sensors and may trigger interferon and inflammatory responses (Rossetti et al., 2012). The purity and composition of reagents (plasmid versus linearized DNA, mutant bases in RNA, high performance liquid chromatography [HPLC] purification of components) also can play a significant role.

Finally, the frequency with which the intended target sequence and related sequences occur in the genome and the local chromatin environment at the target site also can influence the efficiency and specificity of a genome editing approach. All the factors mentioned above are likely to vary according to the treated cell type and modality (ex vivo versus in vivo). Moreover, the ratio of on- to off-target activity also is affected by the intrinsic biology of the targeted cell type, including differences in cell-cycle status, DNA-damage responses, and repair capability.

Preclinical Studies to Assess Efficiency and Specificity

In the development of human genome-editing applications, preclinical studies are undertaken to establish the activity and specificity of each editing nuclease system. The design of these preclinical studies is influenced by the choice of target cells and experimental conditions, and the results should be viewed as providing relative rather than absolute values. An additional caveat is that most of these preclinical studies measure nuclease activity and specificity over a large population of cells, among which nuclease expression will vary. Because the ratio of on- to off-target activity also varies with nuclease expression level, the cells with higher nuclease expression may have a less favorable ratio since the on-target activity will saturate, while activity at off-target sites becomes more evident. On the other hand, cells with lower expression may exhibit a more favorable ratio because activity is evident mainly at the intended target site. This consideration suggests that the dose dependence of on- and off-target rates be considered as part of the process of validating a genome-editing approach.

Assessment of nuclease specificity will continue to evolve as scientific knowledge and techniques improve. From an operational standpoint as of this writing (late 2016), however, the following represents a reasonable approach to conducting this assessment:

- Use both bioinformatics and unbiased screens to identify potential off-target sites (see Appendix A).
- Use deep sequencing of both cell lines and the primary target cell type to determine the frequency of indels at both on- and off-target sites (validation).
- Evaluate validated off-target sites for potential biological effects, and eliminate nucleases that generate off-target activity at sites that could be predicted to have biologic effects. It should be noted that most off-target sites identified to date lie in non-protein-coding regions of the genome, making their functional importance difficult to assess.
- Use assays that measure gross chromosomal integrity, such as karyotyping, single-nucleotide polymorphism (SNP) arrays, and translocation assays. These assays are limited in being relatively insensitive.
- Use diverse functional assays of the target cells of interest to measure the risk of clonal dominance and to assess the actual feasibility, efficiency, and toxicity of the genome-editing manufacturing process.

It is important to note that to develop a genome-editing approach for clinical use, it may not be necessary or feasible to conduct comprehensive efficiency and specificity studies performed at high-enough sensitivity to capture all possible off-target edits. Ongoing work in standard gene therapy, for example, has indicated that uncontrolled lentiviral insertions, which cause even more disruptive changes than nonhomologous repair of a double-strand break, may be relatively safe and well tolerated in several types of cells and tissues. This is true even when large numbers of insertions (up to 10^8 or 10^9 per patient) are introduced. A further consideration is that the off-target activity is dependent on the sequence. Much of the early preclinical testing aimed at establishing targeting efficacy and specificity has been carried out in nonhuman organisms, especially mice. However, the genomes of humans and mice are sufficiently divergent that assessment of the specificity of engineered nucleases in the genomes of mice or other rodents may have somewhat limited predictive power for the same genome-editing approach in humans.

Summary

In summary, genome editing is already being incorporated into somatic gene therapy approaches, and such applications are likely to increase. Genome-editing strategies are in competition with other therapeutic approaches, including small molecule therapies; biologics; and most notably other gene therapy approaches, such as lentiviral vectors and rAAV vectors used for gene replacement. In the end, therefore, each strategy will need to be evaluated against the others in terms of efficacy, risk, cost, and feasibility.

ETHICAL AND REGULATORY ISSUES POSED BY SOMATIC CELL GENOME EDITING

In most respects, somatic cell genome editing will be developed with the benefit of gene therapy's robust base of technical knowledge, and within the existing system of regulatory oversight and ethical norms that have facilitated the current research and clinical development of somatic cell and gene therapy around the world, including the Australia, China, Europe, Japan, and the United States (see Chapter 2). These regulatory systems include a wide range of preclinical models and study designs to support the clinical development of therapies based on edited cells, as well as a roadmap for first-in-human clinical testing and eventual marketing.

Regulatory Oversight in the United States

As described in Chapter 2, clinical testing of somatic cell genome editing could not begin in the United States without the Food and Drug Administration's (FDA's) first having approved an Investigational New Drug (IND) application, and the clinical protocol would require institutional review board (IRB) approval and ongoing review (FDA, 1993). In addition, review by the National Institutes of Health's (NIH's) Recombinant DNA Advisory Committee (RAC) informs the deliberations of the FDA and IRBs and provides a venue for public discussion. Other countries have

similar pathways, as described in Chapter 2, albeit with some variations in
the stage of research at which a cell-based therapeutic can be marketed and
the terms under which it can be withdrawn.

The question of approval for clinical use hinges largely on identifying
when benefits may be expected to outweigh risks when a therapy is used as
labeled and as intended (Califf, 2017). Clinical trial data are increasingly
reviewed within a structured framework that identifies need, alternatives,
areas of uncertainty, and avenues for risk management.[5] According to former FDA Commissioner Robert Califf,

> FDA product review teams must weigh scientific and clinical evidence and
> consider conflicting stakeholder and societal perspectives about the value
> of benefits and the tolerability of risks. They must consider the existence
> and effectiveness of alternative treatments, disease severity, risk tolerance
> of affected patients, and potential for additional insight from postmarket
> data. Such decisions require seeking the appropriate balance between
> high-quality evidence and early access, between benefit and risk, between
> protecting the US public and encouraging innovation that may improve
> health outcomes. (Califf, 2017)

Approval of a gene therapy may depend upon how carefully risks and
benefits can be monitored once it enters clinical use. On this topic, the FDA
has issued an influential (though nonbinding) guidance for gene therapy trials that would have relevance to genome-editing trials as well (FDA, 2006).
Long-term follow-up is not always required, for example, when preclinical data on factors such as vector sequence, integration, and potential for
latency demonstrate that long-term risks are very low. But when long-term
risks are present, "a gene therapy clinical trial must provide for long-term
follow-up observations in order to mitigate those risks" (FDA, 2006, p. 1).
Without such a plan for long-term follow-up observations, the risks would
be unreasonable and (presumably) the trial not approvable. Where merited,
the guidance suggests a 15-year period of posttrial contact, observation,
and physical exams (though this can be shortened based on such factors as
vector persistence, or when subjects are predicted to have only short-term
survival). Prior to enrolling, subjects must give voluntary, informed consent
to long-term follow-up, and while they may withdraw at any time, it is
hoped that they will comply.

Once approved by the FDA for particular populations and indications,
gene-based therapies would be subject to postmarket monitoring and adverse event reporting, and special warnings added. The products would be

[5]Structured Approach to Benefit-Risk Assessment in Drug Regulatory Decision-Making,
PDUFA V Plan (FY 2013-2017). Draft of February 2013. http://www.fda.gov/downloads/
ForIndustry/UserFees/PrescriptionDrugUserFee/UCM329758.pdf (accessed January 30, 2017).

withdrawn completely if shown to be unsafe or ineffective. In addition, postmarket risk evaluation and mitigation strategies (REMSs), such as requiring physicians to have special proficiency or requiring patients to be entered into a registry, could be required if significant safety concerns would preclude approval absent these extra controls.

Off-label use of cells subjected to genome editing would be legal in the United States, in Europe, and in other countries, and is probably to be expected with respect to patient populations (e.g., if approved for adults, use might well be extended off-label to pediatric populations) or for varying degrees of severity of the disease indication.[6] The prospect of off-label use has led to speculation about uncontrolled expansion of the technology into uses that are unsafe, unwise, unnecessary, or unfair. And it is true that off-label use, while an important aspect of innovative medicine, can at times lead to uses that lack a rigorous evidentiary basis. But the specificity of these edited cells may limit the range of off-label uses for unrelated indications more than is the case with many drugs.[7] While one might imagine a cell therapy based on genome editing for muscular dystrophy being of possible interest to those with healthy muscle tissue who wish to become even stronger, other examples are more difficult to envision, at least for the near future. This point is of particular relevance to concerns about uses that go beyond restoration or maintenance of ordinary health (discussed in Chapter 6) because the specificity of edited cells makes such applications less likely at this time.

Several technical challenges faced in moving somatic genome editing toward clinical testing have already been met by conventional somatic gene therapy. Concerning ex vivo strategies, they are based on modifying human cell types and thus can be tested only in in vitro culture models or upon xenotransplant of the modified cells into immunocompromised mice. These studies interrogate cell viability, biodistribution, and biological function in vivo, including self-renewal, multipotency, and clonogenicity, all crucial features of stem cells. In vivo strategies may require preclinical testing of toxicity and biodistribution in nonhuman primates, including evidence that unintentional modification of the germline does not occur. Indeed, the field of gene therapy has determined that in vivo approaches that would lead to unintentional modification of the germline should not be permitted. Note, however, that most assays of germline transmission have low sensitivity, and thus a certain degree of uncertainty may have to be managed in considering clinical development and regulation.

---

[6]The FDA recently held a public hearing to discuss its regulations and policies on manufacturer communications about unapproved or off-label uses of medical products, including cell-based therapies (FDA, 2016a).

[7]Communication, FDA, December 15, 2016.

Several guidance documents have been published by regulatory authorities in the United States and Europe and by the International Conference on Harmonisation (ICH) to illustrate the general principles for investigating and addressing the risks for inadvertent germline integration of gene therapy products in nonclinical studies, and to provide considerations for minimizing this potential risk in humans enrolled in clinical trials (EMA, 2006; FDA, 2012a; ICH, 2006). Such guidelines could be suitably adapted to the design of preclinical studies of somatic genome-editing strategies.

In an effort to speed the development of regenerative medicine, a new public–private partnership has been launched. The International Standards Coordinating Body was established

> to advance process, measurement, and analytical techniques to support the global availability of cell, gene, tissue-engineered, and regenerative medicine products, and cell-based drug discovery products. Creating standards creates a more uniform compliance environment and addresses and assists in future efforts for harmonization internationally of the regulatory framework for submissions across the globe.[8]

The sectors of activity include genetic modification of cells, with specific mention of standards for measuring off-target events in genome editing (Werner and Plant, 2016).

Regulating Somatic Genome Editing by Approach and Indication

An ethical and regulatory assessment of future somatic genome-editing applications may depend on both the technical approach to the editing and the intended indication. Like traditional gene therapy, somatic genome editing could be used to revert an underlying genetic mutation to a variant not associated with disease, which would result in a fraction of the targeted cells regaining normal function. Somatic genome editing also could be used to engineer a cell so that its phenotype differed from that of a normal cell and was better able to resist or prevent disease. For example, a cell could be changed so that it made above-normal amounts of a protein, or so that it was resistant to a viral infection. Both ex vivo and in vivo approaches to genome editing could be applied to treat or prevent a disease. In addition, genome editing could be used to alter a trait not associated with disease (see Chapter 6).

Regardless of the final framework used to assess human somatic cell genome-editing applications, it is vital that the regulatory oversight mechanisms have sufficient legal authority and enforcement capability to identify

---

[8]See http://www.regenmedscb.org (accessed January 10, 2017).

and block unauthorized applications. To date, the existing structures have been successful in preventing unauthorized applications of gene therapy, and the current framework provides guidance on key elements. Although human genome editing may be somewhat more difficult to control than traditional gene therapy because technical advances have made the editing steps easier to perform, the cellular manipulations and delivery of edited cells to the patient continue to demand high-quality laboratory and medical facilities, which generally will ensure that regulatory oversight is in place.

Preventing Premature or Unproven Uses of Genome Editing

The issue of unregulated therapy has been particularly problematic in the field of stem cell/regenerative medicine, with rogue entities around the world making scientifically unfounded claims about stem cell therapies and profiting from desperate patients (Enserink, 2016; FDA, 2016b; Turner and Knoepfler, 2016). In part this is due to some of the past unduly optimistic statements about the near-term prospects of regenerative medicine, in part to the presence of unregulated jurisdictions, and in part to some resistance—at least in the United States—to the regulatory authority of the government. In the United States, federal courts have confirmed the FDA's jurisdiction over the use of manipulated cells, but this is still the subject of some confusion.[9] Edited cells—particularly those taken from a patient and then returned to that patient—may engender the same confusion about whether this is a regulated product or merely the practice of medicine, and the regulatory authority needs to be made clear from the outset. Overall, then, regulatory bodies need the legal authority, leadership commitment, and political support to apply their legal powers to halt the marketing of therapies that use human genome-editing products that have not undergone regulatory review and approval (Charo, 2016a). With regard to stem cell therapies, there has been considerable concern about the absence of vigorous use of enforcement powers by the FDA (Turner and Knoepfler, 2016), although Italy's experience with closing down one clinic has illustrated the level of legal and political power needed to do this (Margottini, 2014).

Special Considerations Associated with Genome Editing in Fetuses

In certain situations, either the most effective or the only approach would be to attempt to edit the somatic cells of a fetus prior to delivery. Diseases for which these special circumstances might apply include those that are multisystemic or have an extremely early onset that would make postnatal intervention too late to benefit the child or are extremely chal-

---

[9]*U.S. v. Regenerative Sciences*, 741 F. 3d 1314 (D.C. Cir 2014).

lenging from a technical standpoint. In addition, because of the tremendous developmental plasticity of the fetus, fetal editing might be more effective than postnatal editing in certain circumstances. An example would be attempting to revert a disease-causing variant that affects every neuron in the brain.

In a more general sense, the therapeutic editing process could be carried out ex vivo in a scenario in which cells could be harvested from the fetus, edited outside the body, and then transplanted back into the fetus. Currently, established methods for isolating and transplanting autologous fetal cells are available for a limited number of cell types, but the range of cell types is likely to increase in the future.

Therapeutic editing in fetuses also could be performed in vivo, in which case the editing machinery would be delivered to the fetus to modify cells in situ. As noted above, the in situ correction of a disease-causing variant early in development has the potential to be more effective than postnatal in vivo editing, when many organ systems are more fully developed. In utero stem cell therapy has been tried (with limited success) (Couzin-Frankel, 2016; Waddington et al., 2005), so the general concept of in utero therapy with emerging areas of medicine has already undergone some ethical analysis. And an International Fetal Transplantation and Immunology Society has been formed, which holds annual meetings to review prospects and progress for fetal gene therapy.[10]

Although fetal genome editing has potential advantages, at least two special ethical issues would need to be addressed: special rules for consent (see Chapter 2) and the increased risk of causing heritable changes to the germline by causing modification of germ cells or germ cell progenitor/stem cells.

With regard to consent, key issues have been addressed by existing oversight mechanisms, fetal surgery has already been used in clinical care, and in utero fetal gene therapy is attracting increasing interest (McClain and Flake, 2016; Waddington et al., 2005). The risk/benefit calculation is shifted relative to a postnatal or adult intervention, with the degree of risk to which a fetus can be subjected being strictly limited when there is no prospect of medical benefit to the future child. When such benefit is possible, however, the more usual standards for risk/benefit balance apply. Decisions about fetal surgery have been made with the understanding that the pregnant woman has the ethical and legal authority to give informed consent. In the United States, as in other countries, maternal consent is required (Alghrani and Brazier, 2011; O'Connor, 2012), and when research is aimed at maternal health as well, maternal consent alone is sufficient.[11]

---

[10]See http://www.fetaltherapies.org (accessed January 30, 2017).
[11]Research Involving Pregnant Women or Fetuses, 45 CFR, Sec. 46.204.

In the United States, however, NIH-funded research is subject to special regulations set forth at 45 CFR Part 46, Subpart B, and paternal consent (if available) also is required if the research holds the prospect of benefit solely to the fetus. Even when not funded by NIH, many studies in the United States employ these same rules.

A second issue is the challenge of assessing whether unintended germline editing has occurred if in vivo somatic editing is attempted in a fetus. A key feature of germline cell development is that the primordial cells that will give rise to germ cells are sequestered from somatic cells at key developmental points. Before this sequestration of germline and somatic cells occurs or has been finalized in early development, germline cells might be edited as efficiently as would be the desired somatic cell targets. As a result, there could be a higher risk of unintentional edits to germline cells early in fetal development compared with performing the same intervention later in fetal development. It might be possible only to assess postnatally whether editing of germ cells or germ cell progenitors had occurred, at which time it would be too late to change the outcome.

CONCLUSIONS AND RECOMMENDATIONS

In general, there is substantial public support for the use of gene therapy (and by extension, gene therapy that uses genome editing) for the treatment and prevention of disease and disability (Robillard et al., 2014). Human genome editing in somatic cells holds great promise for treating or preventing many diseases and for improving the safety, effectiveness, and efficiency of existing gene therapy techniques now in use or in clinical trials. While genome-editing techniques continue to be optimized, however, they are best suited only to treatment or prevention of disease and disability and not to other less pressing purposes.

The ethical norms and regulatory regimes already developed for gene therapy can be applied for these applications. Regulatory assessments associated with clinical trials of somatic cell genome editing will be similar to those associated with other medical therapies, encompassing minimization of risk, analysis of whether risks to participants are reasonable in light of potential benefits, and determining whether participants are recruited and enrolled with appropriate voluntary and informed consent. Regulatory oversight also will need to include legal authority and enforcement capacity to prevent unauthorized or premature applications of genome editing, and regulatory authorities will need to continually update their knowledge of specific technical aspects of the technologies being applied. At a minimum, their assessments will need to consider not only the technical context of the genome-editing system but also the proposed clinical application so that anticipated risks and benefits can be weighed. Because off-target events will vary with the platform technology, cell type, target genome sequence, and other factors, no single standard for somatic genome-editing specificity (e.g., acceptable off-target event rate) can be set at this time.

> RECOMMENDATION 4-1. Existing regulatory infrastructure and processes for reviewing and evaluating somatic gene therapy to treat or prevent disease and disability should be used to evaluate somatic gene therapy that uses genome editing.

> RECOMMENDATION 4-2. At this time, regulatory authorities should authorize clinical trials or approve cell therapies only for indications related to the treatment or prevention of disease or disability.

> RECOMMENDATION 4-3. Oversight authorities should evaluate the safety and efficacy of proposed human somatic cell genome-editing applications in the context of the risks and benefits of intended use, recognizing that off-target events may vary with the platform technology, cell type, target genomic location, and other factors.

> RECOMMENDATION 4-4. Transparent and inclusive public policy debates should precede any consideration of whether to authorize clinical trials of somatic cell genome editing for indications that go beyond treatment or prevention of disease or disability.

5

Heritable Genome Editing

For prospective parents known to be at risk of passing on a serious genetic disease to their children, heritable genome editing[1] may offer a potential means of having genetically related children who are not affected by that disease—a desire shared by many such parents (e.g., Chan et al., 2016; Quinn et al., 2010). Thousands of genetically inherited diseases are caused by mutations in single genes.[2] While individually, many of these genetically inherited diseases are rare, collectively they affect a sizable fraction of the population (about 5-7 percent). The emotional, financial, and other burdens on individual families that result from transmission of such serious genetic disease can be considerable, and for some families could potentially be alleviated by heritable editing. Recent advances in the development of genome-editing techniques have made it realistic to contemplate the eventual feasibility of applying these techniques to the human germline. As discussed elsewhere in this report, improvements in genome-editing techniques are driving increases in the efficiency and accuracy of genome editing while also decreasing the risk of off-target events. Because

---

[1] "Germline editing" refers to all manipulations of germline cells (primordial germ cells [PGCs], gamete progenitors, gametes, zygotes, and embryos) (see Chapter 3). "Heritable genome editing," a form of germline editing that includes transfer of edited material for gestation with the intent to generate a new human being possessing the potential to transmit the "edit" to future generations, is discussed in this chapter. The distinction turns on intent rather than on the technological intervention, which is highly similar in both cases.

[2] See https://www.omim.org (accessed January 3, 2017) and http://www.diseaseinfosearch.org (accessed January 4, 2017).

BOX 5-1
Mitochondrial Replacement Techniques

A technique for mitochondrial replacement already has engendered fresh discussion of heritable genetic modification. All people have DNA in the nuclei of their cells that encodes most of their traits, but also a very small amount of DNA in the mitochondria in their cells. A variety of diseases are caused when mutated mitochondria are passed from parent to child through the mother's egg. Replacing these defective mitochondria with normal mitochondria from another woman's egg would allow for conception of children with vastly reduced risk of inherited disease while satisfying prospective parents' desire for genetically related offspring. Sons could not pass along the donated mitochondria to their own future children, but daughters could, through their now-modified eggs, thus rendering this a potentially heritable form of germline alteration.

A 2016 National Academies committee recommended pursuing a cautious, incremental approach to mitochondrial replacement, with trials limited to situations involving a known risk of passing along serious disease (NASEM, 2016e). It also recommended initially limiting the techniques' use to male embryos, so that any effects of the donation would be experienced only by the first generation of children. With additional research and evidence of safety, the committee concluded, mitochondrial replacement could be expanded to a heritable form that would include female embryos. The United Kingdom's Human Fertilisation and Embryology Authority has also reviewed the mitochondrial replacement procedures and concluded that they are robust enough to proceed with either male or female embryos, although to date the procedures have been approved but not yet performed.

germline genome edits would be heritable, however, their effects could be multigenerational. As a result, both the potential benefits and the potential harms could be multiplied. In addition, the notion of intentional germline genetic alteration has occasioned significant debate about the wisdom and appropriateness of this form of human intervention and speculation about possible cultural effects of the technology. As discussed below, these include concerns about diminishing the dignity of humans and respect for their variety, failing to appreciate the importance of the natural world, and a lack of humility about our wisdom and powers of control when altering that world or the people within it (Skerrett, 2015).

A similar debate is already under way regarding a related set of techniques—mitochondrial replacement—in which genetic disease carried by mitochondrial DNA is avoided by using healthy mitochondria from a donor. Because mitochondria in the egg are passed down maternally through the generations, the effect of these techniques is to make a heritable genetic change, albeit one that does not change the DNA in the nucleus. Mitochondrial replacement has been used in Mexico (Hamzelou, 2016) and Ukraine (Coghlan, 2016) and has been authorized although not yet used in the United Kingdom (HFEA, 2016a,b). A recent National Academies study led to the recommendation that mitochondrial replacement be permitted to proceed to clinical trials in the United States provided it is subject to strict criteria and oversight (NASEM, 2016e) (see Box 5-1). In early 2017, there were reports of a child born after use of the technique in the Ukraine, in this case for an infertility-related condition that would not have met the criteria laid out by either the Human Fertilisation and Embryology Authority (HFEA) or the National Academies report (Coghlan, 2017).

This chapter begins by reviewing potential applications of and alternatives to heritable genome editing. It then describes in turn scientific and technical issues, ethical and social issues, and potential risks associated with these applications. The chapter then turns to the regulation of heritable genome editing. The final section presents conclusions and a recommendation.

POTENTIAL APPLICATIONS AND ALTERNATIVES

Preventing Transmission of Inherited Genetic Disease

Opinions differ as to whether heritable genome editing should be used to prevent the transmission of inherited genetic diseases. Heritable genome editing is not the only way to accomplish this goal. Other options include deciding not to have children; adopting a baby; or using donated embryos, eggs, or sperm. These options, however, do not allow both parents to have a genetic connection to their children, which is of great importance to many people. Alternatively, in vitro fertilization (IVF) with preimplantation genetic diagnosis (PGD) of the embryos can be used to identify affected embryos so that parents can choose to implant only those embryos that are free of the diagnosed mutation. This option is not without potential risks and costs, however, and it also involves discarding affected embryos, which some find unacceptable. One can also avoid transmitting genetic mutations to the next generation by using prenatal genetic diagnosis of the fetus followed by selective abortion of affected fetuses. But as with PGD, some people find it unacceptable to terminate an ongoing pregnancy regardless of the predicted health of the future child.

In these situations, for those who are aware they are at risk of passing on such a mutation, the use of heritable genome editing offers a potential avenue to having genetically related children who are free of the mutation of concern. This form of editing could be done either in gametes (eggs, sperm), in gamete precursors, or in early embryos, but it is important to note that IVF procedures would be required to generate embryos for subsequent genomic modification. In most cases, PGD could be used to identify unaffected embryos to implant.

However, there are some situations where all or a majority of embryos will be affected, rendering PGD difficult or impossible. For example, dominant late-onset genetic diseases, such as Huntington's disease, can occur at high enough frequency in some isolated populations that one parent will be homozygous for the mutation. In such situations, all embryos would carry the dominant disease-causing allele that would cause the disease in the children, so PGD is not useful. In other populations, the frequency of particular disease-causing mutations may be high enough that there is a significant chance that both prospective parents will be carriers of mutations in the same gene. Examples include the tumor suppressor genes BRCA1 and BRCA2, which increase the risk of breast and ovarian cancer even when inherited in a single copy (because of loss of the unaffected copy of the gene) and Tay-Sachs disease and other early-onset lysosomal storage diseases that are caused by the inheritance of two copies of recessive mutations. In these situations, only one in four embryos would be free of a disease-causing mutation. Those unaffected embryos could be identified by PGD, but the number of embryos potentially available for implantation would be significantly reduced. There are also examples of diseases that are caused by pairing of two different mutations in a given gene, known as "co-dominance," and combinations of specific alleles of two or more genes, in which PGD becomes more difficult.

As the survival of people with severe recessive diseases like cystic fibrosis, sickle-cell anemia, thalassemia, and lysosomal storage diseases improves with advances in medical treatments, the possibility cannot be dismissed that there will be an increase in the number of situations in which both prospective parents are homozygous for a mutation. The societal and medical pressures faced by these people often bring them together in social groups where they are more likely to interact and develop close relationships. Similar associations can develop among patients with autosomal dominant genetic diseases that allow development to reproductive age (e.g., achondroplasia, osteogenesis imperfecta), again increasing the likelihood of transmitting disease alleles. As our ability to treat children and adults with serious genetic diseases improves through both conventional and somatic genome-editing therapies, there may be a growing need to address concerns potential parents might have about passing along these diseases to their children. Such situations may well increase interest among carriers and affected individuals in using genome-editing techniques to avoid passing on deleterious genes to their children and subsequent generations.

There can be an additional problem in the case of mutations that compromise fertility, which is the case for women who carry mutations—

such as Fragile X, BRCA-1 (de la Noval, 2016; Oktay et al., 2015), and others—that cause the loss of oocytes during development or postnatally. Beyond inherited mutations, external factors like cancer treatments and environmental chemicals can also reduce ovarian reserve in women who wish to avoid transmission of a genetic disease. In these cases, women have fewer embryos available to screen from each cycle of superovulation, and the chance of establishing a pregnancy with an unaffected embryo (via IVF and PGD) is lower than it is for women without these mutations. As a result, affected women might require multiple superovulation cycles, with their attendant risks, discomforts, and costs, to identify an unaffected embryo.

In all of these situations, if it were safe and efficient to use heritable genome editing (e.g., in gamete progenitors) to correct the mutation, this alternative might be preferred by prospective parents who otherwise would be considering PGD. The number of people in situations like those outlined above might be small, but the concerns of people facing these difficult choices are real.

Treating Diseases That Affect Multiple Tissues

Some genetically inherited diseases affect specific cell types or tissues, such as particular types of blood cells. These diseases can be treated by somatic genome editing, and indeed, some of these treatments are already being used (see Chapter 4). However, somatic genome editing is less well suited to treating other genetic diseases that affect multiple tissues because it may be unable to target all aspects of the disease or may have difficulty reaching a sufficient number of cells in the affected tissues to ameliorate symptoms. Examples of conditions for which somatic genome editing is already being investigated but may not be fully effective include cystic fibrosis, which affects multiple epithelial tissues (tissues of the lungs, gut, and other organs), and muscular dystrophies, which can affect multiple muscle types, including heart muscle, as well as other tissues, such as brain. Couples with such diseases who want to have genetically related children might be future candidates for heritable genome editing because editing the defective gene in the germline could have therapeutic benefit in all tissues.

Duchenne muscular dystrophy (DMD) is an instructive example of the challenges faced by the application of germline genome editing. DMD is an X-linked disease that affects about 1 in 3,600 male births. Symptoms begin to appear within the first few years after birth and progressively worsen. The average life expectancy for a person with DMD is about 25 years. DMD is caused by mutations in one of the largest genes in the genome, dystrophin, which contains multiple repeating similar segments. Both the size of the dystrophin gene and its repeats predispose it to mutation, making this genetic disease relatively common. Somatic genome-editing approaches are already being developed to remove the deleterious alterations in the dystrophin gene in muscle precursors. Such somatic genome-editing approaches will ameliorate the condition but are not expected to correct the symptoms in all tissues.

Once those somatic editing approaches have been tested clinically, one might imagine trying to use germline editing to correct the defect in all tissues. However, women who know they are carriers for a DMD mutation could use PGD to avoid having an affected child. Furthermore, one-third of DMD cases are due to de novo mutations, which would not be recognized until after birth and thus are not amenable to germline genome editing. Somatic editing approaches currently appear to be more useful than germline editing for this disease. However, the pace of advances in genome-editing methods and stem cell biology may alter that situation.

SCIENTIFIC AND TECHNICAL ISSUES

Practically speaking, considerable technical difficulties remain to be overcome in applying genome editing to zygotes and early embryos. Although the efficiency and accuracy of targeting can be extremely high, and there are sound reasons for believing that off-target effects can be greatly reduced (see Chapter 3 and Appendix A), there still would be a need to ensure that only embryos with correctly targeted alleles would be returned to the uterus to complete pregnancy.

Mosaicism

If genome editing were performed in a zygote (fertilized egg) or an early embryo, there would be a significant chance that some of the cells in the resulting early embryo would not have the desired (or even any) edits. This situation is called "mosaicism," and it presents a significant challenge to the application of heritable genome editing in zygotes or embryos. Screening of an edited embryo by PGD to test for mosaicism would not ensure correct editing of the implanted embryo because a single cell may not reflect the genotype of the other cells of the embryo, and removal of multiple cells for testing would destroy the embryo.

The impact of mosaicism depends to some extent on the gene being targeted. Mosaicism is a serious problem if the gene of interest encodes a required cellular function, but if the gene encodes a secreted factor (e.g., growth hormone or erythropoietin), or leads to the secretion of a required molecule (such as a blood clotting factor), then correcting the gene in only a subset of cells may be sufficient. Furthermore, because the germline in the resulting child may also be mosaic, editing only a subset of cells may not solve the problem for succeeding generations. But it may offer a better chance of finding a disease-free embryo after PGD, or allow culture and selection of edited spermatogonial stem cells (see section on potential alternative routes to heritable edits below), thereby enabling those children to have unaffected offspring. Overall, the issue of mosaicism would currently present a serious impediment to the clinical application of heritable genome editing in zygotes or early embryos, although recent progress suggests that this impediment may eventually become surmountable (Hashimoto et al., 2016).

Potential Alternative Routes to Heritable Edits

Editing the embryo genome is not the only potential way to achieve heritable genome modification. Approaches that directly modify the genomes of the gametes (eggs and sperm) or their precursors before fertilization could overcome problems of mosaicism and would potentially allow preselection of appropriately targeted gametes before in vitro fertilization.

There are a number of potential routes to gamete genome editing, some of which are already in use in mice and others of which remain to be fully developed. For example, spermatogonial stem cells (which will give rise to sperm) could be isolated by biopsy from testes, edited in culture, tested for correct gene editing, and then reimplanted into the testes. Alternatively, generating sperm or oocyte progenitors via induced pluripotent stem (iPS) cells would allow genome editing to occur in the stem cell population. Correctly targeted clones could be identified and used to generate spermatids or perhaps sperm, either in vitro or in vivo, and used to fertilize donor eggs. Significant progress on such technologies is being made in mice and other mammals, including nonhuman primates (Hermann et al., 2012; Hikabe et al., 2016; Shetty et al., 2013; Zhou et al., 2016). A future in which this kind of approach could be extended to ensure precise and effective correction of a disease-causing variant in gametes is not unrealistic (see further discussion in Chapter 3 and Appendix A). The future prospects for heritable genome editing in humans will change dramatically if genome editing in progenitors of human eggs and sperm becomes a reality.

Effect on the Human Gene Pool

Another consideration is that some genes that cause serious genetic diseases, like sickle-cell anemia, have been subject to positive selection to maintain the disease-causing allele in the population because it produces some protection against infectious disease when present in one copy (heterozygous) (see Chapter 4). The same might be true for some other disease-causing variants, and there is some evidence suggesting that might be the case for cystic fibrosis, although this has not yet been established

(Poolman and Galvani, 2007). Such examples have led some to question whether heritable genome editing to remove disease-causing variant genes might significantly alter the human gene pool. As discussed earlier, the numbers of cases of human germline editing to treat disease, if it were to be approved, would be very small, and there is little chance of any significant effects on the gene pool in the foreseeable future. It has also been proposed that any heritable genome editing should be restricted to making changes that occur naturally in the human population (i.e., converting deleterious disease-causing variant [mutant] alleles to a common nonpathogenic DNA sequence) to minimize the risk of unexpected effects of the modification in generations to come (see also Chapter 6 for discussion of genome editing for enhancement purposes). Changing a disease-causing mutation to a known existing nonpathogenic sequence would be the case in any currently envisioned therapeutic applications, and thus the effect of any such heritable genome-editing changes for therapeutic purposes is expected to have minimal effect on the human gene pool.

Ability to Select Appropriate Gene Targets

Finally, the issue arises of whether current knowledge of human genes, genomes, and genetic variation and the interactions between genes and the environment is sufficient to enable heritable genome editing to be performed safely. While current knowledge is arguably sufficient for some genes, in many cases it is not. There is uncertainty, for example, about why the APOE4 allele, which clearly correlates with increased risk of Alzheimer's disease, is present in the human gene pool at such a high frequency. One theory is that it may confer an advantage in other respects, similar to the heterozygous advantage of sickle-cell mutations that confer protection against malaria (see Chapter 4). A gene such as APOE4 would not be a good candidate for heritable genome editing because it may confer some protection against liver damage by hepatitis C infection (Kuhlman et al., 2010; Wozniak et al., 2002), and also the fact that its deleterious effects are not fully penetrant. Knowledge of genome–environment interactions will improve over time as large-scale projects linking genomic sequences with details of health, environment, and lifestyle are carried out—such as the 100,000 Genomes Project in the United Kingdom and the Precision Medicine Initiative in the United States. As understanding of the genome progresses and genome-editing/stem cell technologies improve, future possibilities for editing the heritable germline to improve human health and well-being will need to be the subject of ongoing, careful consideration. Each potential target gene would need to be evaluated carefully on both scientific and ethical grounds, and only well-understood genes would be suitable candidates for heritable genome editing.

ETHICS AND REGULATION OF EDITING THE GERMLINE
TO CORRECT DISEASE-CAUSING TRAITS

Nearly half a century ago, Bernard Davis published an essay that presciently outlined discussions still under way today about the promise, the risks, and the roadmaps for genetic research, including research on making heritable changes in the germline (Davis, 1970). He began his article with a call "to assess objectively the prospects for modifying the pattern of genes of a human being by various means" (p. 1279) and continued with a caution: that one must keep in mind that "the most interesting human traits—relating to intelligence, temperament, and physical structure—are highly polygenic" (p. 1280) and therefore depend upon large numbers of genes interacting in complex ways with the environment. This is still true, but more is being learned every year about the genetic regulatory circuits that control complex traits, and there is an ongoing need to consider the potential benefits and risks of heritable genome editing.

Balancing Individual-Level Benefits and Societal-Level Risks

One of the challenging characteristics of debates concerning heritable genome editing is that they require balancing possible benefits that accrue primarily to individuals (such as prospective parents and children) against not only risks to the individuals, but also against possible harms at a social and cultural level. This is a complicated ethical analysis, in no small part because the individual benefits and risks are more immediate and concrete, whereas concerns about social and cultural effects are necessarily more diffuse. In addition, although examination of past technological innovations can help in making predictions about social and cultural changes, these predictions remain necessarily speculative because any such changes resulting from a new technology take time to develop. Thus, the ethical debates become difficult because the arguments can fail to engage each other directly.

In the United States, appropriate consideration of social and cultural concerns is usually resolved within the context of civil rights jurisprudence and legal decisions, which compare the burdens on individual liberties or the discriminatory impact of those burdens to whether there is a rational or compelling need for these particular state restrictions. In these cases, the outcomes are often determined less by the substantive arguments for and against the technology or an individual's choice and more by the level of justification required to uphold the restrictions. When ordinary liberties are restricted, a mere rational basis for the governmental restrictions will be upheld by the courts. If the liberties involved are fundamental, such as those specifically identified in the Bill of Rights or otherwise deemed fundamental by the courts, then a much more compelling and well-crafted justification for the restrictions is required. The contours of the latter category can be uncertain, however, because of enduring debates surrounding the methodology and legitimacy of judicial determinations that some rights are fundamental despite their absence from the Bill of Rights. Procreative rights fall within this disputed area, making it more difficult to predict which level of justification will be needed should there be a challenge to government restrictions on one or more aspects of procreative activities (Murray and Luker, 2015).

Parental Benefits

The possible benefits of heritable genome editing accrue most immediately to individuals: the prospective parents who want to have an unaffected genetically related child (and that child) but fear passing along a disease. The desire for genetic relation is evidenced by the fact that many prospective parents, faced with the choice between foregoing genetically related children or risking the birth of a child with a genetic illness, will choose to risk having an affected child (Decruyenaere et al., 2007; Dudding et al., 2000; Krukenberg et al., 2013). If an edit is made in a gene that is well understood and the change is a conversion to a known, common, nonpathological sequence, heritable genome editing may represent an option that is at times more effective or acceptable than PGD. It would offer benefits to the parents and allow for the birth of a child who would enjoy better health. In the case of some disorders that are lethal at a young age, it would allow for the birth of a child with the prospect of a more ordinary lifespan.

Access to heritable genome editing would be consistent with the broadest legal and cultural interpretations of parental autonomy rights in the United States. The desire to have genetically related children may arise from a variety of factors, ranging from a wish to see one's self or one's ancestors reflected in the appearance of the children to a belief in the need for a biological linkage in order to satisfy a sense of lineage, continuity, or even some form of immortality (Rulli, 2014). Precluding access to this technology could be regarded as limiting parental autonomy, depending upon the country and the culture. Indeed, some people feel they have a religious or historical mandate to have genetically related children. There are others who do not share this view of parental autonomy, and see germline editing as a step toward seeing children as constructed products and an increasing intolerance of their inevitable imperfections and failures to live up to parental expectations (Sandel, 2004). And some would argue that satisfying the desire for genetically related children is not an unalloyed benefit, as it can be seen as reifying what some view as outdated notions of kinship and family precisely at a time when adoption, same-sex marriage, donor gametes, surrogacy, and stepparenting are being normalized (Franklin, 2013).

In the United States, procreative liberty is grounded in legal cases that relate to the right to have children at the time one wishes, and with considerable latitude in rearing practices.[3] Relevant cases focus on a right to rear children and shape their characters largely to fit parental preferences, the right not to have the state involuntarily sterilize persons, the right to use contraception to avoid conceiving, the right to control one's body even if it entails terminating a previable pregnancy, and the right to preserve one's health even if it entails terminating a viable pregnancy. In a related case concerning statutory interpretation of the Americans with Disabilities Act, the U.S. Supreme Court acknowledged that procreation is a major life activity.[4] The broad view of these cases would include methods of achieving pregnancy and a right to use the same technologies to reduce the risk of disease and disability in those children.

However, the constitutional law cases in the United States do not directly address a right to destroy an ex utero embryo, nor do they address PGD or the legality of IVF. The expansive view above remains untested with respect to how broadly it construes procreative liberty, and related cases on parental rights and reproduction do not clearly support this interpretation (Nelson, 2013). Procreative liberty—like all liberties—can be viewed either as a negative right that protects parties from governmental prohibitions or as a positive right that obligates government to facilitate choices or provide services. In the United States, a negative-right analysis of procreation protects parents from government prohibitions on key aspects of reproductive choice (such as use of contraceptives) and parental discretion (such as choice of language of educational instruction). But reasonable regulation of a technology for the protection of the health and well-being of those affected is entirely permissible, even when claims of constitutional rights can be made. And the concept of procreative liberty has never been extended to a positive right to demand that government fund or even approve new reproductive technologies.

Potential Risks

Balanced against the possible benefits of heritable genome editing are a variety of potential risks. As discussed earlier in the chapter, genome-editing technologies in their current state still face technical challenges that would need to be overcome before they could be applied to editing the human

---

[3]*Meyer v. Nebraska*, 262 U.S. 390 (1923); *Pierce v. Society of Sisters*, 268 U.S. 510 (1925); *Farrington v. Tokushige*, 273 U.S. 284 (1927); *Prince v. Massachusetts*, 321 U.S. 158 (1944); *Wisconsin v. Yoder*, 406 U.S. 205 (1972).

[4]*Bragdon v. Abbott*, 524 U.S. 624 (1998).

germline, necessitating caution and careful review of any proposals to proceed to clinical trials.

Unintended Consequences

One concern is that human intervention may have unintended consequences. In the case of heritable genome editing, this concern has two distinct components. The first is the possibility of off-target effects of the editing process, as in the case of somatic genome editing. As discussed elsewhere in this report (in detail in Appendix A but also in other chapters), this technical question is receiving a great deal of scientific attention. Although improvements in genome-editing technology are reducing the incidence of off-target events, and methods for assessing their rate, some approaches already approved for somatic therapies, are being developed, they have not yet reached the point at which clinical trials of heritable genome editing could be authorized. Before any such clinical trials are approved, it will be necessary to demonstrate that the editing procedures will not lead to any significant increase in unintended variants. The required level of such variants will be necessarily lower than for somatic genome editing, but given that heritable genome editing may not go forward for some time, the technology for minimizing and assessing off-target events will undoubtedly have improved significantly. In addition, experience with somatic genome editing will have refined understanding of what might be considered acceptable or unacceptable rates of unintended variants.

Whatever standards are developed for somatic applications, there will be less tolerance for off-target effects in germline applications. By definition, those affected by the edits (future offspring) did not make the decision to be subjects of research or attempts at therapy, and adverse effects might be multiplied by reverberation across generations. Both factors lead to a more conservative approach to the risk/benefit balance.

A second concern is that the intended genome edits themselves might have unintended consequences, even in the absence of off-target effects. In the case of heritable genome editing to convert a well-understood disease-causing variant gene to a widely occurring nonpathological variant, the editing change would be to a version of the gene that is known not to have deleterious consequences. These variants are broadly present in the population already, so the chances that the edit would have some unexpected effects are small. On the other hand, the question of unintended consequences of a targeted edit would arise in the context of edits performed to make a change to a DNA sequence that is not already prevalent in the population, as would be the case for some so-called enhancements. In germline editing, the concern is magnified because the alteration could affect descendants, as discussed further in Chapter 6.

Long-Term Follow-Up

As with any new procedure, carefully monitored clinical trial protocols would be required for heritable genome editing, with attention to monitoring off-target events as well as the efficiency and correctness of the specific edit. Unlike conventional clinical trials, heritable genome-editing trials would likely require long-term prospective follow-up studies across subsequent generations. This follow-up would entail study of the future children affected by the intervention, none of whom would have been party to the initial decision to participate in a research trial. Data of this type would be important for determining whether the techniques had achieved their goals (Friedmann et al., 2015). Even those who have volunteered to be research subjects cannot be compelled to participate in long-term follow-up. Nonetheless, encouragement is permitted. Experience from xenotransplantation and some drug and device trials shows that this encouragement can be successful. And despite the particular challenge of studying offspring rather than those who consented to the research, experience with other reproductive technologies suggests that follow-up can be carried out in numbers sufficient to permit conclusions about many possible long-term effects (Lu et al., 2013).

Societal Effects

Some have argued that germline editing can be justified on grounds that go beyond mere parental choice. There is a line of thought that germline modification could be used to create a level playing field for those whose traits now put their children and descendants at a disadvantage (Buchanan et al., 2001). Others see a public health benefit in access to heritable genome editing because it might somewhat reduce the prevalence of many devastating diseases, such as Tay-Sachs and Huntington's disease. That said, it is important to note that the history of abusive and coercive eugenics (discussed in the section on human dignity and the fear of eugenics below) is intertwined with previous, undoubtedly well-intentioned public health and hygiene movements, which is one reason why discussions of public health benefits often engender some skepticism and unease.

Some contemporary transhumanists point out that the human body is flawed in that it easily becomes diseased, requires a great deal of sleep, has various cognitive limitations, and eventually dies. They suggest that it would make sense to improve the human species by making it more resistant to disease, more moral, and more intelligent (Hughes, 2004). Some, such as philosopher John Harris, say that in certain cases there is a moral obligation to enhance ourselves genetically (Harris, 2007). But these are arguments about enhancement, not the restoration or maintenance of ordinary health. That topic is addressed in more detail in Chapter 6.

A "Natural" Human Genome and the Appropriate Degree of Human Intervention

Among the social and cultural arguments against heritable genome editing are positions that support a preference for a "natural" genome. Although there is wide acceptance of human intervention in agriculture and medicine, some hold the view that the human genome is different and should be free of intentional manipulation because of some aspect of its naturalness, whether defined as "normal," "real," or otherwise determined largely by forces other than human intervention (Nuffield Council, 2015), and some aspect of its "humanness" (Machalek, 2009; Pollard, 2016). However, the human genome is not entirely "human," as it includes Neanderthal and Denisovan DNA (Fu et al., 2015; Pollard, 2016; Vernot et al., 2016). Nor does it exist in any single, static state. As reviewed in Chapter 4, each time a cell divides, numerous changes in the DNA sequence occur, and environmental insults such as radiation and chemicals (both natural and synthetic) also produce sequence changes. Moreover, meiosis combined with fertilization creates in each individual a novel assortment of gene variants. The result is significant variation in genomic DNA sequence among individuals (Kasowski et al., 2010; Zheng et al., 2010) and even within the cells of a single individual. Every human (other than monozygotic twins) begins with a unique genome—actually two genomes that subsequently diversify as cells divide, each of which is "natural." There is no single human genome shared by all of humanity.

The concern then devolves to the view that the human genome should be treated with a sense of humility and that humanity should recognize the limits of wisdom and science, and even that human intervention is more dangerous or more unpredictable than natural processes. This concern often is expressed by the term "playing God," which captures the notion that humans lack a god-like omniscience that would be required to make any changes in the genome safely (and to predict that such changes would actually serve the intended purpose). Even those approaching the issue from a nontheological point of view may use the term to represent a more general notion about appropriate limits of intentional human control of the environment or of the human genome (President's Commission, 1983).

To some extent, this argument implicitly accepts the thesis that the forces of nature and evolution are a better—or at least less problematic—source of genome alteration than human intervention. However, the natural variations in human genomes arise by chance and are selected for or against during evolution by founder effects and according to selection pressures such as climate, nutrition, and infectious disease, some of which may no longer be relevant in the modern world. Accordingly, while it is important to recognize the limits of human understanding and proceed with all due care, this does not necessarily mean that society should forswear any human intervention at all.

Overall, from a scientific viewpoint, some conclusions about likely benefits and risks of heritable genome editing can be supported with a fair degree of certainty, while others remain uncertain and in need of further investigation and societal debate, calling for humility with respect to those conclusions. Assessing the probabilities of efficacy and risk is the focus of clinical trials, which can be viewed as a manifestation of the recognition of the limits of human knowledge.

Beyond the scientific assessment of risks and uncertainties, the question of the proper extent of human intervention in nature has long been discussed in spiritual and religious terms. In the contemporary West, where Christian traditions have had the most influence on what is today a more religiously diverse and often secular culture, these ideas are expressed in the debate about which tasks in improving or stewarding nature are the domain or obligation of humans and which are to be left to God (Cole-Turner, 1993; Vatican, 2015). This thinking reflects beliefs that are present across a variety of traditions and many centuries, including St. Francis' Canticle of Creation and the belief systems among some Native American nations.

In the Jewish tradition, on the other hand, there is an explicit obligation to build and develop the world in any way that is beneficial to people, and such improvements are viewed as a positive collaboration between God and humans, not as an interference with creation (Steinberg, 2006). Similarly, many Muslims and Buddhists view genetic engineering as just one of many welcome interventions to reduce suffering from disease (HDC, 2016; Inhorn, 2012; Pfleiderer et al., 2010). The question will always be how much human-directed intervention in nature and in humans themselves is appropriate or even permissible. This is a spiritual and practical question asked by both religious and nonreligious people, although somewhat more often by the former (Akin et al., 2017). Even among the religious, adherents of different faiths will have varying degrees of interest or concern (Evans, 2010).

Human Dignity and the Fear of Eugenics

International covenants, treaties, and national constitutions, including European treaties focused on banning germline modification, typically invoke the concept of dignity (Hennette-Vauchez, 2011). While this term has many meanings, it is most often invoked in the debate about heritable genome editing to affirm that humans have value simply by virtue of being human and not because of their capacities, and thus cannot be treated as instruments of another's will (Andorno, 2005a; Sulmasy, 2008). Emmanuel Kant viewed human agency and free will as essential aspects of human dignity. The term also can signal a special regard for humans as opposed to other species, an appreciation of the intellectual capacities of humans, and a commitment to promoting autonomy and human flourishing. Since rights and other individualistic arguments cannot easily be used to address concerns about future generations or humanity, "dignity" has been invoked to "provide an ultimate theoretical reason to prevent a misuse of emerging biotechnological powers" (Andorno, 2005b, p. 74). Even if limited to preventing serious disease or disability, the prospect of using heritable genome editing triggers concern that purely voluntary, individual decisions can collectively change social norms regarding the acceptance of less serious disabilities (Sandel, 2004).

The disability rights community is not monolithic, and its attitudes toward genetic technologies such as prenatal screening can vary from supportive to skeptical (Chen and Schiffman, 2000; Saxton, 2000). There has been a long and ongoing debate among different parts of the disability community with regard to the use of screening technologies. These tensions are real, continuing, and unlikely to be resolved entirely. Still, disability activists have been among the most visible critics of using technology to screen for or determine the genetic qualities of children. Jackie Leach Scully writes of a fear that voluntary prenatal diagnostic techniques, which would also apply to genome editing, set us on a "slippery slope" (a concept discussed further below) toward intolerance of disability and even the risk of a return to the coercive practices of the past (Scully, 2009).

Others write that a policy of prevention by genetic screening (and by extension genome editing) "appears to reflect the judgment that lives with disabilities are so burdensome to the disabled child, her family, and society that their avoidance is a health care priority—a judgment that exaggerates and misattributes many or most of the difficulties associated with disability" (Wasserman and Asch, 2006, p. 54). The same observation has been made concerning the differing perceptions of disabled persons and medical professionals about the degree of distress caused by a particular condition (Longmore, 1995). Studies suggest that "many members of the health professions view childhood disability as predominantly negative for children and their families, in contrast to what research on the life satisfaction of people with disabilities and their families has actually shown" (Parens and Asch, 2000, p. 20).

Indeed, there is concern that the availability of the technology might actually lead to a judgment that parents who forego heritable genome editing are negligent, a theory seriously discussed (although ultimately abandoned) with respect to genetic screening when it became a common practice (Malek and Daar, 2012; Sayres and Magnus, 2012; Wasserman and Asch, 2012). Others have cited fears that hard-won successes at developing laws and policies that make the world accessible to those with disabilities will lose support when the number of persons directly affected declines.

One can argue that these concerns reflect a false dichotomy, and that unconditional love for a disabled child once born and respect for all people who are born with or who develop disabilities are not incompatible with intervening to avert disease and disability prior to birth or conception. And the decades that saw the explosion of prenatal diagnosis (accompanied by selective abortion of affected fetuses) and preimplantation diagnostics (accompanied by selective implantation of nonaffected embryos) are the same as those in which public attitudes toward disability became far more accepting (Hernandez et al., 2004; Makas, 1988; Steinbach et al., 2016). It would appear that "encouraging attempts to reduce the incidence of a genetic disease is compatible with continuing respect for those born with the disease and providing support for their distinctive needs" (Kitcher, 1997, p. 85).

The disability community is characterized by a long and ongoing tension with regard to the use of screening technologies. The literature appears to support openly acknowledging that this tension is real, continuing, and unlikely to be resolved entirely, and that any step toward the use of genome editing to eliminate disabilities must be carried out with care and open discussion (Kitcher, 1997). The committee supports this call for continued public deliberation (see Chapter 7).

Public policy has shifted toward eliminating discrimination in employment or public services, and public investment in changing the social, physical, and employment environment to achieve this goal has increased, with measures ranging from accessible buildings to sign language presentations to aural signals for street crossings. The range of measures remains insufficient, however, and one cannot know whether this shift in attitude would have been even more dramatic if genetic screening and abortion laws had not made it easier to reduce the prevalence of birth defects. Nonetheless, this progress does to some extent address the concern that reducing the prevalence of disabilities will necessarily decrease empathy, acceptance, or integration of those who have them.

Economic and Social Justice

Recognizing that heritable genome-editing technology is unlikely to be used widely in the near future and that drastic transformation of the species or immediate changes in cultural norms are unlikely, some social justice arguments focus on the effects of the technology's being accessible only to a few rather than to too many. In this framing, the technology is another example of a society's allocating considerable resources to developing a technology that will benefit only a relatively few wealthy people when this money could be used to relieve the suffering of millions of poor people through already existing technologies (Cahill, 2008). One counterargument is that the research phase may include those less well-off, or that even if treatments for rare but compelling diseases often start with the wealthy, they eventually become more affordable and available for the poor. Moreover, the research that will make heritable genome editing possible will likely provide insights that will lead to health care interventions for other disorders as well. More to the point, perhaps, is the reality that—at least in the United States—health care budgets are not set globally, and therefore the decision to refrain from spending in one area will not necessarily result in the funds being redirected to another area of need.

Another concern is that if heritable genome editing were to become prevalent among those who are wealthier or better insured, it could change the prevalence of avoidable diseases between advantaged and disadvantaged populations and could permanently establish what Harris (2007) calls "parallel populations." While great inequality already exists, the argument continues, heritable genome editing would make a culturally determined inequality into one that is biological. While such a phenomenon already exists in the form of durable effects of better nutrition and use of vaccines among the advantaged populations of the world, some critics are concerned about adding yet another, more durable form of superior access to better health (Center for Genetics and Society, 2015). These concerns apply to a range of health advances, and are not limited to genome editing.

The Slippery Slope

Many scholars who support (or at least are not opposed to) germline modifications align the possible uses of genome editing along a continuum of acceptability. This continuum almost always starts with converting single-gene disorders to a common, nondeleterious sequence at the most-acceptable end, and moves toward enhancements that are unrelated to disease on the least-acceptable end. The slippery slope claim is that taking the first step with single-gene disorders is likely to lead, in some number of years, to the conduct of nondisease enhancements that many would rather see prohibited. As one group involved with somatic modification wrote in the journal *Nature*, "many oppose germline modification on the grounds that permitting even unambiguously therapeutic interventions could start us down a path towards non-therapeutic genetic enhancement" (Lanphier et al., 2015, p. 411).

The slippery slope arguments of most critics do not claim inevitability but are instead probabilistic. They are based on what could be described as predictive sociology about how societies actually function and rejection of the notion that placing barriers and speed bumps on the slippery slope will be a sufficient deterrent to less desirable uses (Volokh, 2003). Many scientific advances in the past—ranging from reconstructive surgery (which has led to plastic surgery for aesthetics) to prenatal screening for lethal disorders (which has led to screening of carriers for disease genes and preimplantation screening for nonlethal, even late-onset disorders)—have raised similar concerns about a slippery slope toward less compelling or even antisocial uses.

An opponent of editing the germline would not necessarily oppose on principle replacing a disease gene variant with a corresponding, common, nondisease variant, as such a change would give offspring no social advantage and is the type of instrumental action directed at future children that is currently part of modern medicine. Many opponents, however, do not believe genome editing would stop there and observe that a number of social processes make the slope more slippery. Parts of the medical profession might become invested in providing the service or patient groups in seeking the service, creating powerful interest groups favoring its maintenance or even expansion. IVF, for example, was originally developed to circumvent fallopian tube blockage. It soon was extended, however, to circumventing naturally age-related decline in fertility and even postmenopausal infertility, and later became an enabling technology for PGD. Likewise, PGD was originally designed to select against embryos with serious deleterious mutations but later was expanded to conditions that not all agree are diseases or disabilities, as well as to sex selection.

On the other hand, slippery slope arguments have their critics, who point to their inherent uncertainty and the fact that many such claims do not come to pass. Indeed, despite predictions to the contrary, neither IVF nor PGD has come to be used for convenience or for selection of trivial traits. Even artificial insemination, which offers an inexpensive way to "optimize" the male genetic contribution, has not become a widespread practice except when the male partner is absent, infertile, or at risk of passing on a seriously deleterious mutation. Furthermore, among those women who already needed to use donor gametes, almost none took advantage of the opportunity to obtain semen from the so-called Nobel Prize sperm bank (Plotz, 2006), although there has been evidence of a stronger tendency to "optimize" when it comes to egg donation (Klitzman, 2016). Those who reject slippery slope arguments often are less concerned than proponents about situations that might be viewed as the bottom of the slope.

Many of the attempts to introduce speed bumps or friction on the slippery slope in the evolution of genetic modification of humans have focused on the easily grasped linguistic/cognitive difference between a body/ individual and offspring/society, thereby establishing the distinction between editing of somatic and germline cells. Critics would claim that the current debate about crossing the cognitive barrier (i.e., crossing the germ-line) is proof of the existence of a slippery slope.

Overall, slippery slope arguments do not depend on universal condemnation of the initial, most compelling applications of heritable genome editing. But while many think that regulation could establish effective speed bumps, proponents of slippery slope arguments raise the question of whether and how society can develop regulations that are sufficiently robust to quell the fear of a progressive move toward less compelling and more controversial applications. Indeed, they would say that regulations would do little to stop the progression down a slippery slope because regulations are based on cultural views, and it is precisely the underlying change in cultural views that is the slippery slope.

REGULATION

Regulation in the United States

In the United States, heritable genome editing would be subject to a complex landscape of state and federal laws and regulations (see Chapter 2). The legality of research, and perhaps even clinical application, would vary from state to state as a result of differing laws on fetal and embryo research. Federal funding for the research would likely be unavailable because of current legislative restrictions on funding research involving human embryos. Should heritable genome editing move into clinical investigations, the U.S. Food and Drug Administration (FDA) would have regulatory jurisdiction. The altered cells—whether gametes or the embryo—would need to be implanted for gestation, and this transfer would trigger the same FDA jurisdiction as that used by the agency in 2001 (FDA, 2009) when it determined that reproductive cloning could not proceed without authorization. This jurisdiction derives from the agency's power to regulate tissue transplantation. While IVF and even PGD were developed before the FDA policy in this area was fully developed and therefore have not been regulated as closely as more recent products, genome editing would fall squarely within FDA jurisdiction.

A careful stepwise process (outlined in more detail in Chapter 2) would include consideration by the National Institutes of Health's (NIH's) Recombinant DNA Advisory Committee (RAC) (with public comment and transparent review), local institutional review board (IRB) and local institutional biosafety committee (IBC) review, and FDA review before any decision about whether to permit clinical trials could be made. If heritable genome editing succeeded in research trials and was approved for marketing, there would also be mechanisms for oversight in the post-approval context.

Because heritable genome editing would involve the use of other assisted reproductive technologies, oversight of its use would likely involve the same statutes and regulations that apply to IVF and PGD. Some of these regulations focus on donor material safety, transparency, and reporting requirements, as is the case with IVF, or on quality control of the laboratories (though not necessarily the actual diagnostics) used for PGD. Heritable genome editing would be performed in conjunction with IVF and PGD, and thus could involve statutes and regulations that apply to those technologies. For example, IVF itself is subject to rules that require registration of facilities, screening of donor gametes for communicable diseases, and compliance with good tissue-handling standards (FDA, 2001). Programs using IVF also must report pregnancy success rates to the Centers for Disease Control and Prevention (CDC).[5]

Following the publication of the National Academies report on mitochondrial replacement techniques, which can result in heritable changes in small amounts of mitochondrial (i.e., nonnuclear) DNA present in the egg, and the publication of genome-editing research in China using nonviable human embryos, NIH made a statement to the effect that it would not fund research involving genome editing of human embryos.[6] Francis Collins, Director of NIH, stated that NIH "will not fund any use of gene-editing technologies in human embryos" (Collins, 2015). He noted that the "concept of altering the human germline in embryos for clinical purposes has been debated over many years from many different perspectives, and has been viewed almost universally as a line that should not be crossed" (Collins, 2015). But this research is already something NIH could not fund because of legal obstacles created by the Dickey-Wicker Amendment (forbidding U.S. Department of Health and Human Services [HHS] funding of such work) and the RAC policy of declining to review such work in accordance with the requirement for NIH-funded projects (see Chapter 2).

The NIH statement also highlighted the requirement for FDA approval of an Investigational New Drug (IND) application for any clinical trials involving transfer and gestation of an edited embryo. The FDA had never received or approved a proposal to modify the germline, but apparently alarmed by the direction of research, the U.S. Congress held hearings in

---

[5]Assisted Reproductive Technology Programs, 42 U.S.C. § 263a-1 (current through Public Law 114-38).

[6]The NIH statement can be accessed at https://www.nih.gov/about-nih/who-we-are/nih-director/statements/statement-nih-funding-research-using-gene-editing-technologies-human-embryos (accessed January 30, 2017).

June 2015 on "The Science and Ethics of Engineered Human DNA."[7]
These hearings were followed by the omnibus spending bill provision, discussed in Chapter 2, that prevents the FDA from using any of its resources
to even consider an application to proceed with clinical trials involving
germline modification.[8] This limitation will last at least through the end of
April 2017. Beyond that date, the prohibition may be extended or deleted,
depending on the details of the next budget exercise. If the prohibition is
lifted, the FDA will once again be permitted to entertain requests to initiate clinical trials in this area, although the restrictions on the use of federal
funds for such research will remain.

Statements and Views from Other Bodies

Heritable genetic engineering has been the subject of public and academic discussion for decades. Salient instruments that have legal effect
include the European Oviedo convention, which allows genetic engineering
only for preventive, diagnostic, or therapeutic purposes and only when it is
not aimed at changing the genetic makeup of a person's descendants, thus
precluding heritable genome editing. Although signed by 35 nations, this
convention is binding only on those 29 that ratified it (6 nations did not
ratify it in full), and even then requires implementation through domestic
legislation (COE, 2016).

More recently, as discussed in Chapter 1, the organizers of the December 2015 International Summit convened by the science and medicine
academies of the United States, the United Kingdom, and China called for
a pause of some undefined duration in any attempt at heritable genome
editing. Their statement read:

> It would be irresponsible to proceed with any clinical use of germline edit-
> ing unless and until
>
> (i) the relevant safety and efficacy issues have been resolved, based on
> appropriate understanding and balancing of risks, potential benefits, and
> alternatives, and
> (ii) there is broad societal consensus about the appropriateness of the
> proposed application. Moreover, any clinical use should proceed only
> under appropriate regulatory oversight.

---

[7]"The Science and Ethics of Engineered Human DNA." Hearing before the Subcommittee
on Research and Technology, of the House Committee on Science, Space and Technology,
June 16, 2015. https://science.house.gov/legislation/hearings/subcommittee-research-and-
technology-hearing-science-and-ethics-genetically (accessed January 30, 2017).
[8]Consolidated Appropriations Act of 2016, HR 2029, 114 Cong., 1st sess. (January 6,
2015) (https://www.congress.gov/114/bills/hr2029/BILLS-114hr2029enr.pdf [accessed January 4, 2017]).

At present, these criteria have not been met for any proposed clinical use: the safety issues have not yet been adequately explored the cases of most compelling benefit are limited and many nations have legislative or regulatory bans on germline modification. However, as scientific knowledge advances and societal views evolve, the clinical use of germline editing should be revisited on a regular basis. (NASEM, 2016d, p. 7)

Similarly, in its 2016 professional guidelines for regenerative medicine research, the International Society for Stem Cell Research included the following statement: "Until further clarity emerges on both scientific and ethical fronts, the ISSCR holds that any attempt to modify the nuclear genome of human embryos for the purpose of human reproduction is premature and should be prohibited at this time" (ISSCR, 2016a, p. 8).

In 2015, a self-organized group of multinational experts called the Hinxton Group published a statement exploring the possibility that heritable genome editing might be acceptable, albeit with many caveats (Hinxton Group, 2015, p. 3). According to that statement, "[p]rior to any movement toward human reproductive applications, a number of crucial scientific challenges and questions must be addressed." The statement proceeds to list a number of technical questions related to safety and efficacy and stresses the need to explore cultural attitudes and whether and how legal limits might be placed on particular uses.

The French National Academy also appears to have taken the position that while heritable genome editing is unacceptable now, one can contemplate a time when it might be permitted, stating that "this research, including that on germline cells and human embryos, should be carried out provided that it is scientifically and medically justified" (ANM, 2016, p. 2).

These statements all recognize that issues of safety and efficacy associated with heritable genome editing are far from resolved and that attempts to apply this form of genome editing should not be made at this time. They all note, however, that the science is continuing to progress rapidly, and they avoid calling for permanent prohibitions. Indeed, the Hinxton Group recommends that "a detailed but flexible roadmap [be] produced to guide the development of standards for safety and efficacy" (Hinxton Group, 2015, p. 3).

CONCLUSIONS AND RECOMMENDATION

In some situations, heritable genome editing would provide the only or the most acceptable option for parents who desire to have genetically related children while minimizing the risk of serious disease or disability in a prospective child. Yet while relief from inherited diseases could accrue from its use, there is significant public discomfort about heritable genome editing, particularly for less serious conditions and for situations in which alternatives exist. These concerns range from a view that it is inappropriate for humans to intervene in their own evolution to anxiety about unintended consequences for the individuals affected and for society as a whole.

More research is needed before any germline intervention could meet the risk/benefit standard for authorizing clinical trials. But as the technical hurdles facing genome editing of progenitors of eggs and sperm are overcome, editing to prevent transmission of genetically inherited diseases may become a realistic possibility.

The primary U.S. entity with authority for the regulation of heritable genome editing—the FDA—does incorporate value judgments about risks and benefits in its decision making. A robust public discussion about the values to be placed on the benefits and risks of heritable genome editing is needed now so that these values can be incorporated as appropriate into the risk/benefit assessments that will precede any decision about whether to authorize clinical trials. But the FDA does not have a statutory mandate to consider public views on the intrinsic morality of a technology when deciding whether to authorize clinical trials. That level of discussion takes place at the RAC, in legislatures, and at other venues for public engagement (see Chapter 7).

Heritable genome-editing trials must be approached with caution, but caution does not mean they must be prohibited. If the technical challenges were overcome and potential benefits were reasonable in light of the risks, clinical trials could be initiated if limited to the most compelling circumstances, if subject to a comprehensive oversight framework that would protect the research subjects and their descendants, and if sufficient safeguards were in place to protect against inappropriate expansion to uses that are less compelling or less well understood.

RECOMMENDATION 5-1. Clinical trials using heritable genome editing should be permitted only within a robust and effective regulatory framework that encompasses
- the absence of reasonable alternatives;
- restriction to preventing a serious disease or condition;
- restriction to editing genes that have been convincingly demonstrated to cause or to strongly predispose to that disease or condition;
- restriction to converting such genes to versions that are prevalent in the population and are known to be associated with ordinary health with little or no evidence of adverse effects;
- the availability of credible preclinical and/or clinical data on risks and potential health benefits of the procedures;

- ongoing, rigorous oversight during clinical trials of the effects of the procedure on the health and safety of the research participants;
- comprehensive plans for long-term, multigenerational follow-up that still respect personal autonomy;
- maximum transparency consistent with patient privacy;
- continued reassessment of both health and societal benefits and risks, with broad ongoing participation and input by the public; and
- reliable oversight mechanisms to prevent extension to uses other than preventing a serious disease or condition.

Given how long modifying the germline has been at the center of debates about moral boundaries, as well as the pluralism of values in society, it would be surprising if everyone were to agree with this recommendation. Even for those who do agree, it would be surprising if they all shared identical reasoning for doing so. For some, the debate is about respecting parental desires for genetically related children. For others, it is primarily about allowing children to be born as healthy as possible. But as noted earlier in this chapter, some do not view heritable genome editing as a benefit to the resulting child, who otherwise might never have been conceived at all. And for others, the desire of parents who carry genetic disease to have a genetically related child through this technology, instead of having a genetically unrelated child, is not sufficient to outweigh the social concerns that have been raised. There are also those who think the final criterion of Recommendation 5-1 cannot be met, and that once germline modification had begun, the regulatory mechanisms instituted could not limit the technology to the uses identified in the recommendation. If it is indeed not possible to satisfy the criteria in the recommendation, the committee's view is that heritable genome editing would not be permissible. The committee calls for continued public engagement and input (see Chapter 7) while the basic science evolves and regulatory safeguards are developed to satisfy the criteria set forth here.

Heritable genome editing raises concerns about premature or unproven uses of the technology, and it is possible that the criteria outlined here for responsible oversight would be achievable in some but not all jurisdictions. This possibility raises the concern that "regulatory havens" could emerge that would tempt providers or consumers to travel to jurisdictions with more lenient or nonexistent regulations to access the restricted procedures (Charo, 2016a). The result could be a "race to the bottom" that would encourage laxer standards in nations seeking revenues from medical tourism, as has happened with both stem cell therapy and mitochondrial replacement techniques (Abbott et al., 2010; Charo, 2016b; Turner and

Knoepfler, 2016; Zhang et al., 2016). The phenomenon of medical tourism, which encompasses the search for faster and cheaper therapeutic options, as well as newer or less regulated interventions, will be impossible to control completely if the technical capabilities exist in more permissive jurisdictions (Cohen, 2015; Lyon, 2017). Thus, it is important to highlight the need for comprehensive regulation.

As of late 2015, the United States was unable to consider whether to begin heritable genome-editing trials, regardless of whether the criteria laid out above could be met. As noted above, a provision (in effect until at least April 2017) included in a congressional budget bill[9] contains the following language:

> None of the funds made available by this Act may be used to notify a sponsor or otherwise acknowledge receipt of a submission for an exemption for investigational use of a drug or biological product under section 505(i) of the Federal Food, Drug, and Cosmetic Act (21 U.S.C. 355(i)) or section 351(a)(3) of the Public Health Service Act (42 U.S.C. 262(a)(3)) in research in which a human embryo is intentionally created or modified to include a heritable genetic modification. Any such submission shall be deemed to have not been received by the Secretary, and the exemption may not go into effect.

The current effect of this provision is to make it impossible for U.S. authorities to review proposals for clinical trials of heritable genome editing, and therefore to drive development of this technology to other jurisdictions, some regulated and others not.

---

[9]Consolidated Appropriations Act of 2016, HR 2029, 114 Cong., 1st sess. (January 6, 2015) (https://www.congress.gov/114/bills/hr2029/BILLS-114hr2029enr.pdf [accessed January 4, 2017]).

6

Enhancement

Somatic gene and cell therapies are widely seen as morally acceptable. Indeed, bone marrow transplantation, in which cells of differing genetic composition are introduced into patients, has been used for decades, and the use of gene therapy to treat children with severe combined immune deficiency, so-called bubble boy disease, is now a part of medical treatment (De Ravin et al., 2016). Beyond issues of safety, efficacy, and informed consent, there has been no concern about the legitimacy of somatic cell and gene therapies among those who generally endorse modern medicine. Genome editing is playing an increasing part in somatic gene therapy to treat and prevent disease (see Chapter 4). Recent advances, however, have increased the possibility that genome editing could also be used for purposes that go beyond the kinds of gene therapy and other medical interventions discussed above. Thus, the question has been raised anew as to whether enhancement should be regulated or prohibited, and whether there are important differences depending on whether the enhancements are somatic or heritable.

This chapter explores the possible applications of genome editing to achieve what is commonly described as "enhancement," a term that itself is problematic; it implies a change from—indeed an improvement upon—an existing condition. Enhancements may range from the mundane, such as cosmetic changes in hair color; to the more physically interventionist, such as elective cosmetic surgery; to the more dangerous and problematic, such as the use of some steroids and other drugs among athletes in competitive settings.

Enhancement is commonly understood to refer to changes that alter what is "normal," whether for humans as a whole or for a particular individual prior to enhancement. The question of what is meant by normal then arises. Is it average? Is it whatever nature has prescribed? Is it whatever luck has wrought? Given the wide range of capabilities exhibited by humans for any particular trait, there is little basis for deeming any one condition normal or any meaningful value in determining an average. Nonetheless, there have been some attempts to describe the range of conditions that, given the right environment, are consistent with an ability to appreciate life and participate in the world.

This chapter begins by reviewing several key issues in genome editing for enhancement. It then addresses in turn somatic (nonheritable) and germline (heritable) genome editing for enhancement purposes. The chapter ends with conclusions and recommendations.

HUMAN GENETIC VARIATION AND DEFINING "NORMAL" AND "NATURAL"

Before beginning to discuss so-called enhancement, it is important to explore how terminology related to human gene therapy and genome editing has the potential to bias judgments unconsciously. Many diseases are associated with DNA variants, and the common term used to describe a variant—"mutation"—has therefore taken on a negative connotation in common parlance. A distinction often is made between "normal" and "mutant" or "disease (causing)" genes, with the latter being viewed negatively. The term "normal" also is applied to phenotype, or the individual traits that result from interaction between the genotype and the environment. Here it is important to note that the "normal" distribution of any given trait (e.g., height, weight, strength, aural or visual acuity) covers a wide spectrum and can be affected by many factors, including but by no means limited to gene variants, which often interact both with each other and with environmental factors. Hence, the term "normal" denotes a range or spectrum, not some ideal state.

The word "natural" has similarly taken on a positive connotation reflecting a common view that nature produces things that are healthier and generally better than anything artificial—this despite evidence demonstrating that "natural" things can be either safe or intrinsically dangerous. In the present context, genetic variants that exist in nature may either support health or cause disease, and the human population contains multiple variants of most genes (see Chapter 4). Thus, there is no single "normal" human genome sequence; rather, there are multiple variant human genomic sequences (IGSR, 2016), all of which occur in the worldwide human gene pool and, in that sense, are "natural," and all of which can be either advantageous or disadvantageous.

At any given position in the genome, some variants are more common than others. Some are beneficial and some detrimental, their effects at times depending on such factors as whether a person has one copy (heterozygosity) or two copies (homozygosity) of the variant, or whether the gene is sex chromosome–linked (hemizygous for a gene on the Y chromosome and either heterozygous or homozygous on the X chromosome). Another factor may be the particular environment in which a person lives. A well-known example is the case of sickle-cell anemia. Hemoglobin is the protein that carries oxygen in red blood cells. The most widespread variant encodes a fully functional protein, whereas the sickle-cell variant can cause the protein to aggregate and distort the red cells into a sickle shape if *both* copies of the gene are this variant (the homozygous state), which in turn causes the symptoms of sickle-cell disease. As noted in Chapter 5, however, being heterozygous for this variant confers some resistance to malaria, and for this reason, the sickle-cell variant has been maintained by natural selection in populations from malaria-prone areas (e.g., Africa, India, and the Mediterranean), the disadvantages of sickle-cell disease at the population level being balanced against the population-level advantages of resistance to malaria. So in this case, which natural variant is advantageous depends on the environment.

In this report, the committee uses the term "variant" and eschews to the extent possible the use of "mutant" or "normal" in referring to gene variants. There is, however, a distinction worth keeping in mind. Many variants are "natural," and changing a gene variant that is associated with disease, such as the sickle-cell variant of hemoglobin, to a variant that is prevalent in the population (i.e., "natural") but not disease-causing can be viewed as a therapeutic or preventive change. It is also possible, however, to envision the possibility of changing a gene to a variant form that does not exist (or is rare) in the human gene pool but has some property that could be viewed as an "enhancement" since it is predicted to have a beneficial effect. Such a change is a more radical step than that of replacing a disease-causing variant with a common human variant known not to cause disease.

UNDERSTANDING PUBLIC ATTITUDES TOWARD ENHANCEMENT

Personal improvements take many forms. They can require significant personal effort, as in taking piano lessons, or they can be largely independent of personal effort, as in wearing teeth-straightening braces. They can be temporary, as in benefiting from the caffeine in morning coffee, or long-lasting, as in immunization against disease. They can be easily reversible, as in hair coloring, or reversible only with difficulty, as in cosmetic surgery. And they can be provided in connection with a corrective intervention, as in removing cataracts and inserting lenses that provide greater acuity than the person ever had naturally. All of these factors influence how improvements are evaluated in terms of fairness and public acceptability.

Although surveys indicate significant support for gene therapy and genetic engineering to improve the health of both existing individuals and unborn children (see Table 6-1), the possibility of "enhancement" in new and potentially more wide-ranging ways can engender anxiety as well as

TABLE 6-1 Summary of Public Attitudes Toward Aspects of Gene Therapy or Genome Editing as Revealed by a Selection of Surveys

Question	Poll (Year)	Percent Affirmative
Attitudes about gene therapy and gene editing in adults and children		
To improve health of the person being treated		
Approve of genetic engineering to cure a disease	Times-CNN-Yankelovich (1993)	79
If it is possible to cure people with fatal diseases by altering their genes, do you feel those people ought to be allowed to do this?	Troika-Lifetime-PSRA (1991)	65
Approve of scientists changing the makeup of human cells to cure a	March of Dimes-Harris (1992)	87
usually fatal genetic disease	OTA-Harris (1986)	83
Approve of scientists changing the makeup of human cells to reduce the	March of Dimes-Harris (1992)	78
risk of developing a fatal disease later in life	OTA-Harris (1986)	77
Government funding and regulation of gene therapy		
Federal government should fund scientific research on developing new gene therapy treatments	STAT-HSPH-SSRS (2016)	64
FDA should approve gene therapy treatments for use in the United States	STAT-HSPH-SSRS (2016)	59

TABLE 6-1 Continued

Question	Poll (Year)	Percent Affirmative
To improve health inherited by the child		
Approve of parents being offered a way to change their own genes to prevent their children from having a genetic disease	Hopkins-PSRA (2002)	59
Approve of scientists changing the makeup of human cells to stop	March of Dimes-Harris (1992)	84
children from inheriting a usually fatal genetic disease	OTA-Harris (1986)	84
Approve of scientists changing the makeup of human cells to stop	March of Dimes-Harris (1992)	66
children from inheriting a nonfatal birth defect	OTA-Harris (1986)	77
If you had a child with a usually fatal genetic disease, willing to have child	March of Dimes-Harris (1992)	88
undergo therapy to have those genes corrected	OTA-Harris (1986)	86
To improve intelligence, physical traits, or appearance		
Approve of genetic engineering to improve a person's intelligence	Times-CNN-Yankelovich (1993)	34
Approve of scientists changing the makeup of human cells to improve the	March of Dimes-Harris (1992)	42
intelligence level that children would inherit	OTA-Harris (1986)	44
Approve of genetic engineering to improve a person's physical appearance	Times-CNN-Yankelovich (1993)	25
Approve of scientists changing the makeup of human cells to improve the	March of Dimes-Harris (1992)	43
physical characteristics that children would inherit	OTA-Harris (1986)	44
Approve of parents being offered a way to change their own genes to have children who would be smarter, stronger, or better looking	Hopkins-PSRA (2002)	20
Approve if scientists offered parents a way to change their genes in order to have smarter or better-looking children	Family Circle-PSRA (1994)	10

continued

TABLE 6-1 Continued

Question	Poll (Year)	Percent Affirmative
Attitudes about changing human genomes before birth		
To improve future health		
Changing the genes of unborn babies to reduce their risk of developing certain serious diseases should be legal	STAT-HSPH-SSRS (2016)	26
Changing a baby's genetic characteristics to reduce the risk of serious diseases is an appropriate use of medical advances	Pew (2014) VCU (2003)	46 41
If future science developed the ability to change a child's inherited characteristics by changing the child's genetic structure in the womb and you were making the decision, would consider doing so to improve his/her general physical health	ABC (1990)	49
To improve intelligence, physical traits, or appearance		
Changing the genes of unborn babies to improve their intelligence or physical characteristics should be legal	STAT-HSPH-SSRS (2016)	11
Changing a baby's genetic characteristics to make the baby more intelligent is an appropriate use of medical advances	Pew (2014)	15
If future science developed the ability to change a child's inherited characteristics by changing the child's genetic structure in the womb and you were making the decision, would consider doing so to improve his/her intelligence	ABC (1990)	28
If future science developed the ability to change a child's inherited characteristics by changing the child's genetic structure in the womb and you were making the decision, would consider doing so to improve his/her body characteristics such as height and weight	ABC (1990)	13

TABLE 6-1 Continued

Question	Poll (Year)	Percent Affirmative
If future science developed the ability to change a child's inherited characteristics by changing the child's genetic structure in the womb and you were making the decision, would consider doing so to improve his/her hair or eye color or facial characteristics	ABC (1990)	8
Government funding of research		
Federal government should fund scientific research on changing the genes of unborn babies to reduce their risk of developing certain diseases	STAT-HSPH-SSRS (2016)	44
Federal government should fund scientific research on changing the genes of unborn babies that aims to improve their characteristics, such as intelligence, or physical traits, such as athletic ability or appearance	STAT-HSPH-SSRS (2016)	14

NOTES: Emphasis added. ABC = American Broadcasting Company; CNN = Cable News Network; FDA = U.S. Food and Drug Administration; HSPS = Harvard T.H. Chan School of Public Health; OTA = Office of Technology Assessment; PSRA = Princeton Survey Research Associates; VCU = Virginia Commonwealth University.
SOURCE: Blendon et al., 2016.

enthusiasm. In 2016, a Pew study of surveys of more than 4,000 individuals revealed that anxiety outpaced enthusiasm not only for enhancement through somatic genome editing, but also for mechanical and transplant-related enhancement (Pew Research Center, 2016). A single study is not definitive, and public opinion on novel interventions in some other controversial areas (such as in vitro fertilization) has become more favorable over time and with evidence of successes. But the Pew study and many others suggest that policy in this area needs to be developed with full attention to public attitudes and understandings.

Sometimes, the lines between therapy, prevention, and enhancement are blurred, and even the definition of a "disease" that is to be cured or prevented can be open to debate. For this reason, the distinctions between preventing or treating disease and disability (i.e., "therapy") and the notion of "enhancement" may not fully capture either public attitudes or public policy options. To the extent that there is any public disquiet about the use of gene therapy for disease prevention as opposed to treatment, it appears to be linked to more generalized concerns about "meddling with nature" or "crossing a line we should not cross" (Macer et al., 1995) (see Chapter 5). This is even more true for interventions that appear unrelated to either disease treatment or prevention. As noted above, Americans appear to be largely unenthusiastic about the idea of "enhancement" (Blendon et al., 2016; Pew Research Center, 2016; see Table 6-1).

It is possible that this lack of enthusiasm is due in part to hesitation concerning innovation, which has been shown to be a common phenomenon throughout history, ranging from things now considered quite ordinary, such as coffee and refrigeration, to things still hotly debated, such as transgenic crops (Juma, 2016). Resistance or skepticism may be an outgrowth of concerns about the degree to which an innovation affects cultural identity or may distort socioeconomic patterns in a fashion that is harmful to at least some part of the population. If and when these concerns are either addressed through remedial measures or shown to be unwarranted, innovations that are needed or perceived as desirable become widely accepted.

What is unclear is whether genome editing for enhancement would follow such a pattern or would be such a disruptive application of a new technology that the resistance would persist over time, or whether new concerns will arise as the technology progressed and new applications emerges. "Status quo bias" is a phenomenon in which the preference for what is familiar can affect the way people form judgments about the merits of an innovation. The predisposition toward the status quo may arise from concerns about transition costs (i.e., how people adapt to the circumstances arising from an innovation), about risk (with innovations assumed to have risks that are less amenable to measurement relative to the status quo), about deviation from what is natural (people holding the unwarranted belief that the past processes of natural evolution have optimized humans for the current environment), and about effects on individuals (concern that technology will diminish the quality of relationships between people).

A means of testing for whether status quo bias is affecting the evaluation of new technology has been suggested. In this "reversal test," one asks, for example, whether those who think people should not have more influence over their traits would also think it would be good if people had less influence (Bostrom and Ord, 2006). The test is intended to distinguish concerns about an innovation itself from concerns about any move away from the status quo. It can be useful when juxtaposed with arguments about a "slippery slope" (see Chapter 5) because it helps distinguish concerns about the technology as it is used today from concerns about future unwanted extensions of the technology.

DRAWING LINES: THERAPY VERSUS ENHANCEMENT

Given the wide range of other interventions people undergo to alter their bodies and their personal circumstances, any discussion of so-called enhancement must begin with a working definition. Enhancement has been variously defined as "boosting our capabilities beyond the species-typical level or statistically normal range of functioning," (Daniels, 2000 in NSF, 2010, p. 3) "a nontherapeutic intervention intended to improve or extend a human trait," (NSF, 2010) or "improvements in the capacities of existing individuals or future generations" (NSF, 2010; President's Council on Bioethics, 2002, p. 1). One definition focuses on interventions that improve bodily condition or function beyond what is needed to restore or sustain health (Parens, 1998). This is a definition that addresses intent as much as the technical intervention, as most interventions can be used either to "enhance" or to restore. For example, under this definition, improving musculature for patients with muscular dystrophy would be restorative, whereas doing so for individuals with no known pathology and average capability would be considered enhancement. Recognizing the importance of intent as an aspect of "enhancement" is helpful, as most biomedical interventions will be subject (in the United States) to regulation by the U.S. Food and Drug Administration (FDA), whose statutory authority explicitly links the initial risk-benefit balance needed for approval to the "intended" use of the product, even though postapproval uses can range beyond that original intended purpose.

Another definitional matter concerns the meaning of "therapy." It is understood to encompass treatment of a disease (the definition of which is itself subject to debate, as discussed in the section on fairness and enhancement below). But prevention of disease also often is viewed as being encompassed by therapy. To reduce the risk of breast cancer in a person of average health and with nondeleterious variants, for example, is not to cure a disease or even to prevent one that is likely to occur, but this boosted resistance is often viewed as therapeutic prevention, akin to immunization against infectious diseases. A similar point pertains with respect to reducing cholesterol in persons at no more than average risk for heart disease; this is already a widespread practice in American society, and statins and aspirin are widely used to enhance resistance to heart disease pharmacologically even for those not at high risk. Genome edits for such purposes could be similarly health-promoting.

Box 6-1 summarizes key efforts to delineate the distinctions between therapy and enhancement.

BOX 6-1
Making Distinctions

In the 1970s, certain central distinctions were drawn (Juengst, 1997; Walters and Palmer, 1997). First, the distinction between somatic and germline genome modifications was established: somatic enhancements affect only a single individual, but heritable enhancements can be passed down through the generations. Discussions of heritable enhancements included concerns about possible effects on the gene pool and fears of a return to some form of eugenics. Second, a distinction was drawn between treating or preventing disease (therapy) and enhancement. Discussions of enhancement focused on issues such as safety and (especially in competitive environments such as sports) unfair advantage, with the definition of "unfair" highly dependent on context.

Available technology and the desire of prominent scientists to mitigate social concerns surrounding genetics—particularly after the Asilomar conference organized by scientists in 1975 to discuss the risks and benefits of recombinant DNA techniques—pushed the debate even further in the direction of the distinction between "medicine" or "therapy" and "enhancement." It is important to note, as well, that somatic therapy to treat very severe diseases was all that any responsible scientist could imagine actually doing with the technology of the time. An influential schematic developed in the early 1970s (depicted in the table below) defined cells 1 and 2 as "medicine" and as the "treatment of hereditary diseases," respectively (Anderson and Kulhavy, 1972, p. 109), as opposed to enhancements (somatic or heritable, respectively) in cells 3 and 4.

TABLE Schematic for Therapy Versus Enhancement

Purpose	Somatic	Germline
Therapeutic Treatment of Disease	Somatic Therapy (Cell 1)	Germline Therapy (Cell 2)
Enhancement of Capabilities	Somatic Enhancement (Cell 3)	Germline Enhancement (Cell 4)

By the mid-1980s, scientists and bioethicists had begun to call for the morally relevant line to be between disease and enhancement rather than somatic and germline. John Fletcher, then head of bioethics at the National Institutes of Health (NIH), wrote that "the most relevant moral distinction is between uses that may relieve real suffering and those that alter characteristics that have little or nothing to do with disease" (Fletcher, 1985, p. 303). Gene therapy pioneer Theodore Friedmann wrote that "the need for efficient disease control or the need to prevent damage early in development or in inaccessible cells may eventually justify germ line therapy" (Friedmann, 1989, p. 1280). In 1991, as the first three somatic gene therapy trials were under way, the chair of the Human Gene Therapy Subcommittee of NIH's Recombinant DNA Advisory Committee (RAC) called for "a detailed public discussion of the ethical issues surrounding germline genetic intervention in humans" (Walters, 1991, p. 118). Disease correction was defined as returning to "normal functioning," but to go beyond that was labeled "eugenics."

Somatic (Nonheritable) Genome Editing, Fairness, and Enhancement

With these distinctions in mind, there appears to be broad international consensus, derived from decades of research and clinical trials for gene therapy, that a somatic intervention undertaken to modify a person's genetic makeup for purposes of treating disease is not only permissible but encouraged, provided it proves to be safe and effective.

Before the modern tools needed to modify DNA were developed, government-supported research was focused on developing solid-organ transplantation to replace damaged or diseased organs and on bone marrow transplantation and reconstitution to cure leukemia and other life-threatening disorders, even though these treatments required substituting donor DNA for the patient's DNA in the solid-organ or blood-forming cells. Those cases fell clearly under what is typically considered medical care. Government-supported research also has been conducted in many countries to advance the fields of gene therapy and regenerative medicine and, more recently, human genome editing to modify the DNA in the blood-forming cells of patients with sickle-cell disease and other blood disorders and some forms of cancer. These precedents, and many others like them, have built robust scientific, regulatory, and ethical oversight structures (see Chapter 4).

As noted above, many discussions of the ethics of enhancement have been based on contrasting the concepts of "therapy" and "enhancement." However, given the evolution of the role of the physician over the past several decades from a healer of the sick to a promoter of health through preventive measures, the therapy–enhancement duality needs to be modified to accommodate a wide range of preventive interventions, such as vaccines, that are neither therapy nor enhancement but blend into each at the edges. For example, while genome editing to lower the cholesterol level of a patient with severe coronary artery disease would likely be viewed as a therapy, and genome editing of a sibling of the patient with high cholesterol who also had other risk factors for coronary artery disease might be viewed as a preventive measure, genome editing to lower the cholesterol of a healthy 21-year-old child of the patient to reduce disease risk below what is average or "normal" in the general population might be viewed as approaching the line between prevention and enhancement. Interventions thus can be viewed as falling on a therapy–prevention–enhancement spectrum, although the boundaries between the three categories are still open to debate and will likely vary with the specifics of the intervention.

With the growth in understanding of the human genome and of which sequence variants are associated with which conditions, the number of traits that could be addressed by genome editing continues to grow. This growing potential again raises the question of what it means to be "normal" and whether deviations from "normality" are really a disease. Everyone would agree that the manifestation of Tay-Sachs disease is not normal and constitutes a disease, but opinions differ as to whether genetically caused deafness should be considered a disease. It is not normal in the sense of being typical or being consistent with the range of capabilities typically associated with the human species, but it can also be associated with membership in a community of persons sharing this characteristic, many of whom reject the notion that deaf people need to be "cured" or otherwise treated to eliminate or circumvent their lack of hearing.

Commentators have noted that the concept of disease is not always objective, but rather can be the result of social agreement influenced by power and prejudice. In the 1950s, for example, homosexuality was considered a disease, and even today it is occasionally the subject of "therapeutic" interventions aimed at "curing" it. In the 1930s, "criminality" was considered a genetic disorder. Some disability activists began to question whether such traits as dwarfism or deafness should be considered diseases instead of variants that enrich human diversity. It is a question that led to discussions about where the line is drawn between normal and pathological, as well as questions about who gets to draw these lines, what authority they have to draw them, which social dimensions are included or excluded, and what provision is made to contest the decisions.

The discovery of variants that simply increase the odds of developing a disease and others that are associated with diseases whose onset is in later life also has blurred the previously bright line demarcating "disease." Early ethical debate built on language used by the pioneers in human genetics, who referred to "inborn errors," noting that most traits targeted for modification were called "errors," as in mistakes from what was supposed to be. The greatest challenge for the normality standard came from some researchers considering what might best be called enhancements for the purpose of relieving disease. This enhancement would not correct errors, but rather instill traits that some lucky minority of humans already have, such as by enhancing immune function or adding cellular receptors to capture cholesterol (Juengst, 1997; Parens, 1998; Walters and Palmer, 1997). Such alterations could be viewed as enhancements or as leveling the playing field for those not fortunate enough to have these traits at birth, and they also complicate the distinction between therapy and enhancement unless one includes prevention as an intermediate concept.

Evolution of the Unfair Social Advantage Demarcation

While both the somatic/germline and disease/enhancement distinctions have been useful, they (like most categories) are imperfect. Some commentators have focused instead on the effect of an intervention and whether that effect is "fair." Changes not made by personal effort (such as exercise or music practice) but by external forces (such as hair coloring and cosmetic surgery) are understood to have the capacity to generate a social advantage, but it is an advantage within the realm of species-typical attributes. For some, such changes are made purely for pleasure; for others they represent an effort to "normalize" or "even the odds" with those who have the most favored appearances. Externally induced changes that offer more significant or unusual advantages, such as those providing greater muscle mass or more acute vision or obviating the need for sleep, raise questions about the authenticity of the resulting capacity and whether the individual newly endowed with these capabilities is somehow diminished by having failed to earn them. Yet people are born with unearned varying capacities, some markedly superior to the norm, which raises the question of whether and when an advantage becomes "unfair."

This is a difficult question to answer precisely because of the highly uneven distribution of abilities in the human population. Unless one assigns great importance to fate, it is difficult to tease out enhancements that allow individuals to fairly match the capacities of others from those that are "unnatural," "abnormal," or "excessive." Furthermore, any attempt to relate enhancement to what is "normal" or "average" risks categorizing efforts to combat widespread "normal" but undesirable aspects of life (e.g., age-related declining eyesight, hearing, and mobility) as a form of "enhancement," with all the pejorative connotations implied by the word.

Society already condones such efforts for many conditions (cataract surgery, hip replacement) using methods other than genome editing. Some respond to inequality in access by favoring interventions that provide more care to more people, and eschew research investment in and insurance coverage for high-cost innovations. This may be a response to economic conditions or a philosophical view of infirmity as a natural part of life, not necessarily in need of every possible measure for treatment and prevention.

Other societies have responded to inequalities that arise from differential access to medical innovations by trying to increase access and insurance coverage, rather than by restricting research or the marketing of new products or technologies. Unpacking such differences requires distinguishing between restrictions on the research itself and decisions about insurance to cover treatments, a topic that in turn requires inquiry into whether insurance is primarily a public good or a privately purchased service.

Even for societies that tend toward expanding access to respond to inequality, a core concern for some is that enhancements are yet another benefit that would accrue primarily to the individual, without benefit to the population as a whole. John Rawls' influential theory of justice emphasizes the idea of equality. He observes that the luck with which someone is born healthy, talented, or in favored social circumstances is neither earned nor deserved. From this he concludes not that all people must be equalized in outcomes but that further distribution of social goods should be designed to account for this initial inequality. This notion leads to so-called equality-based reciprocity, such that inequalities should be tolerated only when they somehow accrue to the population's general advantage, in particular to the advantage of those least well-off (Rawls, 1999).

Some might conclude, therefore, that a problematic enhancement is one that confers a social advantage beyond that which an individual possesses by fate or through personal effort, and that does not benefit the rest of society in any way or undermines the implicit goals of a competition. Using equality of opportunity and societally useful inequality as guides may help distinguish those forms of enhancement that might generally be tolerated (assuming the risks are proportional to the benefits) from those that would be more controversial. Of course, somatic or germline genome editing for enhancement is very unlikely to be the most profound source of inequality in any setting. But those most uncomfortable with using genome editing for enhancement will likely still be concerned regardless of the size of its contribution.

Looking across these themes, one might conclude that enhancement per se is not the focus of concern, but rather the underlying intent and subsequent effect. One response to this concern is to focus on the technologies and applications and to restrict those most likely to be used to unacceptably exacerbate inequalities. A different response is to insist that communities and governments work to make advantageous enhancements available more generally and focus on reducing undesirable inequalities. Within this range of responses lies the choice of governance policy.

Governance of Nonheritable Somatic Editing for Enhancement of the Individual

The governance and ethics of human enhancement have long been the subject of policy reports. Most recently, the U.S. Presidential Commission for the Study of Bioethical Issues focused on human enhancement related to the use of drugs that affect neurological function (Bioethics Commission, 2015), and the European Excellence in Processing Open Cultural Heritage (EPOCH) project summarized the prevailing modes of governance and the roles of academics and bioethicists in these debates, as well as areas of missing evidence needed to identify real possibilities (European Commission, 2012). Earlier efforts include a 2009 report by the U.S. National Science Foundation (NSF) (2010) and a 2003 report by the U.S. President's Council on Bioethics (2003). In the United Kingdom, the Academy of Medical Sciences, British Academy, Royal Academy of Engineering, and The Royal Society came together in 2012 for a policy-focused workshop on emerging technological enhancements that could affect the workplace (AMS et al., 2012). And the French National Advisory Committee on Ethics and the Life Sciences and the Singapore National Bioethics Commission both produced reports in 2013 focused specifically on neuroenhancement (NCECHLS, 2013) and neuroscience research (BAC Singapore, 2013). All of these reports reflect broad input from the medical, bioethical, and academic communities and provide a rich source of information on the concerns that have been raised about enhancements, as well as the profound challenges entailed in clearly delineating the differences among therapy, prevention, and enhancement.

In the United States, governance of enhancement applications of genome editing would fall, as with other gene therapy, to the FDA, the Recombinant DNA Advisory Committee (RAC), institutional biosafety committees (IBCs), and institutional review boards (IRBs), and the legislature (see Chapter 2). The RAC could provide a venue for discussion of somatic enhancement proposals.[1] IRBs and the FDA would look at whether the benefits the enhancement might provide to the individual, to science, and to society are reasonable in light of the risks to the individual, to public health, and to environmental safety. But concerns about culture or societal morals, while important, are generally not within an IRB's remit; the regulations state that an IRB "should not consider possible long-range effects of applying knowledge gained in the research (for example, the possible effects of the research on public policy) as among those research risks that fall within the purview of its responsibility" (45 CFR Sec. 46.111(a)(2)).

Thus, if a protocol holds the potential for great benefit to individuals, and those individuals are willing to accept greater risk, the regulator and IRB might agree that the standard of the possible benefits being reasonable in relation to the risks had been met. If the regulator and IRB decide, however, that there are no real benefits of an enhancement—either to the individual or to science—then even a minimal risk is unjustified. As human genome editing improves technologically, there is every reason to believe that the health and safety risks to individuals will diminish. If these risks become de minimis, one might assume that the potential benefits required to justify the risks also will decline. Thus, as the technology improves, its application could extend from serious illnesses, to less serious illnesses, to prevention, and in the long term to enhancement, however defined.

In the United States, it is also important to keep in mind that once a medical product has been approved for a particular purpose and population, the sponsor is limited to marketing it for these "labeled" indications, but individual physicians are free to use their own judgment and prescribe

---

[1]At the moment, the RAC is not accepting germline editing protocols for review (see Chapters 2 and 5).

the product for other uses and other populations[2] (see Chapter 4). This "off-label" use complicates the question of governance in the United States and in other jurisdictions with similar rules, such as the European Union, because it makes it more difficult to restrict the use of new medical products to those situations that have the best risk/benefit ratios and the general support of the public.

With regard to enhancements, this regulatory scheme has raised concern that some products will be approved for treatment or prevention of disease but then be used off-label for riskier or less well-justified uses. As noted in Chapter 4, however, the specificity of these edited cells will limit the range of off-label uses for unrelated indications far more than is the case with many drugs. While one might imagine a genome-edited cell therapy for muscular dystrophy being of interest to those with healthy muscle tissue who wish to become even stronger, other examples are more difficult to envision. The specificity of edited cells will make such applications less likely for the foreseeable future.

In addition, the FDA has some authority to restrict off-label uses—for example, through requirements for special patient testing or adverse event reporting—and the U.S. Congress can pass legislation to specifically prohibit certain uses, as has been the case for human growth hormone (see Box 6-2). Other jurisdictions have similar powers and choices. Nonetheless, attention to the possible range of off-label uses is necessary, and the need for some control over off-label use can be anticipated.

In conjunction with formal regulatory processes, a number of other aspects of governance will affect whether and how genome editing is used for enhancement. These include professional guidelines, which influence physician behavior directly and set standards against which that behavior is judged in cases of possible malpractice (Campbell and Glass, 2000; Mello, 2001). Insurers that offer malpractice coverage also can influence the willingness of physicians to offer certain services (Kessler, 2011). In another capacity, insurers play a role by choosing to cover the cost of using approved technologies based in part on the purpose for which they are going to be used and whether the use is necessary or elective.

---

[2] 59 *Federal Register* 59, 820, 59, 821 (November 18, 1994). "Once a [drug] product has been approved for marketing, a physician may prescribe it for uses or in treatment regimens of patient populations that are not included in approved labeling." The notice goes on to state that "unapproved" or, more precisely, "unlabeled" uses may be appropriate and rational in certain circumstances, and may in fact reflect approaches to drug therapy that have been extensively reported in medical literature.

HERITABLE GENOME EDITING AND ENHANCEMENT

As noted in Chapter 5, germline genome editing presents the prospect of inducing heritable changes that could affect multiple generations, not just the child who developed from a genome-edited embryo or gametes. In the context of the discussions around enhancement, this prospect may deepen some of the disquiet concerning those applications that are most distant from disease treatment, disease prevention, and correction of significant physical or social disadvantages relative to the norm. This disquiet is influenced not only by the concerns outlined above with respect to somatic genome editing but also by the long and troubling history of eugenics, a history that included coercive measures and even genocide. This history is replete with dogma that creates hierarchies of human quality based on race, religion, national origin, and economic status, and it demonstrates how scientific concepts, such as natural selection, and public welfare measures, such as public hygiene, can be subverted for purposes of cruel and destructive social policies. These considerations lead to the question of whether "enhancement" applications of heritable germline editing should be prohibited entirely or significantly restricted in ways measurably different from those for purely nonheritable somatic editing.

Eugenics

The term "eugenics" was first used in the late 19th century to define the goal of improving the human species by giving "the more suitable races or strains of blood a better chance of prevailing speedily over the less suitable" (Kevles, 1985, p. xiii). The general idea was to create schemes for encouraging people with "good" bloodlines to have more children and those with "bad" bloodlines to have fewer or no children in order to improve the human species. Given their extremely limited understanding of what traits were truly heritable, eugenicists in various societies applied their social biases in ways now deemed unacceptable. In Britain, eugenicists assumed that the "good" traits were those found among the upper classes. They inferred that the fine qualities of the aristocracy were heritable, so the poor should simply produce fewer children. In the United States, the original eugenic impulse involved race or ethnicity. One eugenic goal was to keep races with "bad" traits from immigrating to America. The peak effort in meeting this goal was the 1924 Immigration Control Act, which limited immigrants from Eastern and Southern Europe. It was signed by President Coolidge, who had earlier claimed that "America must be kept American" because "biological laws show that Nordics deteriorate when mixed with other races" (Kevles, 1985, p. 97).

By the 1920s, countries increasingly looked at people's individual qualities independent of their race and class, trying to identify those with sup-
posedly genetic traits such as "feeblemindedness" and "criminality" and
discouraging them from reproducing. These eugenics programs were not
necessarily voluntary, and many felons and women were forcibly sterilized.
Most famously, Justice Oliver Wendell Holmes of the U.S. Supreme Court
wrote the opinion that allowed the sterilization of Carrie Buck, a "feeble-
minded" woman, concluding that sterilization was justified because "[i]t is
better for all the world, if instead of waiting to execute degenerate offspring
for crime, or to let them starve for their imbecility, society can prevent
those who are manifestly unfit from continuing their kind. The principle
that sustains compulsory vaccination is broad enough to cover cutting the
Fallopian tubes. Three generations of imbeciles are enough."[3] Eugenics
programs were part of progressive social reforms and were thought to uplift
the population by improving genetic qualities (Lombardo, 2008).

The logic of eugenics was taken to its extreme conclusion in Nazi
Germany, where those perceived to have genetically derived limitations
were first sterilized and in later years killed. The logic of eugenic purity
was a part of the Holocaust, which resulted in the deaths of millions of
people portrayed as genetic inferiors, primarily Jews, Roma, and those
with disabilities. According to historian Daniel Kevles, after revelation of
the Holocaust, people realized that "a river of blood would eventually run
from the German sterilization law of 1933 to Auschwitz and Buchenwald"
(Kevles, 1985, p. 118).

Reform Eugenics

Revelation of the Holocaust was not the end of eugenics, only the end
of race-based, coercive, state-mandated eugenics. Many scientists had already rejected the mainstream eugenic view, with Hermann Muller writing
in 1935 that eugenics had become "hopelessly perverted" into a pseudo-
scientific facade for "advocates of race and class prejudice, defenders of
vested interests of church and state, Fascists, Hitlerites, and reactionaries
generally" (Kevles, 1985, p. 164). Muller and other prominent scientists,
such as Julian Huxley, would create a "reform" eugenics that sought to
stop the reproduction of people with genetic disease and encourage more
reproduction by people with "superior" genes—from whatever race and
class. People would be encouraged to change their reproductive practices
voluntarily for the good of the species. Most notably for future debates,
these thinkers wanted humanity to seize control of its own evolution and
improve the species in various ways, such as by making humans more intelligent. The ethical debate of the 1950s through the early 1970s was quite

---

[3] *Buck v. Bell*, 274 U.S. 200 (1927).

broad, often focused on what the goals for genetic modification as a species should be. In a theme that would recur from this era forward, some critics of reform eugenics averred that humans should be satisfied with the way they are. In general, the ethical debate was about the genetic goals of the species—or whether to have such goals at all (Evans, 2002).

In 1953, Crick and Watson described the structural basis of how DNA duplicates itself (Watson and Crick, 1953), leading to understanding of how the DNA of genes encodes information. This discovery changed the ethical debate concerning eugenics as people realized that if genes were actually chemicals whose structure could be characterized, society no longer would have to rely on "who mates with whom"; rather, people could be chemically modified to have "more" of the "good" genes. Robert Sinsheimer, a prominent scientist of the time, was typical in his response, writing in 1969 that "the old eugenics would have required a continual selection for breeding of the fit, and a culling of the unfit. The new eugenics would permit in principle the conversion of all of the unfit to the highest genetic level . . . for we should have the potential to create new genes and new qualities yet undreamed in the human species" (Sinsheimer, 1969, p. 13). Theologian Paul Ramsey wrote in 1970 that such proposals would make "man" "his own self-creator" and lead to a new theology of science (Ramsey, 1970, p. 144).

Whether to improve the species and, if so, in what way was the core of the ethical debate until the early 1970s. A discussion then—one continuing today among some transhumanists—is whether human evolution should be left to processes of natural selection, which are random and occur very slowly. For example, Corneliu Giurgea, the Romanian chemist who synthesized Piracetam in 1964 and showed that it might act in cognitive enhancement, said, "Man is not going to wait passively for millions of years before evolution offers him a better brain" (Giurgea, 1981). Indeed, with the specter of climate change on earth and the imagined colonization of Mars, some transhumanists today discuss whether humans need to intervene in their own evolution to cope with the future they are creating (Bostrom, 2005; Rosen, 2014). But in the 1970s, the evident complexity of making changes, let alone determining which changes are desirable, led many to rethink what prominent biologist Bernard Davis would dub "Promethean predictions of unlimited control." He reminded readers of facts now considered obvious, such as that most "enhanced characteristics" are polygenic and thus difficult or impossible to modify (Davis, 1970, p. 1279).

Technological limits of that era also helped shape the debate. It was impossible to imagine somatic enhancements when somatic therapy was not yet successful, so any claim of a somatic enhancement would have been considered too risky, with very little benefit. Similarly, if early attempts at modifying somatic cells through viral vectors were successful in only a small number of the cells, how could sperm, eggs, or zygotes be changed? But where enhancement and heritable change came together, even though not yet technically feasible, public concern was greatest. And the goal of the eugenicists—to make the species better—was placed in this category, thus comingling the rejection of eugenics with the possibilities for germline editing.

Slippery Slope Concerns about Germline Enhancement

Opponents of germline enhancement from the reform eugenics era forward were concerned largely with long-term cultural or social changes that could occur as the result of a sociological slippery slope process (see also Chapter 5). That is, would somatic therapy eventually lead to efforts to enhance the species through germline engineering, a process that might evolve as skill and familiarity with somatic therapy made it easier to imagine other applications as helpful and safe? These opponents were willing to endorse somatic therapy because they thought the somatic/germline distinction was culturally strong, and the public would make a clear distinction between modifying individuals and modifying their offspring (Burgess and Prentice, 2016).

This sort of slippery slope argument emerged in 1981 after a U.S. Supreme Court decision that allowed the patenting of genetically engineered life forms (Evans, 2002). Concerns were raised about "the fundamental nature of human life and the dignity and worth of the individual human being" (President's Commission, 1982, p. 95). The presidential bioethics commission of that era wrote a report entitled *Splicing Life*, in which it reformulated the ethical debate so that the report would be "meaningful to public policy consideration" (President's Commission, 1982, p. 20). To make ethical claims legally actionable meant moving away from arguments about future cultural harms or claims that it is not the role of humanity to modify itself. Consequences needed to be more concrete and near term, not speculative. In the report, the commission stated that it "could find no ground for concluding that any current or planned forms of genetic engineering, whether using human or nonhuman material, are intrinsically wrong or irreligious *per se*" (President's Commission, 1982, p. 77). The report established a framework of risks and benefits and the rights of individuals that would serve as a framework for government regulation of this new science, such as through the human gene therapy subcommittee of the RAC. It was an approach not particularly amenable to consideration of broader and longer-term social effects, for instance slippery slopes, because of its focus on more immediate effects on identifiable persons.

The pre-1980s ethics debate returned in 2001 with the appointment of a federal bioethics commission by President George W. Bush. This commission claimed that it "eschewed a thin utilitarian calculus of costs and benefits, or a narrow analysis based only on individual 'rights.'" Instead, it claimed to ground its reflections "on the broader plane of human procreation and human healing, with their deeper meanings" (President's Council on Bioethics, 2002, p. 10). Most notably, the commission was concerned about the promotion of inequality and about parents having the ultimate power over their children (President's Council on Bioethics, 2003, p. 44). The report did not have a strong impact on policy regarding human genetic modification, but made clear that some in U.S. society viewed germline genetic modification through this particular ethical lens.

The concern of the Bush-era commission that germline enhancement might encourage people to view children as something to be designed and manipulated has long been a concern of some social scientists and humanists. Political theorist Michael Sandel wrote that "to appreciate children as gifts is to accept them as they come, not as objects of our design or products of our will or instruments of our ambition. Parental love is not contingent on the talents and attributes a child happens to have" (Sandel, 2013, p. 349). One implication is that potential parents should refrain from making modifications that would directly benefit their future child, not necessarily because doing so would cause them to see their own child differently, but because it might in a tiny, indirect yet cumulative way promote a culture that would come to see all children differently. Yet critics of this view would argue that the harm is speculative, and that this level of freedom in the relationship of the individual to society is well within the range of what is allowed in liberal democratic societies.

Another concern that has been raised revolves around whether parents might become increasingly viewed as responsible for the qualities of their offspring. According to Sandel, "we attribute less to chance and more to choice. Parents become responsible for choosing, or failing to choose, the right traits for their children" (Sandel, 2004, p. 60).

A similar idea is expressed in the more religious language of making versus begetting. Theologian Gilbert Meilaender describes designing the genetic qualities of one's children as akin to "making" them, whereas nondesign is "begetting" them. More important, and like Sandel, he states that "what we beget is like ourselves. What we make is not; it is the product of our free decision, and its destiny is ours to determine" (Meilaender, 1997, p. 42). By this view, begetting (i.e., nondesign) is critical to human dignity and human rights because "we are equal to each other, whatever our distinctions in excellence of various sorts, precisely because none of us is the 'maker' of another one of us" (Meilaender, 2008, p. 264). These concerns about objectification might possibly apply to germline conversion to genes associated with ordinary health, but would more likely be raised by enhancements, health-related or beyond.

There are other views, of course. One might say that making choices about our genetic future—whether or not they increase the perception that humans are more like objects—is precisely human. As Joseph Fletcher, one of the founders of bioethics, wrote in 1971: "Man is a maker and a selecter and a designer, and the more rationally contrived and deliberate anything is, the more human it is. . . . [T]he real difference is between accidental or random reproduction and rationally willed or chosen reproduction" (Fletcher, 1971, pp. 780-781).

Others have argued that parental discretion allows for a wide range of practices, provided they are not significantly harmful to the physical or psychological development of a child (Robertson, 2008). As discussed in Chapter 5, this view requires a pure reproductive rights framework that must be stretched to its limits to include the right to enhance or diminish traits (Robertson, 2004). It is a vision of parental liberty that already encompasses a wide range of enhancements of infants and children, including such biomedical measures as cosmetic surgeries, the use of growth hormone for short stature of unknown cause (see Box 6-2), and the use of some performance-enhancing drugs. By extension, it could be argued that this liberty encompasses germline enhancements with similar risk/benefit balances. Here again, though, there is very little reason to think that in the United States, the constitutional cases on parenting would prevent the government from banning germline genome editing if it had a rational basis for doing so.

Academic transhumanism has emerged as a contributor to these debates. Transhumanists argue not only for the ethical legitimacy of some forms of enhancement-oriented germline editing, but perhaps even for parental responsibility and an ethical obligation to take advantage of such enhancement possibilities for the benefit of one's children (Persson and Savelescu, 2012). One philosopher has argued that humans are obligated to make the best possible decisions for those who cannot decide for themselves, and this would include future children and their descendants (Harris, 2007). These are arguments about moral obligations, however, as nothing in U.S. statutes or judicial decisions (or those of other countries) imposes them as a matter of law.

Overall, two distinct approaches to evaluating the ethics of germline enhancement have emerged over the past half century. In one, the focus is more societal and philosophical. It encompasses not only the concerns raised about germline editing in general, as described in Chapter 5, but also concerns about altering how children are viewed and about creating or increasing social inequities in a multigenerational fashion as a result of the heritability of the enhancement. Even where the benefits of an individual enhancement might be regarded as justification for an individual intervention, these analyses often feature a concern about the slippery slope and an echo of eugenics movements of the past.

In another approach, the disease/enhancement distinction remains largely useful, as it tracks well to the evaluation of individual risks and benefits. This evaluation is the focus of the regulatory bodies, such as the FDA, that review new medical products for approval and the research oversight bodies that oversee protection of clinical trial participants and others who might be put at physical risk by the trials. When diseases are cured or prevented, the benefit of trials is seen as greater relative to when functional traits are improved beyond what is necessary for a typical life. In turn, this gradation of benefits is balanced against health risks for offspring and future generations, including the potential for disease prevention.

Given that human germline genome editing has not yet been tested clinically for therapeutic or preventive purposes, it appears clear that germline genome editing for purposes of enhancement—that is, not clearly intended to cure or combat disease and disability—is very unlikely at this time to meet the standard of possible benefit and tolerable risk as required to initiate clinical trials. Even as risks recede with greater experience and information, truly discretionary and elective germline edits would be unlikely to have benefits outweighing even minor health risks.

CONCLUSIONS AND RECOMMENDATIONS

Significant scientific progress will be necessary before any genome-editing intervention for indications other than the treatment or prevention of disease or disability can satisfy the risk/benefit standards for initiating a clinical trial. This conclusion holds for both somatic and heritable germline interventions. There is significant public discomfort with the use of genome editing for so-called enhancement of human traits and capacities beyond those typical of adequate health. Therefore, a robust public discussion is needed concerning the values to be placed upon the individual and societal benefits and risks of genome editing for purposes other than treatment or prevention of disease or disability. These discussions would include consideration of the potential for introducing or exacerbating societal inequities, so that these values can be incorporated as appropriate into the risk/benefit assessments that will precede any decision about whether to authorize clinical trials.

RECOMMENDATION 6-1. Regulatory agencies should not at this time authorize clinical trials of somatic or germline genome editing for purposes other than treatment or prevention of disease or disability.

RECOMMENDATION 6-2. Government bodies should encourage public discussion and policy debate regarding governance of somatic human genome editing for purposes other than treatment or prevention of disease or disability.

BOX 6-2
Human Growth Hormone

The experience with human growth hormone (hGH) illustrates the difficulty of finding clear boundaries between therapy and prevention, and between treatment and enhancement. It is also a lesson in how a sudden change in the ease or availability of a technology or intervention can make those boundaries—previously of little importance—suddenly become the subject of professional norms, public opinion, and legal controls.

hGH was a scarce commodity for many years, and its use was limited largely to "treatment" for those who lacked normal levels of the hormone (Ayyar, 2011). With the development of synthetic hGH in 1985, the newly increased supply of affordable hGH triggered a lively debate about whether there ought to be constraints on its use. For example, hGH could now be given to children or adults in good health but with unexplained short stature, ranging from <1st percentile of height for their age to being only slightly shorter than their peers. Some others sought hGH despite being of normal height and growth rate, with an interest in attaining above-average height or strength. Whether or not administration of hGH in these and many other cases reflected a favorable risk/benefit ratio; whether it qualified as treatment, prevention, or enhancement; and which of those uses might be appropriate required careful scientific and ethical investigation. The fact that the hormone would be administered to children too young to make decisions for themselves added to the complexity of the conversation.

The risks and possible benefits of hGH administration were uncertain in the 1980s and 1990s, and the drug was approved only for severe cases of growth hormone deficiency in children. But over time growth hormone therapy was shown to be reasonably safe and effective for patients who had low levels of the hormone in their blood or who experienced severely stunted growth despite normal levels of the hormone; studies showed it bringing children up to the 10th to 25th percentile, depending on dosage and timing of treatment (Allen and Cuttler, 2013; Maiorana and Cianfarani, 2009). But the treatment is not entirely risk free; children can experience relatively minor or moderate adverse events, such as respiratory congestion and headache (Bell et al., 2010; Cohen et al., 2002; Kemp et al., 2005; Lindgren and Ritzen, 1999; Willemsen et al., 2007). In addition, long-term risks have had considerably less study, and there is some evidence to suggest that children who receive hGH may have a slightly increased risk of stroke as adults (Ichord, 2014).

The U.S. Food and Drug Administration (FDA) approved hGH for use in children and adults for a limited and narrowly defined list of indications, including children with growth disorders (e.g., chronic renal insufficiency, Turner's syndrome, Prader-Willi syndrome, Noonan syndrome) or severe unexplained short stature. For adults with severe growth hormone deficiency, treatment can result in modest gains in body composition, exercise capacity, and skeletal integrity (Molitch et al., 2011). They, as well as adults with AIDS-associated wasting syndrome or short bowel syndrome, also qualified for treatment (Ayyar, 2011; Cook and Rose, 2012; Cuttler and Silvers, 2010).

Despite the absence of evidence that hGH supplementation increases muscle strength or aerobic exercise capacity in healthy individuals (Liu et al., 2007), some healthy adults have been drawn to hGH in hopes it would serve as a performance-enhancing drug or would slow the normal aging process. But these uses have been linked to a high risk of serious adverse effects, including diabetes, cancer, hypertension, muscle pain, joint pain, swelling and inflammation of soft tissue, carpal tunnel syndrome, and enlarged breast tissue in men (Liu et al., 2008; Perls and Handelsman, 2015). Additionally, there is some evidence that people with genetic resistance to growth hormone enjoy longer life spans, suggesting that giving hGH to otherwise normally aging adults might actually shorten their lives (Suh et al., 2008). Despite these dangers, hGH was used by some athletes and aging adults (DEA, 2013).

The FDA is responsible for regulation of prescription drugs, and federal law prohibits sponsors from advertising and marketing drugs for uses that go beyond their approved indications. But physicians are generally free to prescribe drugs for other indications not evaluated by the FDA (known as "off-label" prescription), based on their own professional judgment and expertise. This is a common phenomenon with widely acknowledged benefits in cases of evolving information and physician experience, but the slippery slope trend toward off-label so-called enhancement uses of hGH led Congress to take the unusual step of enacting legislative restrictions. According to the Crime Control Act of 1990,* the distribution of hGH for nonapproved indications, such as for antiaging, age-related conditions, or enhancement of athletic performance, is a felony punishable by fines and imprisonment. Both the FDA and the Drug Enforcement Agency interpret this amendment to the Federal Food, Drug, and Cosmetic Act strictly to mean that off-label prescription of hGH is now illegal (Cronin, 2008; FDA, 2012a).

---

*U.S. Code Title 21 § 333(e) Prohibited distribution of human growth hormone
(1) Except as provided in paragraph (2), whoever knowingly distributes, or possesses with intent to distribute, human growth hormone for any use in humans other than the treatment of a disease or other recognized medical condition, where such use has been authorized by the Secretary of Health and Human Services under section 355 of this title and pursuant to the order of a physician, is guilty of an offense punishable by not more than 5 years in prison, such fines as are authorized by title 18, or both.
(2) Whoever commits any offense set forth in paragraph (1) and such offense involves an individual under 18 years of age is punishable by not more than 10 years imprisonment, such fines as are authorized by title 18, or both.
(3) Any conviction for a violation of paragraphs (1) and (2) of this subsection shall be considered a felony violation of the Controlled Substances Act [21 U.S.C. 801 et seq.] for the purposes of forfeiture under section 413 of such Act [21 U.S.C. 853].
(4) As used in this subsection the term "human growth hormone" means somatrem, somatropin, or an analogue of either of them.
(5) The Drug Enforcement Administration is authorized to investigate offenses punishable by this subsection.

7

Public Engagement

The emergence of CRISPR/Cas9 as a research tool in the area of human genome editing has lent new urgency to calls for a broad public dialogue about these technologies and their applications. These calls have come from ethicists and social scientists (e.g., Jasanoff et al., 2015), as well as biomedical scientists (Bosley et al., 2015; Doudna, 2015) and multiple think tanks, bioethics groups, and scientific/professional societies, such as The Hinxton Group (Chan et al., 2015), the Nuffield Council (2016b), and the Center for Genetics and Society (2015).

The idea itself is not new. At the Asilomar Conference in February 1975, an international group of scientists discussed the use of recombinant DNA and decided strict controls should be placed on its use (Berg et al., 1975). The concerns expressed by that group are reflected in a report to the U.S. Senate Committee on Human Resources Subcommittee on Health and Scientific Research. That report argued that it was "increasingly important to society that the serious problems which arise at the interface between science and society be carefully identified, and that mechanisms and models be devised, for the solution of these problems" (Powledge and Dach, 1977, p. 1).

These early efforts have evolved into a "growing political commitment at the highest levels to giving citizens more of a voice in the decisions that affect their lives, and to engaging citizens in making government more responsive and accountable" (Cornwall, 2008, p. 11). In a 2000 report, the U.K. House of Lords recommended that dialogue with the public be a mandatory and integral part of policy processes, including the use of public meetings as a tool for formal citizen engagement (U.K. House of Lords, 2000). Likewise, the 2003 U.S. Nanotechnology Research and Development Act mandated "convening of regular and ongoing public discussions, through mechanisms such as citizens' panels, consensus conferences, and educational events."[1]

These efforts have been motivated in part by the desire to anticipate the reactions of members of the public to potentially controversial technologies and to "avoid unjustifiably inhibiting innovation, stigmatizing new technologies, or creating trade barriers" (Holdren et al., 2011, p. 1). Research also has shown that engaging meaningfully with decision makers and public stakeholders "in processes . . . that incorporate diverse perspectives transparently" can increase public perceptions of the legitimacy of regulatory or policy decisions surrounding emerging technologies (Posner et al., 2016, p. 1760). These findings echo the conclusion of a 2008 National Research Council (NRC) consensus report that public participation in (environmental) assessment and decision making has the potential to improve not only perceptions of legitimacy but also the quality of decisions (Holdren et al., 2011, p. 1; NRC, 2008).

One could argue, for example, that a lack of meaningful engagement with different publics when genetically modified organisms (GMOs) were first introduced did irreparable damage to the emerging scientific field of genetic engineering. Public debates about harmful effects of Bt corn on the larvae of monarch butterflies, for instance, led to "a nearly 10% drop in the value of Monsanto stock, possible trade restrictions by Japan, freezes on the approval process for Bt-transgenic corn by the European Commission (Brussels), and calls for a moratorium on further planting of Bt-corn in the United States" (Shelton and Roush, 1999, p. 832). These debates have also slowed or halted the development and introduction of biofortification of some foods, such as golden rice, which has the potential to reduce disease caused by a vitamin A deficiency. The World Health Organization estimates that 250 million people suffer from vitamin A deficiency (nearly half of them children in the developing world), which is a leading cause of childhood blindness, affecting one-quarter to a half million children worldwide (Achenbach, 2016). A 2016 report from the National Academies argues that increasing micronutrients at appropriate levels in both conventional and genetically engineered crops "could have favorable effects on the health of millions of people" (NASEM, 2016c, p. 228).

Some scholars have argued that human genome editing has raised, and will continue to raise, ethical, regulatory, and sociopolitical questions that go well beyond discussions of technical risks and benefits identified by

---

[1] 21st Century Nanotechnology Research and Development Act, Public Law 108-153 (December 3, 2003).

biologists (Jasanoff et al., 2015) or even philosophical and sociopolitical concerns raised by social scientists and ethicists (Sarewitz, 2015). These scholars argue that the risks and benefits associated with human genome editing should not be defined solely by the scientific community, and that a comprehensive understanding of risks and benefits will require broad public debates that are highly inclusive with respect to the range of voices and how relevant concepts are defined. This argument suggests, as genome-editing technologies and applications develop, the need for ongoing public discussion about how regulatory bodies should draw distinctions between such concepts as therapy and enhancement or disability and disease.

There is considerable variation among countries, and even over time in the same country, with respect to the role of public opinion, world view, and religious affiliation in the formation of public policy. In theocracies, public policy concerning embryo research, germline genome editing, and even somatic therapy may be shaped by explicit reference to religious doctrine. Even in formally secular countries, religious belief may strongly influence individual morality, which in turn is expressed in personal opinions and political preferences. Other countries may have constitutional requirements for various degrees of separation between government programs or policies and religious institutions. For this reason, public engagement is part of public policy formation in a variety of ways across the globe (Pew Research Center, 2008).

In the United States, regulatory agencies such as the U.S. Food and Drug Administration (FDA) have statutory authority to permit or prohibit the marketing of medical products based on technical considerations of risk and benefit. There is no authority to refuse approval for a particular product that is intended for (or might be used for) a purpose that many view as immoral. If such a prohibition were to be enacted, it would emerge from the legislature, subject to limitation where the prohibition would abridge constitutionally protected rights. In matters such as these, public input is an important component of sound decision making.

This chapter begins by delineating the broad concepts encompassed by public engagement. It then reviews in turn U.S. and international public engagement practices. The chapter turns next to lessons learned from past public engagement efforts. The final section presents conclusions and recommendations.

PUBLIC ENGAGEMENT: BROAD CONCEPTS

The broad concepts that guide public engagement have been outlined by Alan Leshner, CEO Emeritus of the American Association for the Advancement of Science:

> We need to engage the public in a more open and honest bidirectional dialogue about science and technology and their products, including not only their benefits but also their limits, perils, and pitfalls. We need to respect the public's perspective and concerns even when we do not fully share them, and we need to develop a partnership that can respond to them. (Leshner, 2003, p. 977)

In the same vein, an editorial in *Nature* called on scientists to participate in these public discussions and bring their expertise to the wider conversation, even when "such public discussions may take many researchers outside their comfort zone" (*Nature*, 2017, p. 5).

In practice, public engagement takes many different forms, and it is beyond the scope of this report to discuss the advantages and disadvantages of different modalities (NRC, 2008; Rowe and Frewer, 2005; Scheufele, 2011). Nonetheless, it is possible to articulate at least three broad principles of engagement that can be applied to guide any effort to broaden the discourse on human genome editing to include the maximum number of relevant viewpoints and stakeholders.

The first principle of public engagement relates to *quality of outcomes.* Previous National Academies reports have identified a host of factors that contribute to high-quality regulatory or policy decisions informed by engagement efforts (NASEM, 2016a; NRC, 1996, 2008). Four such factors are particularly noteworthy for engagement efforts surrounding human genome editing. First is considering and weighing systematically the widest possible range of effects, as well as the uncertainties surrounding them. This includes consideration of risks and benefits that go beyond technical, medical, or scientific questions and encompass the "perspectives and knowledge of [all] interested and affected parties" (NRC, 1996, p. 3). Second is identifying the full range of potential policy or regulatory options. Third is having quality public engagement mechanisms that "deal with both facts and values and in particular with how anticipated changes in the world will affect the things people value" (NRC, 2008, p. 235). And finally, members of the lay public are able to ask questions and suggest solutions that may not have been imagined by regulators or experts.

A second principle of public engagement is the *legitimacy of outcomes.* Legitimacy tends to be connected to a number of related factors. First, processes for public engagement are transparent and perceived by all participants as fair and competent (Hadden, 1995). Second, echoing some of the considerations outlined earlier, public engagement identifies the values, interests, and concerns of all interested or potentially affected parties. Finally, engagement is pursued in a manner consistent with relevant laws and regulations.

These first two engagement principles, however, need to be balanced with a third—*administrative efficiency*. "The goal of full participation needs to be considered in light of the need for administrative efficiency to ensure that decisions are made in a timely manner" (NASEM, 2016c, p. 56), while also guarding against the risk that well-resourced or well-organized constituencies will dominate the public discourse and drown out other voices.

Based on these broad principles, public engagement efforts typically are built around one or more of the following processes (Rowe and Frewer, 2005):

- *Communication/information*—ensuring that decision-relevant information (including ethical, regulatory, and political considerations) effectively reaches maximum cross sections of society. In other words, public engagement efforts—regardless of format—need to focus not only on easy-to-reach audiences (e.g., more educated segments of the population) or highly invested groups (e.g., patient advocacy groups, religious communities, groups concerned with women's rights/gender issues, environmental activists).
- *Consultation*—conveying decision-relevant information from the maximum number of relevant and affected public(s) to the sponsors of the initiative (e.g., regulatory agencies, policy makers at the federal and potentially even state levels). The process of structuring and soliciting this consultation typically is initiated by the sponsor. One possibility for more efficient consultation is to interact with interest and advocacy groups. These groups can be a vehicle for reaching large numbers of people who share a position or goal, although with the caveat that these groups vary widely in how democratically they arrive at their positions or how accurately they reflect the range of views of their members (Seifter, 2015).
- *Participation*—exchanging all decision-relevant information and value considerations among the maximum number of relevant public(s) and policy actors. Dialogue and negotiation transform opinions and increase information and awareness among both sponsors and public participants. Many examples of participatory activities are based at least partially on formal deliberations among (policy) decision makers and members of the public, along the lines of Danish consensus conferences (discussed further below) that provide formal input into policy-making processes (Danish Board of Technology, 2006, 2010a,b).

Regardless of the process, the purpose of engagement efforts is not to create or increase public acceptance of emerging technologies. In this sense, public engagement is a direct response to what is known as the "knowledge deficit model" (Brossard and Lewenstein, 2009)—the notion that it is possible (or desirable) to increase public acceptance of new technologies by closing knowledge deficits and building relevant scientific literacy among nonexpert audiences. Public engagement models deviate from knowledge deficit models in two ways. First, they acknowledge that very limited empirical data support the assumption that more informed citizens will be more accepting of emerging technologies (Scheufele, 2013). Second, such models abandon the notions (1) that building public support for science is, in all cases, desirable; and (2) that public debate or even controversy is always undesirable. Instead, public engagement is designed to facilitate "the sharing and exchange of knowledge, perspectives, and preferences between or among groups who often have differences in expertise, power, and values" (NASEM, 2016b, p. 22). As a result, it "gives all stakeholders opportunities to discuss the potential risks, benefits, and consequences of a technology before it is developed or deployed; can motivate attention to issues important to the public good; and ideally encourages civic participation and expression of views by all the diverse groups that are concerned with an issue" (NASEM, 2016a, pp. 1-7).

Empirical evidence also is limited on how effective different models of public engagement are in achieving these goals, and the existing literature draws mainly on examples of engagement activities from the local and regional levels. As a result, it is difficult either to point to specific structures or processes for effective engagement that are applicable across contexts or to predict how they can be tailored to fit the wide diversity of participants, regulatory questions, and topics (NASEM, 2016a).

U.S. PRACTICES

Across different issues, countries, and jurisdictions, efforts to translate the principles discussed above into practice have varied widely. In the United States, the Obama administration codified the idea of public engagement under the label *responsible development*: "Innovation with respect to emerging technologies—such as nanotechnology, synthetic biology, and genetic engineering, among others—requires not only coordinated research and development but also appropriate and balanced oversight" (Holdren et al., 2011, p. 1). In practice, this concept involves *communication* and *consultation*, as described in the previous section, as two key processes:

- *Communication*: "The Federal Government should actively communicate information to the public regarding the potential benefits and risks associated with new technologies" (Holdren et al., 2011, p. 2).
- *Consultation*: "To the extent feasible and subject to valid constraints (involving, for example, national security and confidential business information), relevant information should be developed with ample opportunities for stakeholder involvement and public participation. [This is] important for promoting accountability, for improving decisions, for increasing trust, and for ensuring that officials have access to widely dispersed information" (Holdren et al., 2011, p. 2).

In the United States, Congress enacts laws governing science, health care, and the like, all of which are influenced by democratic processes that bring public opinion and constituent interests to the attention of elected officials. Specialized agencies generally are empowered to implement law (subject in most cases to overall policy direction from the executive branch) through the use of regulations that are developed with public input.

The nature and extent of this public engagement vary to some degree with the overseeing agency, but all agencies are governed by a set of legal rules that have been outlined in the Administrative Procedures Act and subsequently interpreted by the courts. The engagement techniques include advance notice of proposed rulemaking, an opportunity to comment, and a requirement that the agency explain its rationale for a rule and why it adopted or rejected comments. These formal rulemaking processes include relatively straightforward rules regarding public engagement. Often in the case of a highly complex or rapidly evolving area (such as biotechnology or life sciences), subregulatory, legally nonbinding guidance or agency practices apply, some of which also are subject to formal public comment. Lastly, for new research such as genome editing, there can be additional nonbinding review by the National Institutes of Health's (NIH's) Recombinant DNA Advisory Committee (RAC) or by an expert advisory committee convened by the FDA.

Public engagement in science policy is a global affair. One example is the European Commission's introduction of the concept of responsible research and innovation (RRI) in the Horizon 2020 funding program to increase stakeholder participation and influence in research directions. RRI is about "co-creating the future with citizens and civil society organisations, and also bringing on board the widest possible diversity of actors that would not normally interact with each other, on matters of science and technology" (European Commission, 2016b). It includes an effort to map the ethical issues relevant to innovation and, with the help of the public, to identify the best options for governance, whether in formal law or in voluntary standards and practices (European Commission, 2016b). It also includes the VOICES (Views, Opinions, and Ideas of Citizens in Europe on Science) project, with its thousands of participants in focus groups and other exercises (European Commission, 2016c).

Existing Infrastructure for Public Involvement in Genome-Editing Policy

In addition to the general framework for public engagement in policy, there are some particularly relevant opportunities for public engagement in the current approval process for somatic gene therapy research. To the extent that some policy can be formulated at the state level, as has happened in some states with respect to embryo research, cloning, and funding for stem cell research, the states themselves can be stakeholders that engage with the federal agencies (albeit with complex goals that include concerns about state power and independence) (Seifter, 2014b). In federalist systems, such as those not only of the United States but also of Europe and Australia, it is important to include consideration of regional opportunities for public engagement and policy making as well. Beyond allowing for the possibility that policy making may well occur at the local level, doing so has the potential to increase the perceived legitimacy of centralized, federal policies adopted by administrative rule (Seifter, 2014a).

At the federal level in the United States, opportunities for public engagement exist but tend to be limited and passive, and not the type of fuller public engagement that may be appropriate for an important new technology such as human genome editing, especially as potentially applied to the germline. These opportunities are described below.

National Institutes of Health's Recombinant DNA Advisory Committee

At present, the RAC provides the greatest opportunity for public involvement in the oversight of human gene-transfer or genome-editing protocols. Under the modified procedures enacted in April 2016, the RAC reviews only human gene-transfer protocols that present novel or significant scientific, societal, or ethical concerns. The RAC reviewed the first human CRISPR/Cas9 genome-editing trial in the United States pursuant to these criteria in June 2016. As described in greater detail in Chapter 2, the RAC's process is transparent and provides opportunities for public involvement. RAC meetings are conducted in accordance with the Federal Advisory Committee Act, which requires public advance notice of meetings that are open to the public (unless certain exceptions apply) and in which time is made available for public comment. In addition, recent RAC meetings have been webcast for viewing in real time or from the archives after the meeting, and NIH's Office of Biotechnology Activities has created an email list for individuals who wish to be informed of new RAC meetings and activities.

Although these provisions allow for limited participation by interested members of the public, they are passive in that they apply primarily to a subset of the public that has an existing interest and that seeks out the meeting information. In its current form, the RAC lacks scholarly expertise in public opinion or public engagement research, and is therefore not as well positioned to spearhead efforts to seek input from, or dialogues with, different communities of people at large who have an interest in the issue at hand, often referred to as "publics."

U.S. Food and Drug Administration

The FDA is the second major institutional player in gene therapy approvals in the United States, but as described in more detail in Chapter 2, the Investigational New Drug (IND) application contains confidential business information. Therefore, submissions are proprietary and not available for public review or comment. As noted earlier, however, the website ClinicalTrials.gov has now been amended to increase public access to data on trials and their results, and a product sponsor may elect to make some or all of the IND information publicly available. Furthermore, if a gene therapy or genome-editing protocol is reviewed by an FDA scientific advisory committee, that meeting is open to the public, and a public representative must be included on the advisory committee roster. Once a biological license is approved, additional information is available for public posting. Nonetheless, overall the FDA review process lacks the transparency associated with an advisory body such as the RAC.

The FDA periodically calls informational public meetings, as it did for genetically engineered salmon (FDA, 2010), or hosts a more general public discussion, such as that on how the regulatory system for biotechnology products should be modernized (FDA, 2015c). The FDA's advisory committee meetings, as well as its more generalized meeting mechanisms, would be available for discussion of therapies that depend on genome editing, and they might be particularly useful for discussion of products aimed at or likely to be used off-label for "enhancement."

National Bioethics Commissions

Many nations have bodies to provide advice to their governments or to provide venues for public conversation, and such entities exist on every continent except Antarctica. They are usually appointed by the executive or legislative branches, and offer analyses and policy recommendations on a range of topics in bioethics. In November 1996, a group of national

---

BOX 7-1
U.S. National-Level Bioethics Commissions

Presidential Commission for the Study of Bioethical Issues, 2009-2016
President's Council on Bioethics, 2001-2009
National Bioethics Advisory Commission, 1996-2001
Advisory Committee on Human Radiation Experiments, 1994-1995
Biomedical Ethical Advisory Committee, 1988-1990
President's Commission for the Study of Ethical Problems in Medicine
    and in Biomedical and Behavioral Research, 1978-1983
National Commission for the Protection of Human Subjects of Biomedical
    and Behavioral Research, 1974-1978

---

bioethics commissions met for a summit at the invitation of the American National Bioethics Advisory Commission and the French Comité Consultatif National d'Ethique pour les Sciences de la Vie et de la Santé.[2] Since then, there have been a series of global summits of these bodies, the most recent in Germany and the next to take place in 2018 in Senegal.

Like many other countries, the United States has a long tradition of using bioethics commissions as a venue for both public participation and advice to the government on policy options (see Box 7-1). The tradition began in the 1970s with the creation of the National Commission for the Protection of Human Subjects of Biomedical and Behavioral Research, whose work led to substantial changes in the management of clinical trials. The U.S. federal government has assembled many subsequent commissions to address bioethical issues. Common features of these commissions include opportunities for public testimony, open meetings, the availability of transcripts of commission discussions, and the evident effect of this public participation and observation on both the decisions made at the meetings and the implementation of the resulting recommendations. Although agencies often are restricted by law with regard to what they can consider in their decisions, these venues provide an important outlet for broader considerations that, if necessary, can lead to legislative changes in agency mandates or regulatory approaches.

Institutional Oversight

All gene therapy and genome-editing studies must be approved at the local level by a research institution's institutional review board (IRB)

---

[2]See http://www.who.int/ethics/partnerships/globalsummit/en (accessed January 30, 2017).

and institutional biosafety committee (IBC), both of which are required to include public representatives in their membership. Under current U.S. regulations, an IRB must have at least one member "who is not otherwise affiliated with the institution," and among the types of expertise its membership must represent is sensitivity to "community attitudes."[3] Likewise, an IBC must include at least two members not affiliated with the institution that "represent community attitudes."

INTERNATIONAL PRACTICES

As noted above, in Europe, many of the efforts surrounding public engagement in science have been guided by the idea of *responsible innovation*, that is, a "transparent, interactive process by which societal actors and innovators become mutually responsive to each other with a view to the (ethical) acceptability, sustainability and societal desirability of the innovation process and its marketable products" (Schomberg, 2012, p. 50). This includes elements of *information* and *consultation*, as described above, but also a strong commitment to formal *public participation* in policy formation and decision making in many countries.

An overview of different non-U.S. efforts to engage with public stakeholders is provided in Table 7-1.

TABLE 7-1 Attributes of Public Engagement: Selected Examples

United Kingdom	Denmark	France
• Solicits entities outside of the government, especially specialists in communication and Web resources, to create its public consultation structure • Single-issue focus in its consultation • Wide variety of ways citizens provide input, including workshops, meetings, online questionnaires, and interactive website forums	• Longstanding experience in public consultation • Emergence of ethical issues raised by citizen groups that policy makers have not considered • Report content taken into consideration by policy decision makers via an independent agency that informs and advises the government	• Citizen panels bring attention to new social demands and needs for new legal approaches to novel technologies • Widespread media dissemination of panel discussions • Proliferation of other forums for discussion subsequent to the public consultation

For example, Denmark has a longstanding tradition of consensus conferences for which broad representation is sought, and whose results are

---

[3]21 CFR § 56.107.

taken seriously in the policy-making process. To some extent, however, the emphasis on consensus constrains their ability to present dissenting views (see Table 7-2). Although no country can fully satisfy all the objectives of public engagement in the realm of human germline genome editing, one widely shared objective is to strive to "enrich and expand the scope of traditional debate between experts, politicians, and interested parties by communicating citizens' views and attitudes on controversial technologies" (Scheufele, 2011, p. 11).

TABLE 7-2 Public Engagement in Denmark: Consensus Conferences

Modalities	Strengths	Weaknesses
• These represent one of the earliest and most referenced of consensus conferences (late 1980s). • A representative sample is recruited; around 2,000 randomly selected citizens are invited to apply. • The Danish Board of Technology (DBoT, an independent body created by the Danish Parliament) then selects 14-16 panel members to participate in the conference. • These citizens are introduced to and briefed on the topic(s) at hand by an expert journalist. • They then meet for extensive discussion among themselves. • Finally, they draft a report that expresses their stance on a given issue.	• The final report is taken seriously by the DBoT, which uses it to advise the Danish Parliament. Hence citizens' voices are fully integrated into the debating chambers of the government. • This solicitation of input from selected Danish citizens prior to any form of legislative debate allows policy makers to identify ethical issues they may not even have considered, as well as gives them time to adjust policy proposals in light of the citizen report. • This in turn increases citizens' levels of trust in government. • Many academics, and others as well, consider the Danish consensus conference to be a model unto itself.	• The members of a citizen panel selected through such a top-down system can never be truly representative of the population at large. • The careful monitoring of citizen panel members to minimize imbalances due to age, geographic location, gender, socioeconomic status, and cognitive and personality differences, as well as level of interest in the topic(s), tends to create an "idealized" group of people meant to represent the real world, when such is not the case. • Hence, this highly selective procedure means that those selected already have a pronounced interest in the topic at hand. Thus, inclusion of those who need more exposure to and education on the topic under consideration is neglected. • The final citizens' report must be a consensus; hence no dissension is either allowed or included in the document.

In designing public engagement activities, there are lessons to be learned from previous national efforts. These include the need to avoid having a small or overly selective sample of citizens and viewpoints and having a structure that is overly centralized and controlled in a top-down fashion (a structure that may be difficult to avoid in large, centralized national systems). One way to address these potential pitfalls is to follow the U.K. approach of "outsourcing" many public engagement activities to independent and nongovernmental entities (Sciencewise, 2016; Wilsdon, 2015). However, independent data with which to evaluate the efficacy of these efforts in other countries and their applicability to the U.S. context are limited. Moreover, when the process involves formulating future public policy for a country at large, it may be advantageous to have a central organizer of these types of consultations.

LESSONS LEARNED FROM PUBLIC ENGAGEMENT ACTIVITIES

Public engagement efforts are crucially important for guiding societal and political debates about the social, ethical, legal, and political aspects of applications of human genome editing. Given the infrastructures already in place to engage the public, as well as the general principles for engagement discussed in this chapter, the committee sees particular value in an approach that uses different processes for engagement for different types of questions surrounding genome editing. At the same time, it is essential that all such efforts adhere to all the principles for effective public engagement outlined earlier and that they apply two additional engagement principles to help avoid potential pitfalls.

First, any effort to engage the public broadly needs to distinguish between systematic public opinion research and public engagement exercises. The former uses social scientific methods to measure public opinion in ways that allow for generalization from representative samples to larger populations. Such efforts include quantifiable indicators of how likely it is that certain characteristics observed in a sample occur in the general population (e.g., Dillman et al., 2014). Public opinion research is particularly useful for identifying informational needs, perceptions of risk and benefit, or other attitudinal variables among different publics (Scheufele, 2010). By contrast, public engagement exercises such as consensus conferences or public meetings typically rely on representatives of highly interested and knowledgeable groups that can help policy makers or the scientific community identify ethical, legal, or societal considerations early in the policy-making process. The specific populations on which most engagement exercises draw and the social dynamics that drive conversational settings—even with professional moderators—often limit the ability to generalize findings from such exercises to broader public opinion (Merkle, 1996; Scheufele, 2011). Parallel

efforts with focus groups and broad public surveys of more randomly selected samples may be needed.

A second important principle relates to communicating the specific
types of science on which policy makers or other conveners of engagement
exercises seek input. Human beings interpret new information by using existing frames of reference (Goffman, 1974; Kahneman and Tversky, 1984).
Fairly minor differences in how scientific techniques are described in meeting materials or the examples that are chosen for particular applications
can significantly alter initial attitudes among participants, as well as the
overall nature of discussions (Anderson et al., 2013). Thus, it is important
that written meeting materials or presentations by experts during public
engagement exercises not be developed only by technical experts based on
their perceptions of relevance or appropriateness. Instead, they need to be
systematically pretested using empirical social science to ensure that they
minimize a priori biases and allow for inclusive, broad discussions that
are not constrained artificially to the technical or scientific aspects of the
subject.

MOVING FORWARD

Current infrastructure in the United States adequately includes public
input for current modes of gene therapy, including both commercially
and publicly funded basic research involving human genome editing. As
discussed earlier, science in the United States is subject to well-functioning
quality controls, oversight mechanisms, and ethical controls. Many of
these mechanisms, such as IRBs, already involve public input. Similarly,
the public has a means of providing systematic input on funding priorities,
regulations, and other aspects of basic research through electoral choices
at the federal, state and local levels.

Engagement mechanisms built into current regulatory infrastructures
in the United States are sufficient to address somatic applications of human genome-editing techniques, but this does not mean they cannot be
improved. The engagement processes employed by groups such as the RAC
are communication of relevant information and consultation with affected
or interested parties. In rarer cases, efforts have also been undertaken to
provide for true public *participation* in regulatory rulemaking. Ideally, all
oversight bodies involved in human genome editing would expand their
portfolio of engagement efforts to develop more systematic and sustain-
able modes of public participation. In particular, an expansion of current
modes of public engagement will be necessary to help regulatory bodies
define the definitions of and boundaries between such terms as "therapy"
and "enhancement" or "disease" and "disability." These efforts might be
aided by regulatory agencies' adding members with relevant expertise to

specific committees, such as FDA advisory committees that need to evaluate the benefits of an indication and the degree of unmet need for a new edited cell- or tissue-based product.

For any consideration of applications of genome editing of the human germline, extensive, inclusive, and meaningful public input consistent with the principles of engagement outlined in this chapter would be a necessary condition for moving forward. To this end, ongoing monitoring of public attitudes, information deficits, and emerging concerns would be essential. These public engagement efforts would allow agencies and other policy bodies to (1) communicate effectively by informing different publics and providing policy-relevant scientific information, and (2) identify areas requiring systematic efforts to create infrastructures for public engagement early in the process (NASEM, 2016a). The complex issues surrounding enhancement also would require an ongoing public debate to inform regulators and policy makers about the individual and societal values to be placed on the benefits and risks before clinical trials for such enhancement interventions could be authorized. These ongoing efforts to encourage public engagement would need to be tied directly to the policy-making process (NRC, 2008, p. 19).

To facilitate and monitor the effectiveness of such engagement efforts, federal agencies would need to consider funding programs for research to (1) promote understanding of the long- and short-term sociopolitical, ethical, and legal aspects of human genome editing; (2) evaluate the efficacy of various efforts to build public engagement (communication, consultation, and participation) into regulatory or policy-making infrastructures; and (3) assess how public engagement can and should influence different areas of policy making. Experiences with the genome initiative's program for including consideration of "ethical, legal, and social issues" as part of its overall funding of scientific research, and experiences with the Centers for Nanotechnology in Society, funded by the National Science Foundation, might provide useful frameworks for structuring similar research agendas or funding programs for public engagement for genome editing.[4]

CONCLUSIONS AND RECOMMENDATIONS

Efforts to advance human medicine through genome editing will be strengthened by public engagement informed by technical experts and by social scientists who undertake systematic public opinion research, develop appropriate communication materials, and minimize artificial biases or constraints that would hinder discussion and debate.

---

[4]See https://www.genome.gov/elsi (accessed January 30, 2017); https://www.nsf.gov/news/news_summ.jsp?cntn_id=117862 (accessed January 30, 2017).

Existing public communication and engagement infrastructures in the United States are sufficient to address oversight of basic science and laboratory research on human genome editing. Similarly, mechanisms for public communication and consultation that are part of the current U.S. regulatory infrastructures are also available to address public communication around the development of human somatic cell genome editing.

Weighing the technical and societal benefits and risks of applications of future uses of germline editing will require more formalized efforts to solicit broad public input and encourage public debate than are currently in place. Furthermore, the complex issues surrounding enhancement will require an ongoing public debate to inform regulators and policy makers about the individual and societal values to be placed on the benefits and risks before clinical trials for such enhancement interventions could be authorized.

The practices and principles developed for effective and inclusive public engagement in other emerging areas of science and technology provide a valuable base to inform public engagement on genome editing.

> RECOMMENDATION 7-1. Extensive and inclusive public participation should precede clinical trials for any extension of human genome editing beyond treatment or prevention of disease or disability.

> RECOMMENDATION 7-2. Ongoing reassessment of both health and societal benefits and risks, with broad ongoing participation and input by the public, should precede consideration of any clinical trials of heritable germline genome editing.

> RECOMMENDATION 7-3. Public participation should be incorporated into the policy-making process for human genome editing and should include ongoing monitoring of public attitudes, informational deficits, and emerging concerns about issues surrounding "enhancement."

> RECOMMENDATION 7-4. When funding human genome-editing research, federal agencies should consider including funding to support near-term research and strategies for
> - identifying areas that require systematic and early efforts to solicit public participation,
> - developing the necessary content and communicating it effectively, and
> - improving public engagement within the context of existing infrastructure.

RECOMMENDATION 7-5. When funding human genome-editing research, federal agencies should consider including funding for research aimed at
- understanding the sociopolitical, ethical, and legal aspects of editing the human germline;
- understanding the sociopolitical, ethical, and legal aspects of uses for genome editing that go beyond treatment or prevention of disease or disability; and
- evaluating the efficacy of efforts to build public communication and engagement on these issues into regulatory or policy-making infrastructures.

8

Summary of Principles
and Recommendations

enome editing offers great potential to advance both fundamental science and therapeutic applications. Basic laboratory research applying genome-editing methods to human
cells, tissues, germline cells, and embryos holds promise for
improving understanding of normal human biology, including furthering knowledge of human fertility, reproduction,
and development, as well as providing deeper understanding of disease
and establishing new approaches to treatment. Such research is proceeding
rapidly within existing oversight systems. Genome editing is already entering clinical testing for somatic treatment of certain genetic diseases, subject
to regulatory systems designed to oversee human somatic cell gene therapy
research. Furthermore, recently developed methods offer the future possibility of editing germline cells to prevent heritable transmission of genetic
disease, within the limits of domestic and transnational law. At the same
time, genome-editing technologies challenge regulators and the public to
evaluate existing governance systems to determine whether there are some
genetic alterations that are insufficiently justified, too risky, or too socially
disruptive to be pursued at this time. This chapter summarizes the conclusions of the committee relating the overarching principles and conclusions
to recommendations for the conduct and oversight of this burgeoning area
of research and application.

OVERARCHING PRINCIPLES FOR GOVERNANCE
OF HUMAN GENOME EDITING

Genome editing holds great promise for preventing, ameliorating, or eliminating many human diseases and conditions. Along with this promise comes the need for ethically responsible research and clinical use.

> **RECOMMENDATION 2-1. The following principles should undergird the oversight systems, the research on, and the clinical uses of human genome editing:**
> 1. **Promoting well-being**
> 2. **Transparency**
> 3. **Due care**
> 4. **Responsible science**
> 5. **Respect for persons**
> 6. **Fairness**
> 7. **Transnational cooperation**

In turn, these principles, detailed below, result in a number of responsibilities when devising a governance system for genome editing:

Promoting well-being: *The principle of promoting well-being supports providing benefit and preventing harm to those affected, often referred to in the bioethics literature as the principles of beneficence and nonmaleficence.*
Responsibilities that flow from adherence to this principle include (1) pursuing applications of human genome editing that promote the health and well-being of individuals, such as treating or preventing disease, while minimizing risk to individuals in early applications with a high degree of uncertainty; and (2) ensuring a reasonable balance of risk and benefit for any application of human genome editing.

Transparency: *The principle of transparency requires openness and sharing of information in ways that are accessible and understandable to stakeholders.*
Responsibilities that flow from adherence to this principle include (1) a commitment to disclosure of information to the fullest extent possible and in a timely manner, and (2) meaningful public input into the policymaking process related to human genome editing, as well as other novel and disruptive technologies.

Due care: *The principle of due care for patients enrolled in research studies or receiving clinical care requires proceeding carefully and deliberately, and only when supported by sufficient and robust evidence.*
Responsibilities that flow from adherence to this principle include proceeding cautiously and incrementally, under appropriate supervision and in

ways that allow for frequent reassessment in light of future advances and cultural opinions.

Responsible science: *The principle of responsible science underpins adherence to the highest standards of research, from bench to bedside, in accordance with international and professional norms.*

Responsibilities that flow from adherence to this principle include a commitment to (1) high-quality experimental design and analysis, (2) appropriate review and evaluation of protocols and resulting data, (3) transparency, and (4) correction of false or misleading data or analysis.

Respect for persons: *The principle of respect for persons requires recognition of the personal dignity of all individuals, acknowledgment of the centrality of personal choice, and respect for individual decisions. All people have equal moral value, regardless of their genetic qualities.*

Responsibilities that flow from adherence to this principle include (1) a commitment to the equal value of all individuals, (2) respect for and promotion of individual decision making, (3) a commitment to preventing recurrence of the abusive forms of eugenics practiced in the past, and (4) a commitment to destigmatizing disability.

Fairness: *The principle of fairness requires that like cases be treated alike, and that risks and benefits be equitably distributed (distributive justice).*

Responsibilities that flow from adherence to this principle include (1) equitable distribution of the burdens and benefits of research and (2) broad and equitable access to the benefits of resulting clinical applications of human genome editing.

Transnational cooperation: *The principle of transnational cooperation supports a commitment to collaborative approaches to research and governance while respecting different cultural contexts.*

Responsibilities that flow from adherence to this principle include (1) respect for differing national policies, (2) coordination of regulatory standards and procedures whenever possible, and (3) transnational collaboration and data sharing among different scientific communities and responsible regulatory authorities.

These principles and responsibilities can be fulfilled in the form of specific recommendations for regulation of genome editing, as presented below.

EXISTING U.S. OVERSIGHT MECHANISMS FOR HUMAN GENOME EDITING

In the United States, existing laws and funding policies at the state and federal levels will govern human genome editing at all stages, from laboratory research through preclinical testing and clinical trials to clinical application. The existing systems, while always having room for improvement, can be deployed to manage currently anticipated uses of human genome editing, but some future uses will require stringent criteria and further public debate.

Laboratory Research Using Genome-Editing Methods

The use of genome editing as a laboratory research tool in human somatic cells and tissues would largely be governed in the same way as other types of laboratory research, which are subject to institutional biosafety review and general standards of laboratory practice. Additional policies are also in place to govern the donation and use of human cells, tissues, or embryos for research. These take account of factors such as whether the tissue is left over from a clinical procedure or is obtained through intervention specifically for research. If tissue has information within or linked to it that makes the donor's identity readily ascertainable, then additional human subjects protections, such as the need for some form of consent and an institutional review board (IRB) review, generally will also apply.

Additional considerations apply to the use of genome editing for laboratory research using human embryos (with no aim of establishing a pregnancy). In the United States, federal funding for research using embryos generally is prohibited by the Dickey-Wicker Amendment, but some state and private sources for such research are available. Such uses would be subject to some of the legal regimes governing human reproduction and products of conception. Recommendations of the 1994 National Institutes of Health (NIH) Human Embryo Research Panel; the National Academies of Sciences, Engineering, and Medicine's Guidelines for Human Embryonic Stem Cell Research; and the guidelines of the International Society for Stem Cell Research guidelines continue to shape research practices in this area.

The ethical and regulatory considerations posed by genome-editing research using human embryos in the laboratory have been explored in the past: the moral status of the embryo, the acceptability of making embryos for research or using embryos that would otherwise be discarded, and legal or voluntary limits that apply to the use of embryos in research. These same ethical considerations are raised in other countries. Even with recognition of the scientific value of using human embryos in research, the practice is limited, discouraged, or even prohibited in many jurisdictions. Genome editing of human embryos purely for nonreproductive research purposes will be subject to those same ethical norms and policies. Where permitted, however, oversight procedures already in place for other forms of embryo research should provide assurance of the necessity and quality of the research.

Oversight of laboratory research using human cells and tissues is an expression of the principle of *Responsible Science*, which includes high-quality experimental design and protocol review. Science proceeds by rigorous peer review and publication of results, and also benefits from sharing of and access to data that can support continued development of the field. The principle of *Transparency* supports sharing information to the fullest extent possible consistent with applicable law. Respect for diversity among nations in domestic policy on research using human embryos should not be an obstacle to *Transnational Cooperation*, including data sharing, collaboration by regulatory authorities, and, where possible, harmonization of standards.

Conclusions and Recommendation: Fundamental Laboratory Research

Laboratory research involving human genome editing—that is, research that does not involve contact with patients—follows regulatory pathways that are the same as those for other basic laboratory in vitro research with human tissues, and raises issues already managed under existing ethical norms and regulatory regimes. This includes not only work with somatic cells but also the donation and use of human gametes and embryos for research purposes, where this research is permitted. While there are those who disagree with the policies embodied in some of those rules, the rules continue to be in effect. Important scientific and clinical issues relevant to human fertility and reproduction require continued laboratory research on human gametes and their progenitors, human embryos, and pluripotent stem cells. This research is necessary for medical and scientific purposes that are not directed at heritable genome editing, though it will also provide valuable information and techniques that could be applied if heritable genome editing were to be attempted in the future.

> **RECOMMENDATION 3-1. Existing regulatory infrastructure and processes for reviewing and evaluating basic laboratory genome-editing research with human cells and tissues should be used to evaluate future basic laboratory research on human genome editing.**

Somatic Cell Genome Editing for Treatment or Prevention of Disease and Disability

The most immediate clinical applications of genome editing will be in human somatic cells for the treatment or prevention of disease and disability. Indeed such research is already in clinical trials. In the United States, clinical applications that use somatic cell genome editing fall under the jurisdiction of the U.S. Food and Drug Administration (FDA), which regulates human tissue- and cell-based therapies. Initiation of any genome-editing clinical trial requires prior approval by the FDA, and IRBs will also oversee aspects of these trials such as recruitment, counseling, and adverse-event monitoring for trial participants. Regulatory assessments associated with clinical trials of somatic cell genome editing will be similar to those associated with other medical therapies, including minimization of risk, analysis of whether risks to participants are reasonable in light of potential benefits, and whether participants are recruited and enrolled with appropriate voluntary and informed consent. Additional oversight in the United States includes local safety reviews by institutional biosafety committees and national-level review opportunities under the auspices of the NIH Recombinant DNA Advisory Committee (RAC), for both specific, novel protocols and for general approaches.

The ethical norms and regulatory regimes already developed for other forms of gene therapy are adequate for managing new applications involving somatic genome editing with the purpose of treating or preventing disease and disability. But regulatory oversight should also emphasize prevention of unauthorized or premature applications of genome editing.

In some circumstances, it may also be desirable to consider undertaking genome editing in the somatic cells of a fetus in utero, for example, where fetal editing could be significantly more effective than postnatal intervention for genetic diseases with devastating effects early in development. The potential benefit to the resulting child would be key. But in utero genome editing would also require special attention to issues surrounding consent and to any increased risk of on-target or off-target modifications to fetal germ cells or germ cell progenitors.

Recommendations for regulating somatic cell genome editing are informed by several of the overarching principles. An important goal in both the research and clinical uses of somatic genome editing is *promoting well-being*. *Transparency* and *responsible science* are necessary for advancing the research with confidence in the quality of the work, while *due care* ensures that the applications proceed incrementally with careful attention to risks and benefits, as well as reassessments that allow timely response to changing scientific and clinical information. As therapeutic and preventive medical technologies are developed, *fairness* and *respect for persons* call for attention to equitable access to the benefits of these advances, protection of individual choice to pursue or decline use of these therapies, and respect for the dignity of all persons regardless of that choice.

Conclusions and Recommendations: Somatic Therapy

In general, there is substantial public support for the use of gene therapy (and by extension, gene therapy that uses genome editing) for the treatment and prevention of disease and disability. Human genome editing in somatic cells holds great promise for treating or preventing many diseases and for improving the safety, effectiveness, and efficiency of existing gene therapy techniques now in use or in clinical trials. While genome-editing techniques continue to be optimized, however, they are best suited only to treatment or prevention of disease and disability and not to other, less pressing purposes.

The ethical norms and regulatory regimes already developed for gene therapy can be applied for these applications. Regulatory assessments associated with clinical trials of somatic cell genome editing will be similar to those associated with other medical therapies, encompassing minimization of risk, analysis of whether risks to participants are reasonable in light of potential benefits, and determining whether participants are recruited and enrolled with appropriate voluntary and informed consent. Regulatory oversight also will need to include legal authority and enforcement capacity to prevent unauthorized or premature applications of genome editing, and regulatory authorities will need to continually update their knowledge of specific technical aspects of the technologies being applied. At a minimum, their assessments will need to consider not only the technical context of the genome-editing system but also the proposed clinical application so that anticipated risks and benefits can be weighed. Because off-target events will vary with the platform technology, cell type, target genome sequence, and other factors, no single standard for somatic genome-editing specificity (e.g., acceptable off-target event rate) can be set at this time.

RECOMMENDATION 4-1. Existing regulatory infrastructure and processes for reviewing and evaluating somatic gene therapy to treat or prevent disease and disability should be used to evaluate somatic gene therapy that uses genome editing.

RECOMMENDATION 4-2. At this time, regulatory authorities should authorize clinical trials or approve cell therapies only for indications related to the treatment or prevention of disease or disability.

RECOMMENDATION 4-3. Oversight authorities should evaluate the safety and efficacy of proposed human somatic cell genome-editing applications in the context of the risks and benefits of intended use, recognizing that off-target events may vary with the platform technology, cell type, target genomic location, and other factors.

RECOMMENDATION 4-4. Transparent and inclusive public policy debates should precede any consideration of whether to authorize clinical trials of somatic cell genome editing for indications that go beyond treatment or prevention of disease or disability.

Heritable Genome Editing

Heritable genome editing, which creates genetic changes heritable by future generations, has the potential to alleviate the suffering caused by genetically inherited diseases. However, it also raises concerns that extend beyond consideration of individual risks and benefits. Although heritable editing would not currently be approved given the uncertainty about safety and efficacy, the technology is advancing rapidly, such that it may, in the not-so-distant future, become a realistic possibility that needs serious consideration. There are circumstances in which genome editing in germline cells or embryos might be the only or most acceptable option for prospective parents who wish to have a genetically related child while minimizing the risk of transmitting a serious disease or disability.

There is a history of debate around the possibility of making heritable changes to the human genome. Because the effects of such changes could be multigenerational, both the potential benefits and the potential harms could be multiplied. Benefits from such editing would accrue to any future child born with reduced burden from genetically inherited disease, and to the prospective parents seeking to have a genetically related child without fear of passing along a disease. On the other hand, concerns have been raised about the wisdom and appropriateness of this form of human intervention. The intended genome edits themselves might have unintended consequences which, if inherited, would also affect descendants. As with other forms of advanced medical technologies, questions of equality of access arise. The prospect of heritable genome editing also triggers concerns similar to those raised earlier by preimplantation and prenatal genetic screening, that is to say that purely voluntary, individual decisions might collectively change social norms about the acceptance of disabilities.

Conclusions and Recommendations: Heritable Genome Editing

In some situations, heritable genome editing would provide the only or the most acceptable option for parents who desire to have genetically related children while minimizing the risk of serious disease or disability in a prospective child. Yet while relief from inherited diseases could accrue from its use, there is significant public discomfort with heritable genome editing, particularly for less serious conditions and for situations in which alternatives exist. These concerns range from a view that it is inappropriate for humans to intervene in their own evolution to anxiety about unintended consequences for the individuals affected and for society as a whole. More research is needed before any germline intervention could meet the risk/benefit standard for authorizing clinical trials. But as the technical hurdles facing genome editing of progenitors of eggs and sperm are overcome, editing to prevent transmission of genetically inherited diseases may become a realistic possibility.

The primary U.S. entity with authority for the regulation of heritable genome editing—the FDA—does incorporate value judgments about risks and benefits in its decision making. A robust public discussion about the values to be placed on the benefits and risks of heritable genome editing is needed now so that these values can be incorporated as appropriate into the risk/benefit assessments that will precede any decision about whether to authorize clinical trials. But the FDA does not have a statutory mandate to consider public views on the intrinsic morality of a technology when deciding whether to authorize clinical trials. That level of discussion takes place at the RAC, in legislatures, and at other venues for public engagement, discussed in Chapter 7.

Heritable germline genome-editing trials must be approached with caution, but caution does not mean they must be prohibited. If the technical challenges are overcome and potential benefits are reasonable in light of the risks, clinical trials could be initiated, limited to only the most compelling circumstances and subject to a comprehensive oversight framework that would protect the research subjects and their descendants; and have sufficient safeguards in place to protect against inappropriate expansion to uses that are less compelling or less well understood.

> RECOMMENDATION 5-1. Clinical trials using heritable genome editing should be permitted only within a robust and effective regulatory framework that encompasses
> - the absence of reasonable alternatives;
> - restriction to preventing a serious disease or condition;
> - restriction to editing genes that have been convincingly demonstrated to cause or to strongly predispose to that disease or condition;
> - restriction to converting such genes to versions that are prevalent in the population and are known to be associated with ordinary health with little or no evidence of adverse effects;
> - the availability of credible preclinical and/or clinical data on risks and potential health benefits of the procedures;

- ongoing, rigorous oversight during clinical trials of the effects of the procedure on the health and safety of the research-participants;
- comprehensive plans for long-term, multigenerational follow-up that still respect personal autonomy;
- maximum transparency consistent with patient privacy;
- continued reassessment of both health and societal benefits and risks, with broad ongoing participation and input by the public; and
- reliable oversight mechanisms to prevent extension to uses other than preventing a serious disease or condition.

Given how long modifying the germline has been at the center of debates about moral boundaries, as well as the pluralism of values in society, it would be surprising if everyone were to agree with this recommendation. Even for those who do agree, it would be surprising if they all shared identical reasoning for doing so. There are also those who think the final criterion of Recommendation 5-1 cannot be met, and that once germline modification had begun, the regulatory mechanisms instituted could not limit the technology to the uses identified in the recommendation. If, indeed, it is not possible to satisfy the criteria in the recommendation, the committee's view is that heritable genome editing would not be permissible. The committee calls for continued public engagement and input while the basic science evolves and regulatory safeguards are developed to satisfy the criteria set forth here.

Heritable genome editing also raises concerns about premature or unproven uses of the technology, and it is possible that the criteria outlined here for responsible oversight would be achievable in some but not all jurisdictions. This possibility raises the concern that "regulatory havens" could emerge that would tempt providers or consumers to travel to jurisdictions with more lenient or nonexistent regulations to undergo the restricted procedures. The phenomenon of medical tourism, which encompasses the search for faster and cheaper therapeutic options, as well as newer or less regulated interventions, will be impossible to control completely if the technical capabilities exist in more permissive jurisdictions. Thus, it is important to highlight the need for comprehensive regulation.

As of late 2015, the United States is unable to consider whether to begin heritable genome-editing trials, regardless of whether the criteria laid out above could be met. A provision (in effect until at least April 2017) was passed in a congressional budget bill,[1] in which Congress included the following language:

> None of the funds made available by this Act may be used to notify a sponsor or otherwise acknowledge receipt of a submission for an exemption for investigational use of a drug or biological product under section 505(i) of the Federal Food, Drug, and Cosmetic Act (21 U.S.C. 355(i)) or section 351(a)(3) of the Public Health Service Act (42 U.S.C. 262(a)(3)) in research in which a human embryo is intentionally created or modified to include a heritable genetic modification. Any such submission shall be deemed to have not been received by the Secretary, and the exemption may not go into effect.

The current effect of this provision is to make it impossible for U.S. authorities to review proposals for clinical trials of heritable genome editing, and therefore to drive development of this technology to other jurisdictions, some regulated and others not.

Genome Editing for Purposes Other Than Treating or Preventing Disease or Disability

Both the ongoing development of therapeutic uses of somatic genome editing, and possible future development of therapeutic uses of heritable genome editing, raise the issue of defining disease and disability, and the question of how and where to set appropriate boundaries for treatment and prevention of these conditions. Like other technologies, human genome-editing methods may be applied for a wide range of purposes, including to enhance human capacities beyond the normal range. It is difficult to define the concept of enhancement. The lines between what are considered therapy, prevention, and enhancement are not rigid or easily discernible in all cases, and even the definition of what is considered a disease can be open to debate. For this reason, distinguishing between treating or preventing disease and disability on the one hand, and a notion of enhancement on the other, is challenging. Possible uses of genome editing thus fall along a continuum of acceptability. Addressing serious genetic disorders by converting causative genetic variants to nondeleterious variants generally falls at the most acceptable end of this spectrum, while editing to produce enhancements unrelated to disease typically falls at the least acceptable end. The report draws a distinction between genome editing for the purpose of treating or preventing disease or disability and for other purposes, without

---

[1] Consolidated Appropriations Act of 2016, HR 2029, 114 Cong., 1st sess. (January 6, 2015) (https://www.congress.gov/114/bills/hr2029/BILLS-114hr2029enr.pdf [accessed January 4, 2017]).

concluding that there is, as yet, any general consensus as to how to define the blurry boundaries of enhancement more clearly.

Editing to create a genetic enhancement could, in principle, be undertaken in the context of somatic cell or heritable editing. As with other potential applications of genome editing, individual risks and benefits would be associated with the assessment of such editing. But the possibility of genetic enhancement raises a number of additional ethical and social concerns for which easy answers are not available, and differences of opinion are likely.

Conclusions and Recommendations: Genome Editing for Purposes Other Than Treatment or Prevention of Disease

Significant scientific progress will be necessary before any genome-editing intervention for indications other than the treatment or prevention of disease or disability can satisfy the risk/benefit standards for initiating a clinical trial. This conclusion holds for both somatic and heritable genome-editing interventions. There is significant public discomfort with the use of genome editing for so-called enhancement of human traits and capacities beyond those typical of adequate health. Therefore, a robust public discussion is needed concerning the values to be placed upon the individual and societal benefits and risks of genome editing for purposes other than treatment or prevention of disease or disability. These discussions would include consideration of the potential for introducing or exacerbating societal inequities, so that these values can be incorporated as appropriate into the risk/benefit assessments that will precede any decision about whether to authorize clinical trials.

RECOMMENDATION 6-1. Regulatory agencies should not at this time authorize clinical trials of somatic or germline genome editing for purposes other than treatment or prevention of disease or disability.

RECOMMENDATION 6-2. Government bodies should encourage public discussion and policy debate regarding governance of somatic human genome editing for purposes other than treatment or prevention of disease or disability.

The Role of Public Engagement in Governance of Human Genome Editing

Efforts to advance human medicine through genome editing will be strengthened by public engagement, and this engagement will be particularly critical for the potential uses that are not captured effectively by current regulatory frameworks. In the United States in particular, regulatory authority tends to focus primarily on health and safety of individuals and the public, and not on issues surrounding possible effects on social mores and culture. These latter concerns are regularly addressed in other fora, such as advisory committees, but lack legal force unless reflected in legislation that is grounded in the limited powers granted to government. Other countries have systems that more explicitly account for public attitudes in deciding whether and how to permit new technologies to be developed, with widely varying degrees of legal constraint on governmental authority.

Conclusions and Recommendations: Public Engagement

Efforts to advance human medicine through genome editing will be strengthened by public engagement informed by technical experts and by social scientists who undertake systematic public opinion research, develop appropriate communication materials, and minimize artificial biases or constraints that would hinder discussion and debate.

Existing public communication and engagement infrastructures in the United States are sufficient to address oversight of basic science and laboratory research on human genome editing. Similarly, mechanisms for public communication and consultation that are part of the current U.S. regulatory infrastructures are also available to address public communication around development of human somatic cell genome editing.

Weighing the technical and societal benefits and risks of applications of future uses of heritable genome editing will require more formalized efforts to solicit broad public input and encourage public debate than are currently in place. Furthermore, the complex issues surrounding enhancement will require an ongoing public debate to inform regulators and policy makers about the individual and societal values to be placed on the benefits and risks before clinical trials for such enhancement interventions could be authorized.

The practices and principles developed for effective and inclusive public engagement in other emerging areas of science and technology provide a valuable base to inform public engagement on genome editing.

RECOMMENDATION 7-1. Extensive and inclusive public participation should precede clinical trials for any extension of human genome editing beyond treatment or prevention of disease or disability.

RECOMMENDATION 7-2. Ongoing reassessment of both health and societal benefits and risks, with broad ongoing participation and input by the public, should precede consideration of any clinical trials of heritable germline genome editing.

RECOMMENDATION 7-3. Public participation should be incorporated into the policy-making process for human genome editing and should include ongoing monitoring of public attitudes, informational deficits, and emerging concerns about issues surrounding "enhancement."

RECOMMENDATION 7-4. When funding human genome-editing research, federal agencies should consider including funding to support near-term research and strategies for
- identifying areas that require systematic and early efforts to solicit public participation,
- developing the necessary content and communicating it effectively, and
- improving public engagement within the context of existing infrastructure.

RECOMMENDATION 7-5. When funding human genome-editing research, federal agencies should consider including funding for research aimed at
- understanding the sociopolitical, ethical, and legal aspects of editing the human germline;
- understanding the sociopolitical, ethical, and legal aspects of uses for genome editing that go beyond treatment or prevention of disease or disability; and
- evaluating the efficacy of efforts to build public communication and engagement on these issues into regulatory or policy-making infrastructures.

References

AAP (American Academy of Pediatrics). 2014. Off-label use of drugs in children. *Pediatrics* 133(3):563-567.

Abbott, K. W. A., D. J. Sylvester, and G. E. Marchant. 2010. Transnational regulation: Reality or romanticism? In *International handbook on regulating nanotechnologies*, edited by G. Hodge, D. Bowman, and A. Maynard. Cheltenham, UK: Edward Elgar Publishing. Pp. 525-544.

Abudayyeh, O. O., J. S. Gootenberg, S. Konermann, J. Joung, I. M. Slaymaker, D. B. Cox, S. Shmakov, K. S. Makarova, E. Semenova, L. Minakhin, K. Severinov, A. Regev, E. S. Lander, E. V. Koonin, and F. Zhang. 2016. C2c2 is a single-component programmable RNA-guided RNA-targeting CRISPR effector. *Science* 353(6299):aaf5573.

Achenbach, J. 2016. 107 Nobel laureates sign letter blasting Greenpeace over GMOs. *The Washington Post*, June 29. https://www.washingtonpost.com/news/speaking-of-science/wp/2016/06/29/more-than-100-nobel-laureates-take-on-greenpeace-over-gmo-stance/?utm_term=.feb89580ad48 (accessed October 18, 2016).

Akin, H., K. M. Rose, D. A. Scheufele, M. Simis-Wilkinson, D. Brossard, M. A. Xenos, and E. A. Corley. 2017. Mapping the landscape of public attitudes on synthetic biology. *Bioscience* 67(3):290-300.

Alghrani, A., and M. Brazier. 2011. What is it? Whose it? Re-positioning the fetus in the context of research. *The Cambridge Law Journal* 70(1):51-82.

Allen, D. B., and L. Cuttler. 2013. Short stature in childhood—challenges and choices. *New England Journal of Medicine* 368(13):1220-1228.

American Cancer Society. 2015. *Off-label drug use: What is off-label drug use?* http://www.cancer.org/treatment/treatmentsandsideeffects/treatmenttypes/chemotherapy/off-label-drug-use (accessed January 5, 2017).

AMS (Academy of Medical Sciences), British Academy, Royal Academy of Engineering, and The Royal Society. 2012. *Human enhancement and the future of work.* https://www.acmedsci.ac.uk/viewFile/publicationDownloads/135228646747.pdf (accessed January 5, 2017).

AMS, AMRC (Association of Medical Research Charities), BBSRC (Biotechnology and Biological Sciences Research Council), MRC (Medical Research Center), and Wellcome Trust. 2015. *Genome editing in human cells—initial joint statement.* https://wellcome. ac.uk/sites/default/files/wtp059707.pdf (accessed January 4, 2017).

Anderson, A. A., J. Kim, D. A. Scheufele, D. Brossard, and M. A. Xenos. 2013. What's in a name? How we define nanotech shapes public reactions. *Journal of Nanoparticle Research* 15(2):1-5.

Anderson, R. C., and R. W. Kulhavy. 1972. Learning concepts from definitions. *American Educational Research Journal* 9(3):385-390.

Andorno, R. 2005a. The Oviedo convention: A European legal framework at the intersection of human rights and health law. *Journal of International Biotechnology Law* 2(4):133-143.

Andorno, R. 2005b. Human dignity and the UNESCO Declaration on the Human Genome. In *Ethics, Law and Society*, Vol. 1, edited by J. Gunning and S. Holm. Burlington, VT: Ashgate Publishing Company. Pp. 73-84.

Anguela, X. M., R. Sharma, Y. Doyon, J. C. Miller, H. Li, V. Haurigot, M. E. Rohde, S. Y. Wong, R. J. Davidson, and S. Zhou. 2013. Robust ZFN-mediated genome editing in adult hemophilic mice. *Blood* 122(19):3283-3287.

ANM (Académie Nationale de Médecine). 2016. *Genome editing of human germline cells and embryos.* http://www.academie-medecine.fr/wp-content/uploads/2016/05/report-genome-editing-ANM-2.pdf (accessed January 4, 2017).

Arras, J. 2016. Theory and bioethics. In *The Stanford encyclopedia of philosophy*, edited by E. N. Zalta. http://plato.stanford.edu/archives/sum2016/entries/theory-bioethics (accessed January 4, 2017).

Au, P., D. A. Hursh, A. Lim, M. C. Moos, S. S. Oh, B. S. Schneider, and C. M. Witten. 2012. FDA oversight of cell therapy clinical trials. *Science Translational Medicine* 4(149): 149fs31.

Ayyar, V. S. 2011. History of growth hormone therapy. *Indian Journal of Endocrinology and Metabolism* 15(Suppl. 3):S162-S165.

BAC (Bioethics Advisory Committee) Singapore. 2013. *Ethical, legal and social issues in neuroscience research: A consultation paper.* http://www.bioethics-singapore.org/index/publications/consultation-papers.html (accessed November 4, 2016).

Baltimore, D., P. Berg, M. Botchan, D. Carroll, R. A. Charo, G. Church, J. E. Corn, G. Q. Daley, J. A. Doudna, M. Fenner, H. T. Greely, M. Jinek, G. S. Martin, E. Penhoet, J. Puck, S. H. Sternberg, J. S. Weissman, and K. R. Yamamoto. 2015. A prudent path forward for genomic engineering and germline gene modification. *Science* 348(6230):36-38.

Bamford, K. B., S. Wood, and R. J. Shaw. 2005. Standards for gene therapy clinical trials based on pro-active risk assessment in a London NHS Teaching Hospital Trust. *QJM: Monthly Journal of the Association of Physicians* 98(2):75-86.

Barrangou, R., and E. G. Dudley. 2016. CRISPR-based typing and next-generation tracking technologies. *Annual Review of Food Science and Technology* 7:395-411.

BBAW (Berlin-Brandenburg Academy of Sciences and Humanities). 2015. *Human genome surgery—towards a responsible evaluation of a new technology.* http://www.gentechnologiebericht.de/bilder/BBAW_Human-Genome-Surgery_PDF-A1b-1.pdf (accessed January 4, 2017).

Bell, J., K. L. Parker, R. D. Swinford, A. R. Hoffman, T. Maneatis, and B. Lippe. 2010. Long-term safety of recombinant human growth hormone in children. *Journal of Clinical Endocrinology & Metabolism* 95(1):167-177.

Berg, P., and J. E. Mertz. 2010. Personal reflections on the origins and emergence of recombinant DNA technology. *Genetics* 184(1):9-17.

Berg, P., D. Baltimore, S. Brenner, R. O. Roblin, and M. F. Singer. 1975. Asilomar conference on DNA recombinant molecules. *Science* 188(4192):991-994.

Bertero, A., M. Pawlowski, D. Ortmann, K. Snijders, L. Yiangou, M. C. de Brito, S. Brown, W. G. Bernard, J. D. Cooper, E. Giacomelli, L. Gambardella, N. R. F. Hannan, D. Iyer, F. Sampaziotis, F. Serrano, M. C. F. Zonneveld, S. Sinha, M. Kotter, and L. Vallier. 2016. Optimized inducible shRNA and CRISPR/Cas9 platforms for in vitro studies of human development using hPSCs. *Development* 143:4405-4418.

Beumer, K. J., and D. Carroll. 2014. Targeted genome engineering techniques in Drosophila. *Methods* 68(1):29-37.

Bioethics Commission. 2015. *Gray matters: Topics at the intersection of neuroscience, ethics, and society* (Vol. 2). Washington, DC: Presidential Commission for the Study of Bioethical Issues.

Blakeley, P., N. M. Fogarty, I. del Valle, S. E. Wamaitha, T. X. Hu, K. Elder, P. Snell, L. Christie, P. Robson, and K. K. Niakan. 2015. Defining the three cell lineages of the human blastocyst by single-cell RNA-seq. *Development* 142(18):3151-3165.

Blendon, R. `J., M. T. Gorski, and J. M. Benson, M.A. 2016. The public and the gene-editing revolution. *New England Journal of Medicine* 374(15):1406-1411.

Boggio, A. 2005. Italy enacts new law on medically assisted reproduction. *Human Reproduction* 20(5):1153-1157.

Booth, C., H. B. Gaspar, and A. J. Thrasher. 2016. Treating immunodeficiency through HSC gene therapy. *Trends in Molecular Medicine* 22(4):317-327.

Borg, J. J., G. Aislaitner, M. Pirozynski, and S. Mifsud. 2011. Strengthening and rationalizing pharmacovigilance in the EU: Where is Europe heading to? A review of the new EU legislation on pharmacovigilance. *Drug Safety* 34(3):187-197.

Bosley, K. S., M. Botchan, A. L. Bredenoord, D. Carroll, R. A. Charo, E. Charpentier, R. Cohen, J. Corn, J. Doudna, G. Feng, H. T. Greely, R. Isasi, W. Ji, J.-S. Kim, B. Knoppers, E. Lanphier, J. Li, R. Lovell-Badge, G. S. Martin, J. Moreno, L. Naldini, M. Pera, A. C. F. Perry, J. C. Venter, F. Zhang, and Q. Zhou. 2015. CRISPR germline engineering: The community speaks. *Nature Biotechnology* 33(5):478-486.

Bostrom, N. 2005. In defense of posthuman dignity. *Bioethics* 19(3):202-214.

Bostrom, N., and T. Ord. 2006. The reversal test: Eliminating status quo bias in applied ethics. *Ethics* 116(4):656-679.

Brossard, D., and B. Lewenstein. 2009. A critical appraisal of model of public understanding of science: Using practice to inform theory. In *Understanding science: New agendas in science communication*, edited by L. Kahlor and P. Stout. New York: Routledge. Pp. 11-39.

Brown, K. V. 2016. Inside the garage labs of DIY gene hackers, whose hobby may terrify you. *Fusion*, March 29. http://fusion.net/story/285454/diy-crispr-biohackers-garage-labs (accessed January 9, 2016).

Buchanan, A., D. W. Brock, N. Daniels, and D. Wikler. 2001. *From chance to choice: Genetics and justice*. New York: Cambridge University Press.

Burgess M., and D. Prentice. 2016. Let Congress know to take it slow on human gene editing. *Dallas News*, December 28.

Cahill, L. S. 2008. *Germline genetics, human nature, and social ethics*. Cambridge, MA: MIT Press.

Califf, R. M. 2017. Benefit-risk assessments at the U.S. Food and Drug Administration: Finding the balance. *Journal of the American Medical Association*. http://jamanetwork.com/journals/jama/fullarticle/2599251 (accessed February 3, 2017).

Califf, R. M., and R. Nalubola. 2017. FDA's science-based approach to genome edited products. *FDA Voice*, January 18. http://blogs.fda.gov/fdavoice/index.php/2017/01/fdas-science-based-approach-to-genome-edited-products (accessed February 2, 2017).

Campbell, A., and K. C. Glass. 2000. Legal status of clinical and ethics policies, codes, and guidelines in medical practice and research. *McGill Law Journal* 46(2):473-489.

Carroll, D. 2014. Genome engineering with targetable nucleases. *Annual Review of Biochemistry* 83:409-439.

Center for Genetics and Society. 2015. *Extreme genetic engineering and the human future: Reclaiming emerging biotechnologies for the common good.* http://www.geneticsandsociety.org/downloads/Human_Future_Exec_Sum.pdf (accessed January 6, 2017).

Chan, J. L., L. N. C. Johnson, M. D. Sammel, L. DiGiovanni, C. Voong, S. M. Domchek, and C. R. Gracia. 2016. Reproductive decision-making in women with BRCA1/2 mutations. *Journal of Genetic Counseling* 1-10.

Chan, S., P. J. Donovan, T. Douglas, C. Gyngell, J. Harris, R. Lovell-Badge, D. J. Mathews, and A. Regenberg. 2015. Genome editing technologies and human germline genetic modification: The Hinxton Group consensus statement. *The American Journal of Bioethics* 15(12):42-47.

Chapman, K. M., G. A. Medrano, P. Jaichander, J. Chaudhary, A. E. Waits, M. A. Nobrega, J. M. Hotaling, C. Ober, and F. K. Hamra. 2015. Targeted germline modifications in rats using CRISPR/Cas9 and spermatogonial stem cells. *Cell Reports* 10(11):1828-1835.

Charo, R. A. 2016a. On the road (to a cure?)—stem-cell tourism and lessons for gene editing. *New England Journal of Medicine* 374(10):901-903.

Charo, R. A. 2016b. The legal and regulatory context for human gene editing. *Issues in Science and Technology* 32(3):39.

Charpentier, E., and J. A. Doudna. 2013. Biotechnology: Rewriting a genome. *Nature* 494(7439):50-51.

Chen, E. A., and J. F. Schiffman. 2000. Attitudes toward genetic counseling and prenatal diagnosis among a group of individuals with physical disabilities. *Journal of Genetic Counseling* 9(2):137-152.

Cho, S. W., S. Kim, J. M. Kim, and J.-S. Kim. 2013. Targeted genome engineering in human cells with the Cas9 RNA-guided endonuclease. *Nature Biotechnology* 31(3):230-232.

Choulika, A., A. Perrin, B. Dujon, and J.-P. Nicolas. 1995. Induction of homologous recombination in mammalian chromosomes by using the I-SceI system of *Saccharomyces cerevisiae. Molecular and Cellular Biology* 15(4):1968-1973.

CIOMS (Council for International Organizations of Medical Sciences). 2012. *Bioethics.* http://www.cioms.ch/index.php/2012-06-07-19-16-08/about-us/bioethics (accessed January 4, 2017).

CIOMS. 2017. *International Ethical Guidelines for Health-Related Research Involving Humans.* http://apps.who.int/bookorders/anglais/detart1.jsp?codlan=1&codcol=84&codcch=35 (accessed May 9, 2017).

CIRM (California Institute for Regenerative Medicine). 2015. *Scientific and medical accountability standards.* https://www.cirm.ca.gov/our-funding/chapter-2-scientific-and-medical-accountability-standards (accessed January 4, 2017).

Cockburn, K., and J. Rossant. 2010. Making the blastocyst: Lessons from the mouse. *Journal of Clinical Investigation* 120(4):995-1003.

COE (Council of Europe). 2016. *Chart of signatures and ratifications of Treaty 164.* http://www.coe.int/en/web/conventions/full-list/-/conventions/treaty/164/signatures (accessed November 3, 2016).

Coghlan, A. 2016. Exclusive: "3-parent" baby method already used for infertility. *New Scientist*, October 10. https://www.newscientist.com/article/2108549-exclusive-3-parent-baby-method-already-used-for-infertility (accessed November 3, 2016).

Coghlan, A. 2017. First baby born using three-parent technque to treat infertility. *New Scientist*, January 18. https://www.newscientist.com/article/2118334-first-baby-born-using-3-parent-technique-to-treat-infertility (accessed January 19, 2017).

Cohen, I. G. 2015. *Patients and passports: Medical tourism, law, and ethics*, 1st ed. New York: Oxford University Press.

Cohen, P., G. M. Bright, A. D. Rogol, A. M. Kappelgaard, and R. G. Rosenfeld. 2002. Effects of dose and gender on the growth and growth factor response to GH in GH-deficient children: Implications for efficacy and safety. *Journal of Clinical Endocrinology & Metabolism* 87(1):90-98.

Cole-Turner, R. 1993. *The new genesis: Theology and the genetic revolution*. Louisville, KY: Westminster/John Knox Press.

Collins, F.S. 2015. *Statement of NIH Funding of Research Using Gene-Editing Technologies in Human Embryos*. https://www.nih.gov/about-nih/who-we-are/nih-director/statements/statement-nih-funding-research-using-gene-editing-technologies-human-embryos (accessed May 9, 2017).

Cong, L., F. A. Ran, D. Cox, S. Lin, R. Barretto, N. Habib, P. D. Hsu, X. Wu, W. Jiang, and L. A. Marraffini. 2013. Multiplex genome engineering using CRISPR/Cas systems. *Science* 339(6121):819-823.

Cook, D. M., and S. R. Rose. 2012. A review of guidelines for use of growth hormone in pediatric and transition patients. *Pituitary* 15(3):301-310.

Cornwall, A. 2008. *Democratising engagement: What the U.K. can learn from international experience*. London, U.K.: Demos.

Corrigan-Curay, J. 2013. *NIH Recombinant DNA Advisory Committee (RAC) and gene transfer research*. Presentation at the First Meeting on Independent Review and Assessment of the Activities of the NIH Recombinant DNA Advisory Committee, Washington, DC, June 4. https://www.nationalacademies.org/hmd/Activities/Research/ReviewNIHRAC/2013-JUN-04.aspx (accessed November 4, 2016).

Corrigan-Curay, J., M. O'Reilly, D. B. Kohn, P. M. Cannon, G. Bao, F. D. Bushman, D. Carroll, T. Cathomen, J. K. Joung, and D. Roth. 2015. Genome editing technologies: Defining a path to clinic. *Molecular Therapy* 23(5):796-806.

Council of Europe. 2015. *Statement on genome editing technologies*. http://www.coe.int/en/web/bioethics/-/gene-editing (accessed October 21, 2016).

Couzin-Frankel, J. 2016. Ailing fetuses to be treated with stem cells. *Science*, April 14. http://www.sciencemag.org/news/2016/04/ailing-fetuses-be-treated-stem-cells (accessed January 5, 2017).

Cox, D. B. T., R. J. Platt, and F. Zhang. 2015. Therapeutic genome editing: Prospects and challenges. *Nature Medicine* 21(2):121-131.

Cronin, R. 2008. Bureaucrats vs. physicians: Have doctors been stripped of their power to determine the proper use of human growth hormone in treating adult disease. *Washington University Journal of Law & Policy* 27:191. http://openscholarship.wustl.edu/cgi/viewcontent.cgi?article=1141&context=law_journal_law_policy (accessed January 6, 2017).

Cuttler, L., and J. Silvers. 2010. Growth hormone and health policy. *The Journal of Clinical Endocrinology & Metabolism* 95(7):3149-3153.

Cyranoski, D. 2016. Chinese scientists to pioneer first human CRISPR trial. *Nature* 535:476-477.

Daniels, N. 2000. Normal functioning and the treatment-enhancement distinction. *Cambridge Quarterly of Healthcare Ethics* 9(3):309-322.

Danish Board of Technology. 2006. *The consensus conference*. http://www.tekno.dk/subpage.php3?article=468&toppic=kategori12&language=uk (accessed December 10, 2016).

Danish Board of Technology. 2010a. *A clear message from world citizens to COP15 politicians*. http://www.tekno.dk/article/offentliggrelse-af-policy-rapport-om-wwviews-resultater-19-november/ (accessed December 11, 2016).

Danish Board of Technology. 2010b. *Profile of the Danish Board of Technology*. http://www.tekno.dk/about-dbt-foundation/?lang=en (accessed December 11, 2016).

Davis, B. D. 1970. Prospects for genetic intervention in man. *Science* 170(3964):1279-1283.

de la Noval, B. D. 2016. Potential implications on female fertility and reproductive lifespan in BRCA germline mutation women. *Archives of Gynecology and Obstetrics* 294(5): 1099-1103.

De Ravin, S. S., X. Wu, S. Moir, L. Kardava, S. Anaya-O'Brien, N. Kwatemaa, P. Littel, N. Theobald, U. Choi, and L. Su. 2016. Lentiviral hematopoietic stem cell gene therapy for x-linked severe combined immunodeficiency. *Science Translational Medicine* 8(335):335ra357.

DEA (Drug Enforcement Administration). 2013. *Human growth hormone (trade names: Genotropin®, Humatrope®, Norditropin®, Nutropin®, Saizen®, Serostim®).* http://www. deadiversion.usdoj.gov/drug_chem_info/hgh.pdf (accessed January 4, 2017).

Decruyenaere, M., G. Evers-Kiebooms, A. Boogaerts, K. Philippe, K. Demyttenaere, R. Dom, W. Vandenberghe, and J. P. Fryns. 2007. The complexity of reproductive decision-making in asymptomatic carriers of the Huntington mutation. *European Journal of Human Genetics: EJHG* 15(4):453-462.

Deglincerti, A., G. F. Croft, L. N. Pietila, M. Zernicka-Goetz, E. D. Siggia, and A. H. Brivanlou. 2016. Self-organization of the in vitro attached human embryo. *Nature* 533(7602):251-254.

Dever, D. P., R. O. Bak, A. Reinisch, J. Camarena, G. Washington, C. E. Nicolas, M. Pavel-Dinu, N. Saxena, A. B. Wilkens, S. Mantri, N. Uchida, A. Hendel, A. Narla, R. Majeti, K. I. Weinberg, and M. H. Porteus. 2016. CRISPR/Cas9 β-globin gene targeting in human haematopoietic stem cells. *Nature* 539:384-389.

Devereaux, M., and M. Kalichman. 2013. ESCRO committees—not dead yet. *The American Journal of Bioethics* 13(1):59-60.

DeWitt, M. A., W. Magis, N. L. Bray, T. Wang, J. R. Berman, F. Urbinati, S.-J. Heo, T. Mitros, D. P. Muñoz, and D. Boffelli. 2016. Selection-free genome editing of the sickle mutation in human adult hematopoietic stem/progenitor cells. *Science Translational Medicine* 8(360):360ra134.

Dillman, D. A., J. D. Smyth, and L. M. Christian. 2014. *Internet, phone, mail, and mixed-mode surveys: The tailored design method* (4th Edition). Hoboken, NJ: Wiley.

Ding, Y., H. Li, L.-L. Chen, and K. Xie. 2016. Recent advances in genome editing using CRISPR/Cas9. *Frontiers in Plant Science* 7:703.

Doudna, J. 2015. Perspective: Embryo editing needs scrutiny. *Nature* 528(7580):S6-S6.

Doudna, J. A., and E. Charpentier. 2014. The new frontier of genome engineering with CRISPR-Cas9. *Science* 346(6213).

DRZE (Deutsche Referenzzentrum für Ethik in den Biowissenschaften). 2016. *Selected national and international laws and regulations.* http://www.drze.de/in-focus/stem-cell-research/laws-and-regulations (accessed October 25, 2016).

Dudding, T., B. Wilcken, B. Burgess, J. Hambly, and G. Turner. 2000. Reproductive decisions after neonatal screening identifies cystic fibrosis. *ADC Fetal & Neonatal Edition* 82(2):F124-F127.

East-Seletsky, A., M. R. O'Connell, S. C. Knight, D. Burstein, J. H. Cate, R. Tjian, and J. A. Doudna. 2016. Two distinct RNase activities of CRISPR-C2c2 enable guide-RNA processing and RNA detection. *Nature* 538(7624):270-273.

Editing humanity. 2015. *The Economist*, August 22.

EGE (European Group on Ethics in Science and New Technologies). 2016. *Statement on gene editing.* https://ec.europa.eu/research/ege/pdf/gene_editing_ege_statement.pdf (accessed January 5, 2017).

EMA (European Medicines Agency). 2006. *Guideline on non-clinical testing for inadvertent germline transmission of gene transfer vectors.* http://www.ema.europa.eu/docs/en_GB/document_library/Scientific_guideline/2009/10/WC500003982.pdf (accessed February 2, 2017).

Enserink, M. 2016. Swedish academy seeks to stem "crisis of confidence" in wake of Macchiarini scandal. *Science Magazine*, February 11. http://www.sciencemag.org/news/2016/02/swedish-academy-seeks-stem-crisis-confidence-wake-macchiarini-scandal (accessed January 5, 2017).

European Commission. 2012. *Ethics in public policy making: The case of human enhancement.* http://cordis.europa.eu/result/rcn/153896_en.html (accessed November 4, 2016).

European Commission. 2016a. *Horizon 2020 Work Programme 2016-2017.* http://ec.europa.eu/research/participants/data/ref/h2020/wp/2016_2017/main/h2020-wp1617-swfs_en.pdf (accessed January 6, 2017).

European Commission. 2016b. *Public engagement in responsible research and innovation.* https://ec.europa.eu/programmes/horizon2020/en/h2020-section/public-engagement-responsible-research-and-innovation (accessed January 6, 2017).

European Commission. 2016c. *Voices.* http://www.ecsite.eu/activities-and-services/projects/voices (accessed January 6, 2017).

Evans, J. H. 2002. *Playing God?: Human genetic engineering and the rationalization of public bioethical debate.* Chicago, IL: University of Chicago Press.

Evans, J. H. 2010. *Contested reproduction: Genetic technologies, religion, and public debate.* Chicago, IL: University of Chicago Press.

Ezkurdia, I., D. Juan, J. M. Rodriguez, A. Frankish, M. Diekhans, J. Harrow, J. Vazquez, A. Valencia, and M. L. Tress. 2014. Multiple evidence strands suggest that there may be as few as 19,000 human protein-coding genes. *Human Molecular Genetics* 23(22):5866-5878.

FDA (U.S. Food and Drug Administration). 1991. Points to consider in human somatic cell therapy and gene therapy. *Human Gene Therapy* 2(3):251-256.

FDA. 1993. Application of current statutory authorities to human somatic cell therapy products and gene therapy products; notice. *Federal Register* 58(197):53248-53251. http://www.fda.gov/downloads/BiologicsBloodVaccines/SafetyAvailability/UCM148113.pdf (accessed January 5, 2017).

FDA. 2000. *Guidance for industry: Formal meetings with sponsors and applicants for PDUFA products.* Rockville, MD: FDA. http://www.fda.gov/OHRMS/DOCKETS/98fr/990296g2.pdf (accessed November 4, 2016).

FDA. 2001. *IND meetings for human drugs and biologics: Chemistry, manufacturing, and controls information.* Rockville, MD: FDA. http://www.fda.gov/downloads/Drugs/GuidanceComplianceRegulatoryInformation/Guidances/ucm070568.pdf (accessed September 1, 2013).

FDA. 2006. *Guidance for industry: Gene therapy clinical trials—observing subjects for delayed adverse events.* Rockville, MD: FDA. http://www.fda.gov/downloads/BiologicsBloodVaccines/GuidanceComplianceRegulatoryInformation/Guidances/CellularandGeneTherapy/ucm078719.pdf (accessed September 1, 2013).

FDA. 2009. *Cloning.* http://www.fda.gov/BiologicsBloodVaccines/CellularGeneTherapyProducts/Cloning/default.htm (accessed January 5, 2017).

FDA. 2010. *Background document: Public hearing on the labeling of food made from the AquAdvantage salmon.* http://www.fda.gov/downloads/Food/GuidanceRegulation/GuidanceDocumentsRegulatoryInformation/LabelingNutrition/UCM223913.pdf (accessed January 5, 2017).

FDA. 2012a. *Guidance for industry: Preclinical assessment of investigational cellular and gene therapy products.* http://www.fda.gov/BiologicsBloodVaccines/GuidanceCompliance RegulatoryInformation/Guidances/CellularandGeneTherapy/ucm376136.htm (accessed February 3, 2017).

FDA. 2012b. *Import alert #66-71: Detention without physical examination of human growth hormone (HGH), also known as Somatropin.* http://www.accessdata.fda.gov/cms_ia/ importalert_204.html (accessed January 6, 2017).

FDA. 2015a. *Fast track, breakthrough therapy, accelerated approval, priority review.* http:// www.fda.gov/forpatients/approvals/fast/ucm20041766.htm (accessed January 4, 2017).

FDA. 2015b. *Guidance for industry: Considerations for the design of early-phase clinical trials of cellular and gene therapy products.* Rockville, MD: FDA. http://www.fda.gov/ downloads/Biologi.../UCM359073.pdf (accessed February 1, 2017).

FDA. 2015c. *Modernizing the regulatory system for biotechnology products: First public meeting.* http://www.fda.gov/NewsEvents/MeetingsConferencesWorkshops/ucm463783. htm (accessed October 19, 2016).

FDA. 2016a. *Manufacturer communications regarding unapproved uses of approved or cleared medical products.* http://www.fda.gov/NewsEvents/MeetingsConferences Workshops/ucm489499.htm (accessed October 25, 2016).

FDA. 2016b. *Public hearing; request for comments—draft guidances relating to the regulation of human cells, tissues or cellular or tissue-based products.* http://www.fda.gov/ BiologicsBloodVaccines/NewsEvents/WorkshopsMeetingsConferences/ucm462125.htm (accessed October 26, 2016).

FEAM (Federation of European Academies of Medicine), UKAMS (United Kingdom Academy of Medical Sciences), and ANM (Académie Nationale de Médecine. 2017. *Human genome editing in the EU: Report of a workshop held on 28th April 2016.* http://www. feam-site.eu/cms/docs/humangenomeeditingworkshop2016report.pdf (accessed March 10, 2017).

Fletcher, J. 1971. Ethical aspects of genetic controls: Designed genetic changes in man. *New England Journal of Medicine* 285(14):776-783.

Fletcher, J. C. 1985. Ethical issues in and beyond prospective clinical trials of human gene therapy. *Journal of Medicine and Philosophy* 10(3):293-310.

Frankel, M. S., and A. R. Chapman. 2000. *Human inheritable genetic modifications: Assessing scientific, ethical, religious, and policy issues.* Washington, DC: American Association for the Advancement of Science. https://www.aaas.org/sites/default/files/migrate/uploads/ germline.pdf (accessed January 6, 2017).

Franklin, S. 2013. *Biological relatives: IVF, stem cells, and the future of kinship.* http://www. oapen.org/download?type=document&docid=469257 (accessed January 4, 2017).

Friedmann, T. 1989. Progress toward human gene therapy. *Science* 244(4910):1275-1281.

Friedmann, T., P. Noguchi, and C. Mickelson. 2001. The evolution of public review and oversight mechanisms in human gene transfer research: Joint roles of the FDA and NIH. *Current Opinion in Biotechnology* 12(3):304-307.

Friedmann, T., E. C. Jonlin, N. M. P. King, B. E. Torbett, N. A. Wivel, Y. Kaneda, and M. Sadelain. 2015. ASGCT and JSGT joint position statement on human genomic editing. *Molecular Therapy* 23(8):1282.

Frum, T., and A. Ralston. 2015. Cell signaling and transcription factors regulating cell fate during formation of the mouse blastocyst. *Trends in Genetics* 31(7):402-410.

Fu, Q., M. Hajdinjak, O. T. Moldovan, S. Constantin, S. Mallick, P. Skoglund, N. Patterson, N. Rohland, I. Lazaridis, and B. Nickel. 2015. An early modern human from Romania with a recent Neanderthal ancestor. *Nature* 524(7564):216-219.

Gaj, T., S. J. Sirk, S.-L. Shui, and J. Liu. 2016. Genome-editing technologies: Principles and applications. *Cold Spring Harbor Perspectives in Biology.*

Gardner, R. L., and J. Rossant. 1979. Investigation of the fate of 4-5 day post-coitum mouse inner cell mass cells by blastocyst injection. *Journal of Embryology & Experimental Morphology* 52:141-152.

Genovese, P., G. Schiroli, G. Escobar, T. Di Tomaso, C. Firrito, A. Calabria, D. Moi, R. Mazzieri, C. Bonini, and M. C. Holmes. 2014. Targeted genome editing in human repopulating haematopoietic stem cells. *Nature* 510(7504):235-240.

George, B. 2011. Regulations and guidelines governing stem cell based products: Clinical considerations. *Perspectives in Clinical Research* 2(3):94-99.

Giurgea, C. E. 1981. *Fundamentals to a pharmacology of the mind.* American lecture series, publication no. 1041. Springfield, IL: Thomas.

Goffman, E. 1974. *Frame analysis: An essay on the organization of experience.* New York: Harper & Row.

Green, R. 1994. The ethics of embryo research. *The Washington Post,* October 18.

Hadden, S. G. 1995. Regulatory negotiation as citizen participation: A critique. In *Fairness and competence in citizen participation,* edited by O. Renn, T. Webler, and P. Wiedemann. Dordrecht, Netherlands: Springer Science. Pp. 239-252.

Halevy, T., J. C. Biancotti, O. Yanuka, T. Golan-Lev, and N. Benvenisty. 2016. Molecular characterization of down syndrome embryonic stem cells reveals a role for RUNX1 in neural differentiation. *Stem Cell Reports* 7(4):777-786.

Hamzelou, J. 2016. Exclusive: World's first baby born with new "3 parent" technique. *New Scientist,* September 27. https://www.newscientist.com/article/2107219-exclusive-worlds-first-baby-born-with-new-3-parent-technique (accessed November 3, 2016).

Harris, J. 2007. *Enhancing evolution: The ethical case for making people better.* Princeton, NJ: Princeton University Press.

Hashimoto, M., Y. Yamashita, and T. Takemoto. 2016. Electroporation of Cas9 protein/sgRNA into early pronuclear zygotes generates non-mosaic mutants in the mouse. *Developmental Biology* 418(1):1-9.

Hayakawa, K., E. Himeno, S. Tanaka, and T. Kunath. 2014. Isolation and manipulation of mouse trophoblast stem cells. *Current Protocols in Stem Cell Biology* 1:1E.4.

Hayashi, K., S. Ogushi, K. Kurimoto, S. Shimamoto, H. Ohta, and M. Saitou. 2012. Offspring from oocytes derived from in vitro primordial germ cell-like cells in mice. *Science* 338(6109):971-975.

HDC (Halal Industry Development Corporation). 2016. *How does Islam view genetic engineering?* http://www.hdcglobal.com/publisher/pid/b368dc7b-039b-4335-9df3-8c015cbb33af/container/contentId/cc170e96-408d-485d-8ec3-f63644df412c (accessed November 3, 2016).

Health Canada. 2016. *News release—government of Canada plans to introduce regulations to support the Assisted Human Reproduction Act.* http://news.gc.ca/web/article-en.do?nid=1131339&tp=1 (accessed January 5, 2017).

Hennette-Vauchez, S. 2011. A human dignitas? Remnants of the ancient legal concept in contemporary dignity jurisprudence. *International Journal of Constitutional Law* 9(1):32-57.

Hermann, B. P., M. Sukhwani, F. Winkler, J. N. Pascarella, K. A. Peters, Y. Sheng, H. Valli, M. Rodriguez, M. Ezzelarab, G. Dargo, K. Peterson, K. Masterson, C. Ramsey, T. Ward, M. Lienesch, A. Volk, D. K. Cooper, A. W. Thomson, J. E. Kiss, M. C. Penedo, G. P. Schatten, S. Mitalipov, and K. E. Orwig. 2012. Spermatogonial stem cell transplantation into rhesus testes regenerates spermatogenesis producing functional sperm. *Cell Stem Cell* 11(5):715-726.

Hernandez, B., C. B. Keys, and F. E. Balcazar. 2004. Disability rights: Attitudes of private and public sector representatives. *Journal of Rehabilitation* 70(1):28-37.

HFEA (Human Fertilisation and Embryology Authority). 2014. *Third scientific review of the safety and efficacy of methods to avoid mitochondrial disease through assisted conception: Update.* http://www.hfea.gov.uk/docs/Third_Mitochondrial_replacement_scientific_review.pdf (accessed January 5, 2017).

HFEA. 2016a. *Guidance: Mitochondrial donation.* http://www.hfea.gov.uk/9931.html (accessed November 3, 2016).

HFEA. 2016b. *U.K.'s independent expert panel recommends "cautious adoption" of mitochondrial donation in treatment.* http://www.hfea.gov.uk/10559.html (January 4, 2017).

HHS (U.S. Department of Health and Human Services). 1979. *The Belmont Report.* https://www.hhs.gov/ohrp/regulations-and-policy/belmont-report (January 5, 2017).

Hikabe, O., N. Hamazaki, G. Nagamatsu, Y. Obata, Y. Hirao, N. Hamada, S. Shimamoto, T. Imamura, K. Nakashima, and M. Saitou. 2016. Reconstitution in vitro of the entire cycle of the mouse female germ line. *Nature* 539:299-303.

Hinxton Group. 2015. *Statement on genome editing technologies and human germline genetic modification.* http://www.hinxtongroup.org/hinxton2015_statement.pdf (accessed July 21, 2016).

Hirsch, F., Y. Levy, and H. Chneiweiss. 2017. CRISPR-Cas9: A European position on genome editing. *Nature* 541(7635):30.

Hoban, M. D., S. H. Orkin, and D. E. Bauer. 2016. Genetic treatment of a molecular disorder: Gene therapy approaches to sickle cell disease. *Blood* 127(7):839-848.

Hockemeyer, D., and Jaenisch, R. 2016. Induced pluripotent stem cells meet genome editing. *Cell Stem Cell* 18(5):573-586.

Holdren, J. P., C. R. Sunstein, and I. A. Siddiqui. 2011. *Memorandum: Principles for regulation and oversight of emerging technologies.* https://www.whitehouse.gov/sites/default/files/omb/inforeg/for-agencies/Principles-for-Regulation-and-Oversight-of-Emerging-Technologies-new.pdf (accessed January 6, 2017).

Howden, S. E., B. McColl, A. Glaser, J. Vadolas, S. Petrou, M. H. Little, A. G. Elefanty, and E. G. Stanley. 2016. A Cas9 variant for efficient generation of indel-free knockin or gene-corrected human pluripotent stem cells. *Stem Cell Reports* 7(3):508-517.

Hsu, P. D., E. S. Lander, and F. Zhang. 2014. Development and applications of CRISPR-Cas9 for genome engineering. *Cell* 157(6):1262-1278.

Huang, K., T. Maruyama, and G. Fan. 2014. The naive state of human pluripotent stem cells: A synthesis of stem cell and preimplantation embryo transcriptome analyses. *Cell Stem Cell* 15(4):410-415.

Hubbard, N., D. Hagin, K. Sommer, Y. Song, I. Khan, C. Clough, H. D. Ochs, D. J. Rawlings, A. M. Scharenberg, and T. R. Torgerson. 2016. Targeted gene editing restores regulated CD40L function in X-linked hyper-IgM syndrome. *Blood* 127(21):2513-2522.

Hughes, J. 2004. *Citizen cyborg: Why democratic societies must respond to the redesigned human of the future.* Cambridge, MA: Westview Press.

ICH (International Council for Harmonisation of Technical Requirements for Pharmaceuticals for Human Use). 2006. *General principles to address the risk of inadvertent germline integration of gene therapy vectors.* http://www.ich.org/fileadmin/Public_Web_Site/ICH_Products/Consideration_documents/GTDG_Considerations_Documents/ICH_Considerations_General_Principles_Risk_of_IGI_GT_Vectors.pdf (accessed February 2, 2017).

Ichord, R. N. 2014. Adult stroke risk after growth hormone treatment in childhood. First do no harm. *Neurology* 83(9):776-777.

IGSR (Institute for Governmental Service and Research). 2016. *About the IGSR and the 1000 Genomes Project.* http://www.internationalgenome.org/about (accessed November 4, 2016).

ILAR (Institute for Animal Laboratory Research) Roundtable. 2015. *Gene editing to modify animal genomes for research scientific and ethical considerations.* Presented at National Academies of Sciences, Engineering, and Medicine, Washington, DC, December 7-8. http://nas-sites.org/ilar-roundtable/roundtable-activities/gene-editing-to-modify-animal-genomes-for-research (accessed October 21, 2016).

Inhorn, M. C. 2012. *The new Arab man: Emergent masculinities, technologies, and Islam in the Middle East.* Princeton, NJ: Princeton University Press.

IOM (Institute of Medicine). 2005. *Guidelines for human embryonic stem cell research* (Vol. 23). Washington, DC: The National Academies Press.

IOM. 2014. *Oversight and review of clinical gene transfer protocols: Assessing the role of the Recombinant DNA Advisory Committee.* Washington, DC: The National Academies Press.

Irie, N., L. Weinberger, W. W. Tang, T. Kobayashi, S. Viukov, Y. S. Manor, S. Dietmann, J. H. Hanna, and M. A. Surani. 2015. SOX17 is a critical specifier of human primordial germ cell fate. *Cell* 160(1-2):253-268.

Ishikura, Y., Y. Yabuta, H. Ohta, K. Hayashi, T. Nakamura, I. Okamoto, T. Yamamoto, K. Kurimoto, K. Shirane, H. Sasaki, M. Saitou. 2016. In vitro derivation and propagation of spermatogonial stem cell activity from mouse pluripotent stem cells. *Cell Reports* 17(10):2789-2804.

ISSCR (International Society for Stem Cell Research). 2015. *Statement on human germline genome modification.* http://www.isscr.org/home/about-us/news-press-releases/2015/2015/03/19/statement-on-human-germline-genome-modification (accessed June 15, 2016).

ISSCR. 2016a. *Guidelines for stem cell research and clinical translation.* http://www.isscr.org/docs/default-source/guidelines/isscr-guidelines-for-stem-cell-research-and-clinical-translation.pdf?sfvrsn=2 (accessed January 5, 2017).

ISSCR. 2016b. *Updated guidelines for stem cell research and clinical translation.* http://www.isscr.org/home/about-us/news-press-releases/2016/2016/05/12/isscr-releases-updated-guidelines-for-stem-cell-research-and-clinical-translation (accessed November 4, 2016).

Jasanoff, S., J. B. Hurlbut, and K. Saha. 2015. CRISPR democracy: Gene editing and the need for inclusive deliberation. *Issues in Science and Technology* 32(1):25-32.

Jasin, M. 1996. Genetic manipulation of genomes with rare-cutting endonucleases. *Trends in Genetics* 12(6):224-228.

Jinek, M., K. Chylinski, I. Fonfara, M. Hauer, J. A. Doudna, and E. Charpentier. 2012. A programmable dual-RNA-guided DNA endonuclease in adaptive bacterial immunity. *Science* 337(6096):816-821.

Jinek, M., A. East, A. Cheng, S. Lin, E. Ma, and J. Doudna. 2013. RNA-programmed genome editing in human cells. *eLife* 2:e00471.

Juengst, E. T. 1991. Germ-line gene therapy: Back to basics. *Journal of Medicine and Philosophy* 16(6):587-592.

Juengst, E. T. 1997. Can enhancement be distinguished from prevention in genetic medicine? *Journal of Medicine and Philosophy* 22(2):125-142.

Juma, C. 2016. *Innovation and its enemies: Why people resist new technologies.* New York: Oxford University Press.

Kahneman, D., and A. Tversky. 1984. Choices, values, and frames. *American Psychologist* 39(4):341-350.

Kajaste-Rudnitski, A., and L. Naldini. 2015. Cellular innate immunity and restriction of viral infection: Implications for lentiviral gene therapy in human hematopoietic cells. *Human Gene Therapy* 26(4):201-209.

Kasowski, M., F. Grubert, C. Heffelfinger, M. Hariharan, A. Asabere, S. M. Waszak, L. Habegger, J. Rozowsky, M. Shi, and A. E. Urban. 2010. Variation in transcription factor binding among humans. *Science* 328(5975):232-235.

Kemp, S. F., J. Kuntze, K. M. Attie, T. Maneatis, S. Butler, J. Frane, and B. Lippe. 2005. Efficacy and safety results of long-term growth hormone treatment of idiopathic short stature. *Journal of Clinical Endocrinology & Metabolism* 90(9):5247-5253.

Kessler, D. P. 2011. Evaluating the medical malpractice system and options for reform. *The Journal of Economic Perspectives* 25(2):93-110.

Kessler, D. A., J. P. Siegel, P. D. Noguchi, K. C. Zoon, K. L. Feiden, and J. Woodcock. 1993. Regulation of somatic-cell therapy and gene therapy by the Food and Drug Administration. *New England Journal of Medicine* 329(16):1169-1173.

Kevles, D. J. 1985. *In the name of eugenics: Genetics and the uses of human heredity.* Cambridge, MA: Harvard University Press.

Kitcher, P. 1997. *The lives to come: The genetic revolution and human possibilities.* New York: Simon & Shuster.

Kleinstiver, B.P., V. Pattanayak, M.S. Prew, S.Q. Tsai, N.T. Nguyen, Z. Zheng, and J.K. Joung. 2016. High-fidelity CRISPR–Cas9 nucleases with no detectable genome-wide off-target effects. *Nature* 529(7587):490-495.

Klitzman, R. 2016. Buying and selling human eggs: Infertility providers' ethical and other concerns regarding egg donor agencies. *BMC Medical Ethics* 17(1):71.

KNAW (Koninklijke Nederlandse Academie van Wetenschappen). 2016. *Genome Editing: Position Paper of the Royal Netherlands Academy of Arts and Science.* https://www.knaw.nl/shared/resources/actueel/publicaties/pdf/genome-editing-position-paper-knaw-november-2016 (accessed May 9, 2017).

Kohn, D. B., M. H. Porteus, and A. M. Scharenberg. 2016. Ethical and regulatory aspects of genome editing. *Blood* 127(21):2553-2560.

Konermann, S., M. D. Brigham, A. E. Trevino, J. Joung, O. O. Abudayyeh, C. Barcena, P. D. Hsu, N. Habib, J. S. Gootenberg, H. Nishimasu, O. Nureki, and F. Zhang. 2015. Genome-scale transcriptional activation by an engineered CRISPR-Cas9 complex. *Nature* 517:583-588.

Krukenberg, R. C., D. L. Koller, D. D. Weaver, J. N. Dickerson, and K. A. Quaid. 2013. Two decades of Huntington disease testing: Patient's demographics and reproductive choices. *Journal of Genetic Counseling* 22(5):643-653.

Kuhlmann, I., A. M. Minihane, P. Huebbe, A. Nebel, and G. Rimbach. 2010. Apolipoprotein E genotype and hepatitis C, HIV and herpes simplex disease risk: A literature review. *Lipids in Health and Disease* 9:8.

Lanphier, E., F. Urnov, S. E. Haecker, M. Werner, and J. Smolenski. 2015. Don't edit the human germ line. *Nature* 519(7544):410-411.

Lazaraviciute, G., M. Kauser, S. Bhattacharya, P. Haggarty, and S. Bhattacharya. 2014. A systematic review and meta-analysis of DNA methylation levels and imprinting disorders in children conceived by IVF/ICSI compared with children conceived spontaneously. *Human Reproduction Update* 20(6):840-852.

Ledford, H. 2015. Biohackers gear up for genome editing. *Nature* 524(7566):398-399.

Leshner, A. I. 2003. Public engagement with science. *Science* 299(5609):977. http://www.sciencemag.org/content/299/5609/977.short (accessed January 6, 2017).

Lindgren, A. C., and E. M. Ritzen. 1999. Five years of growth hormone treatment in children with Prader-Willi syndrome. Swedish National Growth Hormone Advisory Group. *Acta Paediatrica Supplement* 88(433):109-111.

Liu, H., D. M. Bravata, I. Olkin, S. Nayak, B. Roberts, A. M. Garber, and A. R. Hoffman. 2007. Systematic review: The safety and efficacy of growth hormone in the healthy elderly. *Annals of Internal Medicine* 146(2):104-115.

Liu, H., D. M. Bravata, I. Olkin, A. Friedlander, V. Liu, B. Roberts, E. Bendavid, O. Saynina, S. R. Salpeter, and A. M. Garber. 2008. Systematic review: The effects of growth hormone on athletic performance. *Annals of Internal Medicine* 148(10):747-758.

Lomax, G. P., and A. O. Trounson. 2013. Correcting misperceptions about cryopreserved embryos and stem cell research. *Nature Biotechnology* 31(4):288-290.

Lombardo, P. A. 2008. *Three generations, no imbeciles: Eugenics, the Supreme Court, and Buck v. Bell*. Baltimore, MD: Johns Hopkins University Press.

Long, C., J. R. McAnally, J. M. Shelton, A. A. Mireault, R. Bassel-Duby, and E. N. Olson. 2014. Prevention of muscular dystrophy in mice by CRISPR/Cas9-mediated editing of germline DNA. *Science* 345(6201):1184-1188.

Long, C., L. Amoasii, A. A. Mireault, J. R. McAnally, H. Li, E. Sanchez-Ortiz, S. Bhattacharyya, J. M. Shelton, R. Bassel-Duby, and E. N. Olson. 2016. Postnatal genome editing partially restores dystrophin expression in a mouse model of muscular dystrophy. *Science* 351(6271):400-403.

Longmore, P. K. 1995. Medical decision making and people with disabilities: A clash of cultures. *Journal of Law, Medicine & Ethics* 23(1):82-87.

Lu, Y.-H., N. Wang, and F. Jin. 2013. Long-term follow-up of children conceived through assisted reproductive technology. *Journal of Zhejiang University. Science B* 14(5):359-371.

Lyon, J. 2017. Sanctioned U.K. trial of mitochondrial transfer nears. *Journal of the American Medical Association*. http://jamanetwork.com/journals/jama/fullarticle/2599746 (accessed February 3, 2017).

Macer, D. R., S. Akiyama, A. T. Alora, Y. Asada, J. Azariah, H. Azariah, M. V. Boost, P. Chatwachirawong, Y. Kato, V. Kaushik, F. J. Leavitt, N. Y. Macer, C. C. Ong, P. Srinives, and M. Tsuzuki. 1995. International perceptions and approval of gene therapy. *Human Gene Therapy* 6(6):791-803.

Machalek, A. Z. 2009. *Comparing genomes to find what makes us human*. https://publications. nigms.nih.gov/computinglife/compare_genome.htm (accessed November 3, 2016).

Maiorana, A., and S. Cianfarani. 2009. Impact of growth hormone therapy on adult height of children born small for gestational age. *Pediatrics* 124(3):e519-e531.

Mak, T. W. 2007. Gene targeting in embryonic stem cells scores a knockout in Stockholm. *Cell* 131(6):1027-1031.

Makas, E. 1988. Positive attitudes toward disabled people: Disabled and nondisabled persons' perspectives. *Journal of Social Issues* 44(1):49-61.

Malek, J., and Daar, J. 2012. The case for a parental duty to use preimplantation genetic diagnosis for medical benefit. *American Journal of Bioethics* 12(4):3-11.

Mali, P., L. Yang, K. M. Esvelt, J. Aach, M. Guell, J. E. DiCarlo, J. E. Norville, and G. M. Church. 2013. RNA-guided human genome engineering via Cas9. *Science* 339(6121): 823-826.

Malkki, H. 2016. Huntington disease: Selective deactivation of Huntington disease mutant allele by CRISPR-Cas9 gene editing. *Nature Reviews Neurology* 12(11):614-615.

Maresca, M., V. G. Lin, N. Guo, and Y. Yi Yang. 2013. Obligate Ligation-Gated Recombination (ObLiGaRe): Custom-designed nuclease-mediated targeted integration through nonhomologous end joining. *Genome Research* 23(3):539-546.

Margottini, L. 2014. Final chapter in Italian stem cell controversy? *Science*, October 7.

Maxmen, A. 2015. Easy DNA editing will remake the world. Buckle up. *Wired*, July.

McClain, L. E., and A. W. Flake. 2016. In utero stem cell transplantation and gene therapy: Recent progress and the potential for clinical application. *Best Practice & Research Clinical Obstetrics & Gynaecology* 31:88-98.

Meilaender, G. 1997. Begetting and cloning. *First Things (New York, NY)* 74:41-43.

Meilaender, G. 2008. *Human dignity: Exploring and explicating the council's vision*. https:// bioethicsarchive.georgetown.edu/pcbe/reports/human_dignity/chapter11.html (accessed January 6, 2017).

Mello, M. M. 2001. Of swords and shields: The role of clinical practice guidelines in medical malpractice litigation. *University of Pennsylvania Law Review* 149(3):645-710.

Merkle, D. M. 1996. The polls—review—the National Issues Convention deliberative poll. *Public Opinion Quarterly* 60(4):588-619.

Molitch, M. E., D. R. Clemmons, S. Malozowski, G. R. Merriam, and M. L. Vance. 2011. Evaluation and treatment of adult growth hormone deficiency: An Endocrine Society clinical practice guideline. *The Journal of Clinical Endocrinology & Metabolism* 96(6):1587-1609.

Mullin, E. 2016. Despite the hype over gene therapy, few drugs are close to approval. *MIT Technology Review*, September 29. https://www.technologyreview.com/s/602467/despite-the-hype-over-gene-therapy-few-drugs-are-close-to-approval (accessed January 22, 2017).

Murray, M., and K. Luker. 2015. *Cases on reproductive rights and justice*. St. Paul, MN: West Academic Publishing.

Naldini L. 2015. Gene therapy returns to centre stage. *Nature* 526(7573):351-360.

NASEM (National Academies of Sciences, Engineering, and Medicine). 2016a. *Communicating science effectively: A research agenda*. Washington, DC: The National Academies Press.

NASEM. 2016b. *Gene drives on the horizon: Advancing science, navigating uncertainty, and aligning research with public values*. Washington, DC: The National Academies Press.

NASEM. 2016c. *Genetically engineered crops: Experiences and prospects*. Washington, DC: The National Academies Press.

NASEM. 2016d. *International summit on human gene editing: A global discussion*. Washington, DC: The National Academies Press.

NASEM. 2016e. *Mitochondrial replacement techniques: Ethical, social, and policy considerations*. Washington, DC: The National Academies Press.

NASEM. 2017. *Future biotechnology products and opportunities to enhance capabilities of the biotechnology regulatory system*. http://nas-sites.org/biotech (accessed October 21, 2016).

National Academy of Sciences Leopoldina, Deutsche Akademie der Technikwissenshaften (National Academy of Science and Engineering: "acatech"), Deutsche Forschungsgemeinschaft (German Research Foundation: DFG), and Union der deutschen Akademien der Wissenschaften (Union of German Academies of Sciences and Humanities: Academien Union). 2015. *The opportunities and limits of genome editing*. http://www.leopoldina.org/nc/en/publications/detailview/?publication%5bpublication%5d=699&cHash=4d49c84a36e655feacc1be6ce7f98626 (accessed January 6, 2017).

Nature. 2017. Why researchers should resolve to engage in 2017. *Nature* 541(5). http://www.nature.com/news/why-researchers-should-resolve-to-engage-in-2017-1.21236?WT.mc_id=FBK_NatureNews (accessed January 12, 2017).

NCECHLS (National Consultative Ethics Committee for Health and Life Sciences). 2013. *Opinion no. 122: The use of biomedical techniques for "neuroenhancement" in healthy individuals: Ethical issues*. http://www.ccne-ethique.fr/sites/default/files/publications/ccne.avis_ndeg122eng.pdf (accessed January 5, 2017).

NCSL (National Conference of State Legislatures). 2016. *Embryonic and fetal research laws, January 1, 2016*. http://www.ncsl.org/research/health/embryonic-and-fetal-research-laws.aspx (accessed October 31, 2016).

Nelson, C. E., C. H. Hakim, D. G. Ousterout, P. I. Thakore, E. A. Moreb, R. M. C. Rivera, S. Madhavan, X. Pan, F. A. Ran, and W. X. Yan. 2016. In vivo genome editing improves muscle function in a mouse model of Duchenne muscular dystrophy. *Science* 351(6271):403-407.

Nelson, E. 2013. *Law, policy and reproductive autonomy*. Portland, OR: Hart Publishing.

NIH (National Institutes of Health). 1994. *Report of the Human Embryo Research Panel*. https://repository.library.georgetown.edu/bitstream/handle/10822/559352/human_embryo_vol_1.pdf?sequence=1&isAllowed=y (accessed January 5, 2017).

NIH. 2004. NIH and FDA launch new human gene transfer research data system. *Journal of Investigative Medicine* 52(5):286. http://jim.bmj.com/content/jim/52/5/286.1.full.pdf (accessed November 4, 2016).

NIH. 2011. *Charter: Recombinant DNA Advisory Committee.* Bethesda, MD: NIH. http://oba.od.nih.gov/oba/RAC/Signed_RAC_Charter_2011.pdf (accessed October 1, 2013).

NIH. 2013a. *Frequently asked questions about the NIH review process for human gene transfer trials.* Bethesda, MD: NIH. http://oba.od.nih.gov/oba/ibc/FAQs/NIH_Review_Process_HGT.pdf (accessed September 1, 2013).

NIH. 2013b. *Frequently asked questions of interest to IBCs.* Bethesda, MD: NIH. http://oba.od.nih.gov/oba/ibc/FAQs/IBC_Frequently_Asked_Questions7.24.09.pdf (accessed October 1, 2013).

NIH. 2013c. *NIH guidelines for research involving recombinant or synthetic nucleic acid molecules.* Bethesda, MD: NIH.

NIH. 2015a. *NIH research involving introduction of human pluripotent cells into non-human vertebrate animal pre-gastrulation embryos.* NOT-OD-15-158. https://grants.nih.gov/grants/guide/notice-files/NOT-OD-15-158.html (accessed January 5, 2017).

NIH. 2015b. *Statement on NIH funding of research using gene-editing technologies in human embryos.* https://www.nih.gov/about-nih/who-we-are/nih-director/statements/statement-nih-funding-research-using-gene-editing-technologies-human-embryos (accessed January 5, 2017).

NIH. 2016a. *NIH guidelines for research involving recombinant or synthetic nucleic acid molecules.* Washington, DC: HHS.

NIH. 2016b. *Request for public comment on the proposed changes to the NIH guidelines for human stem cell research and the proposed scope of an NIH steering committee's consideration of certain human-animal chimera research.* https://grants.nih.gov/grants/guide/notice-files/NOT-OD-16-128.html (accessed November 4, 2016).

NIH. 2016c. *State initiatives for stem cell research.* https://stemcells.nih.gov/research/state-research.htm (accessed October 25, 2016).

NRC (National Research Council). 1996. *Understanding risk: Informing decisions in a democratic society.* Edited by P. C. Stern and H. V. Fineberg. Washington, DC: National Academy Press.

NRC. 2002. *Scientific and medical aspects of human reproductive cloning.* Washington, DC: The National Academies Press.

NRC. 2008. *Public participation in environmental assessment and decision making.* Washington, DC: The National Academies Press.

NRC. 2010. *Final report of the National Academies' Human Embryonic Stem Cell Research Advisory Committee and 2010 amendments to the National Academies' guidelines for human embryonic stem cell research.* Washington, DC: The National Academies Press.

NRC and IOM. 2007. *2007 amendments to the National Academies' guidelines for human embryonic stem cell research.* Washington, DC: The National Academies Press.

NRC and IOM. 2008. *2008 amendments to the National Academies' guidelines for human embryonic stem cell research.* Washington, DC: The National Academies Press.

NRC and IOM. 2010. *Final report of the National Academies' Human Embryonic Stem Cell Research Advisory Committee and 2010 amendments to the National Academies' guidelines for human embryonic stem cell research.* Washington, DC: The National Academies Press.

NSF (National Science Foundation). 2010. Ethics of human enhancement: 25 questions & answers. *Studies in Ethics, Law, and Technology* 4(1):1-49.

Nuffield Council. 2015. *Naturalness.* http://nuffieldbioethics.org/project/naturalness (accessed November 3, 2016).

Nuffield Council. 2016a. *Genome editing: An ethical review.* http://nuffieldbioethics.org/project/genome-editing/ethical-review-published-september-2016 (accessed January 6, 2017).

Nuffield Council. 2016b. *Public dialogue on genome editing: Why? When? Who?* http://nuffield bioethics.org/wp-content/uploads/Public-Dialogue-on-Genome-Editing-workshop-report. pdf (accessed January 6, 2017).

OBA (Office of Biotechnology Activities). 2013. *Office of Biotechnology Activities welcome page.* http://oba.od.nih.gov (accessed September 1, 2013).

O'Connor, K. 2012. Ethics of fetal surgery. In *The Embryo Project Encyclopedia.* Tempe: The Embryo Project at Arizona State University.

Oktay, K., V. Turan, S. Titus, R. Stobezki, and L. Liu. 2015. BRCA mutations, DNA repair deficiency, and ovarian aging. *Biology of Reproduction* 93(3):67.

O'Reilly, M., A. Shipp, E. Rosenthal, R. Jambou, T. Shih, M. Montgomery, L. Gargiulo, A. Patterson, and J. Corrigan-Curay. 2012. NIH oversight of human gene transfer research involving retroviral, lentiviral, and adeno-associated virus vectors and the role of the NIH Recombinant DNA Advisory Committee. In *Gene Transfer Vectors for Clinical Application*, Vol. 507, edited by F. Theodore. Bethesda, MD: Academic Press. Pp. 313-335.

Orr-Weaver, T. L., J. W. Szostak, and R. J. Rothstein. 1981. Yeast transformation: A model system for the study of recombination. *Proceedings of the National Academy of Sciences of the United States of America* 78(10):6354-6358.

Parens, E. 1995. Should we hold the (germ) line? *The Journal of Law, Medicine & Ethics* 23(2):173-176.

Parens, E. 1998. *Enhancing human traits: Ethical and social implications.* Washington, DC: Georgetown University Press.

Parens, E., and A. Asch. 2000. *Prenatal testing and disability rights.* Washington, DC: Georgetown University Press.

Pera, M. F. 2014. In search of naivety. *Cell Stem Cell* 15(5):543-545.

Perls, T., and D. J. Handelsman. 2015. Disease mongering of age-associated declines in testosterone and growth hormone levels. *Journal of the American Geriatrics Society* 63(4):809-811.

Persson, I., and J. Savulescu. 2012. *Unfit for the future: The need for moral enhancement.* Oxford, U.K.: Oxford University Press.

Petropoulos, S., D. Edsgard, B. Reinius, Q. Deng, S. P. Panula, S. Codeluppi, A. Plaza Reyes, S. Linnarsson, R. Sandberg, and F. Lanner. 2016. Single-cell RNA-seq reveals lineage and X chromosome dynamics in human preimplantation embryos. *Cell* 165(4):1012-1026.

Pew Research Center. 2008. Stem cell research at the crossroads of religion and politics. *Pew Forum on Religion & Public Life*, July 17. http://www.pewforum.org/2008/07/17/stem-cell-research-at-the-crossroads-of-religion-and-politics (accessed July 17, 2008).

Pew Research Center. 2016. *U.S. public wary of biomedical technologies to enhance human abilities.* http://www.pewinternet.org/2016/07/26/u-s-public-wary-of-biomedical-technologies-to-enhance-human-abilities (accessed January 5, 2015).

Pfleiderer, G., G. Brahier, and K. Lindpaintner. 2010. *GenEthics and religion.* Basel, Switzerland: Karger Medical and Scientific Publishers.

Plotz, D. 2006. *The genius factory: The curious history of the Nobel Prize sperm bank.* New York: Random House, Inc.

Poirot, L., B. Philip, C. Schiffer-Mannioui, D. Le Clerre, I. Chion-Sotinel, S. Derniame, P. Potrel, C. Bas, L. Lemaire, and R. Galetto. 2015. Multiplex genome-edited t-cell manufacturing platform for "off-the-shelf" adoptive t-cell immunotherapies. *Cancer Research* 75(18):3853-3864.

Pollard, K. S. 2016. Decoding human accelerated regions. *The Scientist*, August 1. http://www.the-scientist.com/?articles.view/articleNo/46643/title/Decoding-Human-Accelerated-Regions (accessed November 3, 2016).

Poolman, E. M., and A. P. Galvani. 2007. Evaluating candidate agents of selective pressure for cystic fibrosis. *Journal of the Royal Society, Interface* 4(12):91-98.

Porteus, M. 2016. Genome editing: A new approach to human therapeutics. *Annual Review of Pharmacology and Toxicology* 56:163-190.

Posner, S. M., E. McKenzie, and T. H. Ricketts. 2016. Policy impacts of ecosystem services knowledge. *Proceedings of the National Academy of Sciences of the United States of America* 113(7):1760-1765.

Powledge, T. M., and L. Dach, eds. 1977. *Biomedical research and the public: Report to the Subcommittee on Health and Scientific Research, Committee on Human Resources, U.S. Senate.* Washington, DC: U.S. Government Printing Office.

Präg, P., and M. C. Mills. 2015. Assisted reproductive technology in Europe. Usage and regulation in the context of cross-border reproductive care. *Families and Societies* 43(1-23). http://www.familiesandsocieties.eu/wp-content/uploads/2015/09/WP43PragMills2015.pdf (accessed January 6, 2017).

President's Commission. 1982. *Splicing life: A report on the social and ethical issues of genetic engineering with human beings.* Washington, DC: President's Commission for the Study of Ethical Problems in Medicine and Biomedical and Behavioral Research. https://bioethics.georgetown.edu/documents/pcemr/splicinglife.pdf (accessed January 6, 2017).

President's Commission. 1983. *Deciding to forego life-sustaining treatment: A report on the ethical, medical and legal issues in treatment decisions.* Washington, DC: U.S. Government Printing Office.

President's Council on Bioethics. 2002. *Human Genetic Enhancement.* Staff background paper. https://bioethicsarchive.georgetown.edu/pcbe/background/humangenetic.html (accessed May 9, 2015).

President's Council on Bioethics. 2003. *Beyond therapy.* Washington, DC: President's Council on Bioethics.

Qasim, W., H. Zhan, S. Samarasinghe, S. Adams, P. Amrolia, S. Stafford, K. Butler, C. Rivat, G. Wright, and K. Somana. 2017. Molecular remission of infant B-ALL after infusion of universal TALEN gene-edited CAR T cells. *Science Translational Medicine* 9(374):eaaj2013.

Qi, L. S., M. H. Larson, L. A. Gilbert, J. A. Doudna, J. S. Weissman, A. P. Arkin, and W. A. Lim. 2013. Repurposing CRISPR as an RNA-guided platform for sequence-specific control of gene expression. *Cell* 152(5):1173-1183.

Qiao, J., and H. L. Feng. 2014. Assisted reproductive technology in China: Compliance and non-compliance. *Translational Pediatrics* 3(2):91.

Quinn, G. P., S. T. Vadaparampil, S. Tollin, C. A. Miree, D. Murphy, B. Bower, and C. Silva. 2010. BRCA carriers' thoughts on risk management in relation to preimplantation genetic diagnosis and childbearing: When too many choices are just as difficult as none. *Fertility and Sterility* 94(6):2473-2475.

Rainsbury, J. 2000. Biotechnology on the RAC-FDA/NIH regulation of human gene therapy. *Food and Drug Law Journal* 55:575-600.

Ramsey, P. 1970. *Fabricated man: The ethics of genetic control*, Vol. 6. New Haven, CT: Yale University Press.

Rawls, J. 1999. *A Theory of Justice*, 2nd ed. Cambridge, MA: Belknap Press.

Reardon, S. 2016. First CRISPR clinical trial gets green light from U.S. panel. *Nature News*, June 22. http://www.nature.com/news/first-crispr-clinical-trial-gets-green-light-from-us-panel-1.20137 (accessed June 22, 2016).

Reeves, R. 2016. Second gene therapy wins approval in Europe. *BioNews*, Issue 854. http://www.bionews.org.uk/page_656625.asp (accessed February 2, 2017).

Rine, J., and A. P. Fagen. 2015. The state of federal research funding in genetics as reflected by members of the Genetics Society of America. *Genetics* 200(4):1015-1019.

Robertson, J. A. 2004. Procreative liberty and harm to offspring in assisted reproduction. *American Journal of Law & Medicine* 30(1):7-40.

Robertson, J. A. 2008. Assisting reproduction, choosing genes, and the scope of reproductive freedom. *George Washington Law Review* 76(6):1490-1513.

Robillard, J. M., D. Roskams-Edris, B. Kuzeljevic, and J. Illes. 2014. Prevailing public perceptions of the ethics of gene therapy. *Human Gene Therapy* 25(8):740-746.

Rosen, L. 2014. What Mars One needs is genetically altered human colonists. *h+ Magazine*, April 14. http://hplusmagazine.com/2014/04/14/what-mars-one-needs-is-genetically-altered-human-colonists (accessed January 4, 2017).

Rossant, J. 2015. Mouse and human blastocyst-derived stem cells: Vive les differences. *Development* 142(1):9-12.

Rossetti, M., M. Cavarelli, S. Gregori, and G. Scarlatti. 2012. HIV-derived vectors for gene therapy targeting dendritic cells. In *HIV interactions with dendritic cells*. New York: Springer. Pp. 239-261.

Roux, P., F. Smih, and M. Jasin. 1994a. Expression of a site-specific endonuclease stimulates homologous recombination in mammalian cells. *Proceedings of the National Academy of Sciences of the United States of America* 91(13):6064-6068.

Roux, P., F. Smih, and M. Jasin. 1994b. Introduction of double-strand breaks into the genome of mouse cells by expression of a rare-cutting endonuclease. *Molecular and Cellular Biology* 14(12):8096-8106.

Rowe, G., and L. J. Frewer. 2005. A typology of public engagement mechanisms. *Science Technology & Human Values* 30(2):251-290.

Rulli, T. 2014. Preferring a genetically-related child. *Journal of Moral Philosophy* 13(6):669-698.

Saitou, M., and H. Miyauchi. 2016. Gametogenesis from pluripotent stem cells. *Cell Stem Cell* 18(6):721-735.

Sandel, M. 2004. The case against perfection. *The Atlantic Monthly* 293(3):51-62.

Sandel, M. 2013. The case against perfection. In *Society, ethics, and technology*, 5th ed., edited by M. Winston and R. Edelbach. Boston, MA: Wadsworth, Cengage Learning. Pp. 343-354.

Sander, J. D., and J. K. Joung. 2014. CRISPR-Cas systems for editing, regulating and targeting genomes. *Nature Biotechnology* 32(4):347-350.

Sarewitz, D. 2015. Science can't solve it. *Nature* 522(7557):413-414.

Sasaki, K., S. Yokobayashi, T. Nakamura, I. Okamoto, Y. Yabuta, K. Kurimoto, H. Ohta, Y. Moritoki, C. Iwatani, H. Tsuchiya, S. Nakamura, K. Sekiguchi, T. Sakuma, T. Mori, K. Woltjen, M. Nakagawa, T. Yamamoto, K. Takahashi, S. Yamanaka, and M. Saitou. 2015. Robust in vitro induction of human germ cell fate from pluripotent stem cells. *Cell Stem Cell* 17(2):178-194.

Saxton, M. 2000. Why members of the disability community oppose prenatal diagnosis and selective abortion. In *Prenatal testing and disability rights*, edited by E. Parenz and A. Ash. Washington, DC: Georgetown University Press. Pp. 147-165.

Sayres, L. C., and D. Magnus. 2012. Duty-free: The non-obligatory nature of preimplantation genetic diagnosis. *American Journal of Bioethics* 12(4):1-2.

Scharschmidt, T., and B. Lo. 2006. Clinical trial design issues raised during Recombinant DNA Advisory Committee review of gene transfer protocols. *Human Gene Therapy* 17(4):448-454.

Scheufele, D. A. 2010. Survey research. In *Encyclopedia of science and technology communication*, Vol. 2, edited by S. H. Priest. Thousand Oaks, CA: SAGE Publications. Pp. 853-856.

Scheufele, D. A. 2011. *Modern citizenship or policy dead end? Evaluating the need for public participation in science policy making, and why public meetings may not be the answer.* Joan Shorenstein Center on the Press, Politics and Public Policy Research Paper Series (#R-43). http://shorensteincenter.org/wp-content/uploads/2012/03/r34_scheufele.pdf (accessed January 6, 2017).

Scheufele, D. A. 2013. Communicating science in social settings. *Proceedings of the National Academy of Sciences of the United States of America* 110(Suppl. 3):14040-14047.

Schomberg, R. 2012. Prospects for technology assessment in a framework of responsible research and innovation. In *Technikfolgen abschätzen lehren: Bildungspotenziale transdisziplinärer methoden*, edited by M. Dusseldorp and R. Beecroft. Wiesbaden: VS Verlag für Sozialwissenschaften. Pp. 39-61.

Sciencewise. 2016. *Sciencewise—the U.K.'s national centre for public dialogue in policy making involving science and technology issues.* http://www.sciencewise-erc.org.uk/cms (accessed October 19, 2016).

Scully, J. L. 2009. Towards a bioethics of disability and impairment. In *The handbook of genetics and society: Mapping the new genomic era*, edited by P. Atkinson, P. Glasner, and M. Lock. London, U.K.: Routledge. Pp. 367-381.

Seifter, M. 2014a. States, agencies, and legitimacy. *Vanderbilt Law Review* 67(2):443-504.

Seifter, M. 2014b. States as interest groups in the administrative process. *Virginia Law Review* 100:953-1025.

Seifter, M. 2015. Second-order participation in administrative law. *UCLA Law Review* 1301-1363. http://www.uclalawreview.org/second-order-participation-in-administrative-law (accessed January 4, 2017).

Shahbazi, M. N., A. Jedrusik, S. Vuoristo, G. Recher, A. Hupalowska, V. Bolton, N. M. Fogarty, A. Campbell, L. G. Devito, and D. Ilic. 2016. Self-organization of the human embryo in the absence of maternal tissues. *Nature Cell Biology* 18(6):700-708.

Shalala, D. 2000. Protecting research aubjects—what must be done. *New England Journal of Medicine* 343(11):808-810.

Sharma, R., X. M. Anguela, Y. Doyon, T. Wechsler, R. C. DeKelver, S. Sproul, D. E. Paschon, J. C. Miller, R. J. Davidson, and D. Shivak. 2015. In vivo genome editing of the albumin locus as a platform for protein replacement therapy. *Blood* 126(15):1777-1784.

Shelton, A. M., and R. T. Roush. 1999. False reports and the ears of men. *Nature Biotechnology* 17(9):832.

Shetty, G., R. K. Uthamanthil, W. Zhou, S. H. Shao, C. C. Weng, R. C. Tailor, B. P. Hermann, K. E. Orwig, and M. L. Meistrich. 2013. Hormone suppression with GnRH antagonist promotes spermatogenic recovery from transplanted spermatogonial stem cells in irradiated cynomolgus monkeys. *Andrology* 1(6):886-898.

Sinsheimer, R. L. 1969. The prospect for designed genetic change. *American Scientist* 57(1):134-142.

Skerrett, P. 2015. A debate: Should we edit the human germline? *STAT*, November 30. https://www.statnews.com/2015/11/30/gene-editing-crispr-germline (accessed January 5, 2017).

Slaymaker, I. M., L. Gao, B. Zetsche, D. A. Scott, X. Winston, W. X. Yan, and F. Zhang. 2016. Rationally engineered Cas9 nucleases with improved specificity. *Science* 351(6268):84-88.

Specter, M. 2015. The gene hackers. *The New Yorker*, November 16.

Steinbach, R. J., M. Allyse, M. Michie, E. Y. Liu, and M. K. Cho. 2016. "This lifetime commitment": Public conceptions of disability and noninvasive prenatal genetic screening. *American Journal of Medical Genetics* 170(2):363-374.

Steinberg, A. 2006. Introduction, Ch. 3. In *Halakhic-Medical Encyclopedia* (Hebrew), 2nd ed., Vol. 1. Pp. 158-163.

Steinbrook, R. 2002. Improving protection for research subjects. *New England Journal of Medicine* 346(18):1425-1430.

Steinbrook, R. 2004. Science, politics, and federal advisory committees. *New England Journal of Medicine* 350(14):1454-1460.

Suh, Y., G. Atzmon, M.-O. Cho, D. Hwang, B. Liu, D. J. Leahy, N. Barzilai, and P. Cohen. 2008. Functionally significant insulin-like growth factor I receptor mutations in centenarians. *Proceedings of the National Academy of Sciences of the United States of America* 105(9):3438-3442.

Sulmasy, D. P. 2008. *Dignity and bioethics: History, theory, and selected applications.* Essays commissioned by the President's Council on Bioethics. https://bioethicsarchive. georgetown.edu/pcbe/reports/human_dignity/chapter18.html (accessed January 6, 2017).

Suzuki, K., Y. Tsunekawa, R. Hernandez-Benitez, J. Wu, J. Zhu, E. J. Kim, F. Hatanaka, M. Yamamoto, T. Araoka, Z. Li, M. Kurita, T Hishida, M. Li, E. Aizawa, S. Guo, S. Chen, A. Goebl, R. D. Soligalla, J. Qu, T. Jiang, X. Fu, M. Jafari, C. R. Esteban, W. T. Berggren, J. Lajara, E. Nuñez-Delicado, P. Guillen, J. M. Campistol, F. Matsuzaki, G. H. Liu, P. Magistretti, K. Zhang, E. M. Callaway, K. Zhang, and J. C. Belmonte. 2016. In vivo genome editing via CRISPR/Cas9 mediated homology-independent targeted integration. *Nature* 540:144-149.

Tabebordbar, M., K. Zhu, J. K. Cheng, W. L. Chew, J. J. Widrick, W. X. Yan, C. Maesner, E. Y. Wu, R. Xiao, and F. A. Ran. 2016. In vivo gene editing in dystrophic mouse muscle and muscle stem cells. *Science* 351(6271):407-411.

Takahashi, K., and S. Yamanaka. 2006. Induction of pluripotent stem cells from mouse embryonic and adult fibroblast cultures by defined factors. *Cell* 126(4):663-676.

Takahashi, K., K. Tanabe, M. Ohnuki, M. Narita, T. Ichisaka, K. Tomoda, and S. Yamanaka. 2007. Induction of pluripotent stem cells from adult human fibroblasts by defined factors. *Cell* 131(5):861-872.

Takefman, D. 2013. *The FDA review process.* Presentation at the first meeting on independent review and assessment of the activities of the NIH Recombinant DNA Advisory Committee, Washington, DC, June 4. https://www.nationalacademies.org/hmd/Activities/ Research/ReviewNIHRAC/2013-JUN-04.aspx (accessed November 4, 2016).

Takefman, D., and W. Bryan. 2012. The state of gene therapies: The FDA perspective. *Molecular Therapy* 20(5):877-878.

Taylor, T. H., S. A. Gitlin, J. L. Patrick, J. L. Crain, J. M. Wilson, and D. K. Griffin. 2014. The origin, mechanisms, incidence and clinical consequences of chromosomal mosaicism in humans. *Human Reproduction Update* 20(4):571-581.

Tebas, P., D. Stein, W. W. Tang, I. Frank, S. Q. Wang, G. Lee, S. K. Spratt, R. T. Surosky, M. A. Giedlin, and G. Nichol. 2014. Gene editing of CCR5 in autologous CD4 T cells of persons infected with HIV. *New England Journal of Medicine* 370(10):901-910.

The 1000 Genomes Project Consortium. 2015. A global reference for human genetic variation. *Nature* 526(7571):68-74.

The Washington Post. 1994. Embryos: Drawing the line. *The Washington Post,* October 2.

Turner, L., and P. Knoepfler. 2016. Selling stem cells in the USA: Assessing the direct-to-consumer industry. *Cell Stem Cell* 19(2):154-157.

U.K. House of Lords. 2000. *Select committee on science and technology—third report.* http:// www.publications.parliament.uk/pa/ld199900/ldselect/ldsctech/38/3801.htm (accessed December 14).

UN (United Nations). 1948. *Universal Declaration of Human Rights.* http://www.un.org/en/ universal-declaration-human-rights/index.html (accessed January 5, 2017).

UN. 2006. *Convention on the Rights of Persons with Disabilities (CRPD)*. https://www.un.org/development/desa/disabilities/convention-on-the-rights-of-persons-with-disabilities.html (accessed January 5, 2017).

UNESCO (UN Educational, Scientific and Cultural Organization). 2004a. International declaration on human genetic data. *European Journal of Health Law* 11:93-107.

UNESCO. 2004b. *National legislation concerning human reproductive and therapeutic cloning.* http://unesdoc.unesco.org/images/0013/001342/134277e.pdf (accessed January 5, 2017).

UNESCO. 2005. *Universal declaration on bioethics and human rights.* Paris, France: UNESCO. http://www.unesco.org/new/en/social-and-human-sciences/themes/bioethics/bioethics-and-human-rights (accessed January 4, 2017).

UNESCO. 2015. *Report of the International Bioethics Committee on updating its reflection on the human genome and human rights.* http://www.coe.int/en/web/bioethics/-/gene-editing (accessed October 21, 2016).

UNICEF (UN Children's Fund). 1990. *Convention on the Rights of the Child.* https://www.unicef.org/crc (accessed January 5, 2017).

Urnov, F. D., E. J. Rebar, M. C. Holmes, H. S. Zhang, and P. D. Gregory. 2010. Genome editing with engineered zinc finger nucleases. *Nature Reviews Genetics* 11(9):636-646.

van Delden, J. J. M., and R. van der Graaf. 2016. Revised CIOMS international ethical guidelines for health-related research involving humans. *The JAMA Network*, December 6. http://jamanetwork.com/journals/jama/fullarticle/2592245 (accessed January 4, 2017).

Vatican. 2015. *Encyclical letter Laudato si' of the Holy Father Francis on care for our common home.* http://w2.vatican.va/content/francesco/en/encyclicals/documents/papa-francesco_20150524_enciclica-laudato-si.html (accessed January 4, 2017).

Vernot, B., S. Tucci, J. Kelso, J. G. Schraiber, A. B. Wolf, R. M. Gittelman, M. Dannemann, S. Grote, R. C. McCoy, and H. Norton. 2016. Excavating Neanderthal and Denisovan DNA from the genomes of Melanesian individuals. *Science* 352(6282):235-239.

Volokh, E. 2003. The mechanisms of the slippery slope. *Harvard Law Review* 116(4):1026-1137.

Waddington, S. N., M. G. Kramer, R. Hernandez-Alcoceba, S. M. Buckley, M. Themis, C. Coutelle, and J. Prieto. 2005. In utero gene therapy: Current challenges and perspectives. *Molecular Therapy* 11(5):661-676.

Wailoo, K., A. Nelson, and C. Lee. 2012. *Genetics and the unsettled past: The collision of DNA, race, and history.* New Brunswick, NJ: Rutgers University Press.

Walters, L. 1991. Human gene therapy: Ethics and public policy. *Human Gene Therapy* 2(2):115-122.

Walters, L., and J. G. Palmer. 1997. *The ethics of human gene therapy.* New York: Oxford University Press.

Wasserman, D., and A. Asch. 2006. The uncertain rationale for prenatal disability screening. *The Virtual Mentor: VM* 8(1):53-56.

Wasserman, D., and A. Asch. 2012. A duty to discriminate? *American Journal of Bioethics* 12(4):22-24.

Watson, J. D., and F. H. Crick. 1953. Molecular structure of nucleic acids. *Nature* 171(4356):737-738.

Werner, M., and A. Plant. 2016. Collaboration between National Institute of Standards and Technology and the Standards Coordinating Body for Regenerative Medicines. Presentation of the Alliance for Regenerative Medicine, National Academy of Sciences, Engineering, and Medicine Regenerative Medicine Forum, Washington, DC, October 14.

Willemsen, R. H., M. van Dijk, Y. B. de Rijke, A. W. van Toorenenbergen, P. G. Mulder, and A. C. Hokken-Koelega. 2007. Effect of growth hormone therapy on serum adiponectin and resistin levels in short, small-for-gestational-age children and associations with cardiovascular risk parameters. *Journal of Clinical Endocrinology & Metabolism* 92(1):117-123.

Wilsdon, J. 2015. Let's keep talking: Why public dialogue on science and technology matters more than ever. *The Guardian*, March 20. https://www.theguardian.com/science/political-science/2015/mar/27/lets-keep-talking-why-public-dialogue-on-science-and-technology-matters-more-than-ever (accessed October 19, 2016).

WMA (World Medical Association). 2013. World Medical Association Declaration of Helsinki: Ethical principles for medical research involving human subjects. *Journal of the American Medical Association* 310(20):2191-2194.

Wolf, S. M., R. Gupta, and P. Kohlhepp. 2009. Gene therapy oversight: Lessons for nanobiotechnology. *Journal of Law, Medicine and Ethics* 37(4):659-684.

Wozniak, M. A., R. F. Itzhaki, E. B. Faragher, M. W. James, S. D. Ryder, and W. L. Irving. 2002. Apolipoprotein E-epsilon 4 protects against severe liver disease caused by hepatitis C virus. *Hepatology* 36(2):456-463.

Wright, A. V., J. K. Nunez, and J. A. Doudna. 2016. Biology and applications of CRISPR systems: Harnessing nature's toolbox for genome engineering. *Cell* 164(1-2):29-44.

Wu, Y., D. Liang, Y. Wang, M. Bai, W. Tang, S. Bao, Z. Yan, D. Li, and J. Li. 2013. Correction of a genetic disease in mouse via use of CRISPR-Cas9. *Cell Stem Cell* 13(6):659-662.

Wu, Y., H. Zhou, X. Fan, Y. Zhang, M. Zhang, Y. Wang, Z. Xie, M. Bai, Q. Yin, D. Liang, W. Tang, J. Liao, C. Zhou, W. Liu, P. Zhu, H. Guo, H. Pan, C. Wu, H. Shi, L. Wu, F. Tang, and J. Li. 2015. Correction of a genetic disease by CRISPR-Cas9-mediated gene editing in mouse spermatogonial stem cells. *Cell Research* 25(1):67-79.

Yin, H., W. Xue, S. Chen, R. L. Bogorad, E. Benedetti, M. Grompe, V. Koteliansky, P. A. Sharp, T. Jacks, and D. G. Anderson. 2014. Genome editing with Cas9 in adult mice corrects a disease mutation and phenotype. *Nature Biotechnology* 32(6):551-553.

Zetsche, B., J. S. Gootenberg, O. O. Abudayyeh, I. M. Slaymaker, K. S. Makarova, P. Essletzbichler, S. E. Volz, J. Joung, J. van der Oost, A. Regev, E. V. Koonin, and F. Zhang. 2015. Cpf1 is a single RNA-guided endonuclease of a class 2 CRISPR-Cas system. *Cell* 163(3):759-771.

Zhang, J., H. Liu, S. Luo, A. Chavez-Badiola, Z. Liu, S. Munne, M. Konstantinidis, D. Wells, and T. Huang. 2016. First live birth using human oocytes reconstituted by spindle nuclear transfer for mitochondrial DNA mutation causing leigh syndrome. *Fertility and Sterility* 106(3):e375-e376.

Zheng, W., H. Zhao, E. Mancera, L. M. Steinmetz, and M. Snyder. 2010. Genetic analysis of variation in transcription factor binding in yeast. *Nature* 464(7292):1187-1191.

Zhou, Q., M. Wang, Y. Yuan, X. Wang, R. Fu, H. Wan, M. Xie, M. Liu, X. Guo, Y. Zheng, G. Feng, Q. Shi, X. Y. Zhao, J. Sha, and Q. Zhou. 2016. Complete meiosis from embryonic stem cell-derived germ cells in vitro. *Cell Stem Cell* 18(3):330-340.

Zhu, Y.-Y., and R. Rees. 2012. *Vaccines, blood, & biologics: Clinical review, October 2, 2012—Ducord.* http://www.fda.gov/BiologicsBloodVaccines/CellularGeneTherapyProducts/ApprovedProducts/ucm326333.htm (accessed September 24, 2013).

A

The Basic Science of Genome Editing

This appendix provides technical and historical context for a number of issues related to the basic science of gene therapy and gene editing. Although an effort has been made to maximize the accessibility of this material, a simpler summary of this material can be found in Chapters 3 and 4. This appendix includes detailed material on the following topics:

- breakage and repair of DNA
- precursors of the clustered regularly interspersed short palindromic repeats (CRISPR) system/CRISPR-associated endonuclease (Cas9) gene editing—meganucleases, zinc fingers, and transcription activator-like effector nucleases (TALENs)
- development of CRISPR/Cas9
- the accuracy of gene editing
- enhancing the specificity of CRISPR/Cas9
- quality control and quality assurance for gene editing
- use of dead Cas9 (dCas9) to regulate transcription or to make epigenetic modifications
- gene targeting in transgenic animals
- gene editing in embryos
- alternative routes to heritable germline editing
- editing the mitochondrial genome

GENE THERAPY AND GENOME EDITING

The potential for gene therapy to address human disease has been evident for some years, and much progress has been made in its applications (Cox et al., 2015; Naldini, 2015). Gene therapy refers to the replacement of faulty genes, or the addition of new genes as a means to cure disease or improve the ability to fight disease. Genome editing is one aspect of gene therapy. Established approaches to gene therapy have been based on the results of extensive prior laboratory research on individual cells and on nonhuman organisms, establishing the means to add, delete, or modify genes in living organisms. Key advances include the development of techniques for generating molecular tools for cutting the DNA of genomes in specific places to allow targeted alterations in the DNA sequence. Over recent years, several such methods have been introduced and used effectively in clinical applications.

Within the past 5 years, a completely novel system has been developed based on fundamental research on bacterial systems of immunity to viral infections. The first such system to be developed for use in genome editing of human cells, known as CRISPR/Cas9, is based on RNA-guided targeting and is much simpler, faster, and cheaper than earlier methods. The ease of design, together with the remarkable specificity and efficiency of the CRISPR/Cas9 system has revolutionized the field of genome editing and reignited interest in the potential for editing of the human genome. The development of the CRISPR/Cas9 system as a programmable genome-editing tool was built on a firm foundation of earlier research.

BREAKAGE AND REPAIR OF GENOMIC DNA

Genomes and their constituent genes are made of double-stranded DNA; this DNA can be broken accidentally (e.g., by radiation) or purposefully, using proteins called endonucleases (often called nucleases) that can generate double-strand breaks (DSBs) in DNA.

Cells have mechanisms to repair DSBs in DNA, and these mechanisms can be used to generate alterations in the DNA sequence. Groundbreaking work in bacteria, yeast, and mammalian systems shows that DSBs dramatically stimulate the rate of DNA repair by nonhomologous end joining (NHEJ), in which the broken ends are reattached (see Figure A-1). Such NHEJ repair often results in the deletion or insertion of DNA sequences of varying length, which can disrupt gene function (Rouet et al., 1994).

However, if a homologous stretch of DNA is introduced into the cell as a donor template, homology-directed repair (HDR) can lead to more accurate repair or, if specific alterations are included in the homologous stretch, it can introduce specific precise changes into the recipient genomic

FIGURE A-1 Genome-editing outcomes are mediated by repair of nuclease-induced double-strand DNA breaks by NHEJ or HDR.
NOTE: DSB = double-strand break; HDR = homology-directed repair; NHEJ = nonhomologous end joining.
SOURCE: Modified from Sander and Joung, 2014.

DNA (see Figure A-1). These cellular DNA repair mechanisms have been used to develop several methods that allow genes or the genome to be edited in a very precise manner.

PRECURSORS OF CRISPR/CAS9 GENE EDITING

Three distinct strategies based on nuclease systems for generating targeted cleavages in DNA preceded the development of CRISPR/Cas9— meganucleases, zinc finger nucleases (ZFNs), and TALENs (see Figure A-2). All three have already enabled major advances in establishing the feasibility of using such targeted nucleases both to eliminate disease-causing genes as well as to repair damaged or mutated genes, ushering in a new era in biology and medicine.

Zinc Finger Nucleases

Zinc fingers are segments of protein that have evolved to recognize and bind to specific DNA sequences. Knowledge gained from natural zinc fingers led to the development of ZFNs as designer DNA-cutting enzymes (see Figure A-2), and their use in genome engineering represents pioneering, even heroic, protein engineering. Two major advances in protein engineering enabled the development of ZFNs: (1) the engineering of zinc finger proteins with designed DNA-binding specificity pioneered by Berg (Desjarlais and Berg, 1992), Pabo (Rebar and Pabo, 1994), and Wells (Jamieson et al., 1994); and (2) the generation of fusions between such designer zinc fingers

Nuclease Type	Recognition rules
Meganuclease	Complex
ZFN	1 module per 3 bp
TALENs	1 module per 1 bp
CRISPR/Cas	1 base per 1 bp

FIGURE A-2 Schematic of targetable nucleases discussed in this appendix. The meganuclease is a schematic of the crystal structure of E-DreI (Engineered I-DmoI/CreI). For the zinc-finger nucleases (ZFNs) and transcription activator-like effector nucleases (TALENs) illustrations, DNA is represented horizontally in black, purple ovals represent the FokI nuclease domains, and other modules of the nucleases are multi-colored to indicate that they recognize different bases in the DNA. For the CRISPR/Cas system, the Cas9 protein is represented by an orange oval, DNA is in blue, and guide RNA (chimera of spacer and tracr RNAs—see text) is shown in green. Arrowheads point to the sites of DNA cleavage.
SOURCES: Carroll, 2014. (Modified with permission from the Annual Review of Biochemistry, Volume 83 © 2014 by Annual Reviews, http://www.annualreviews.org); Chevalier et al., 2002.

and a DNA-cleaving protein, FokI nuclease (Kim et al., 1996), yielding "artificial restriction enzymes" that could be used to promote site-specific genome engineering by creating DSBs at defined locations in the genome (Bibikova et al., 2001, 2002, 2003).

Using these findings, Sangamo Therapeutics developed ZFNs from laboratory tools into therapeutic agents that could be used to disable disease-causing genes (by NHEJ) or to correct errors in existing genes (by HDR). The latter goal is particularly challenging, as the efficiency of HDR is usually much lower than the imprecise and mutagenic repair by NHEJ. By overcoming some of these difficult challenges, Sangamo now has several ongoing human clinical trials, the most advanced of which is in the treatment of HIV/AIDS where deletion of the CCR5 HIV coreceptor has the potential to enable the elimination of HIV following bone-marrow transplantation. Other applications of ZFNs have also been, or are being, tested in clinical trials (NCT02695160 [hemophilia B] and NCT02702115 [in vivo editing MPS1]).

Transcription Activator-Like Effector Nucleases

Like ZFNs, TALENs are composed of a DNA-binding protein that recognizes particular DNA sequences fused to a nuclease effector domain to achieve the cleavage (Joung and Sander, 2013) (see Figure A-2). TALEs are secreted bacterial proteins with DNA-binding domains that contain a series of conserved blocks of sequence 32-34 residues long, each with two divergent amino acids. These divergent amino acids are largely responsible for determining the DNA-binding specificity for a single DNA base pair, which allows engineering of specific DNA-binding domains by choosing combinations of repeat segments containing appropriate amino acids. The biotech firm Cellectis reported the successful conduct of the first-ever TALEN-based gene-editing clinical trial in the United Kingdom on a girl with incurable acute lymphoblastic leukemia (ALL) (Qasim et al, 2017). Although the applications of ZFNs and TALENs are largely overlapping, TALENS have the advantage of relative ease of design because of the robust recognition code.

Meganucleases

Meganucleases are nucleases with very long DNA-binding recognition sites, up to 40 nucleotides (Silva et al., 2011) (see Figure A-2). As a result of their length, it is exceedingly unlikely that natural sites would be present by chance even in complex human genomes. The challenge with meganucleases is the difficulty in designing new nucleases to target a sequence of interest at will. Some success has been achieved by designed changes to DNA-binding sites and combining meganucleases with TALE DNA-binding elements. However, meganucleases are unlikely to be much used in human genome editing given the relative simplicity of the alternative methods.

DEVELOPMENT OF CRISPR/CAS9

CRISPR as a Bacterial Adaptive Immunity System

The discovery that CRISPR systems provide adaptive immunity to bacteria represents a major conceptual advance in its own right. This discovery was also critical to the development of CRISPR/Cas9 genome engineering. A brief synopsis of the key findings is provided below (for a more complete review, see Doudna and Charpentier, 2014).

CRISPR loci were first identified based on analyses of bacterial genomes. From these studies, it was inferred that the spacer (i.e., nonrepetitive) regions of CRISPR loci were derived from the genomic DNA of bacteriophages (viruses that infect bacteria) leading to the hypothesis that CRISPR provided a defense mechanism against foreign genetic elements (Makarova et al., 2006; Mojica et al., 2005; Pourcel et al., 2005). The key experimental breakthrough came from research showing that CRISPR allowed bacteria to acquire resistance to bacteriophages by integrating segments of the bacteriophage genome into the CRISPR loci, demonstrating that CRISPR was a new form of adaptive immunity (Barrangou et al., 2007). In 2010, type II CRISPR/Cas systems were shown to mediate cleavage of invading bacteriophage DNA (Garneau et al., 2010). And in 2011, an associated RNA, tracrRNA, was identified (Deltcheva et al., 2011), and the CRISPR-associated gene, Cas9, was shown to be the only protein-coding gene in the type II Cas locus required for the defense function (Sapranauskas et al., 2011).

Development of Cas9 as a Programmable Endonuclease

The critical advance in the development of the CRISPR/Cas9-based genome-editing method came in 2012 from the laboratories of Doudna and Charpentier. They established that the CRISPR-associated protein Cas9, in complex with two small RNAs, CRISPR RNA (crRNA) transcribed from the CRISPR locus, and a trans-activating crRNA (tracrRNA), yields a site-specific endonuclease in which the site of cleavage is defined by base pairing of crRNA to the target DNA. This laid the groundwork for establishing that Cas9 is an endonuclease that can be programmed with a single "guide RNA" (gRNA, a chimera of crRNA transcribed from the CRISPR locus and the tracrRNA) to cleave at specific DNA sites (Jinek et al., 2012) (see Figure A-3a). Concurrent with the Jinek et al. (2012) manuscript, Siksnys and coworkers (Gasiunas et al., 2012) demonstrated that purified complexes containing Cas9 and a crRNA could mediate cleavage of double-stranded DNA in vitro at sites complementary to the crRNA. While this was clearly

FIGURE A-3 Schematic of Cas9 and different Cas9 variants. (a) Unmodified Cas9 with a guide RNA (gRNA) targeting a specific DNA sequence; DNA cut sites are indicated. (b) Paired Cas9 nickases (Cas9n). One of the two nuclease domains of Cas9 is catalytically inactivated to make an enzymatically active nickase. (c) Dimeric RNA-guided FokI–dCas9 nucleases (RFNs). Catalytically inactivated "dead" Cas9 (dCas9) is fused to the dimerization-dependent FokI non-specific nuclease domain. A pair of FokI–dCas9 monomers oriented in a PAM-out orientation mediates efficient DSBs.
SOURCE: Modified from Tsai and Joung, 2016.

an important advance, a key missing element was the identification of the requirement for the tracrRNA to form an active endonuclease.

The Jinek et al. (2012) paper made the key breakthrough of the use of a single chimeric guide RNA (gRNA) that can fulfill the role of both the crRNA and tracrRNA (see Figure A-3a). Thus, mechanistically, the CRISPR/

Cas9 system is superior to both ZFNs and TALENs in terms of ease of use; all that is required to generate a site-specific nuclease is design and synthesis of a single gRNA to target the Cas9 nuclease to the desired site of editing. Although not all predicted guide RNAs work, their synthesis is easy and multiple possible candidates can be synthesized easily and cheaply.

In Vivo Application of the Cas9 Programmable Nuclease

Within months of the publication of the Jinek et al. (2012) and Siksnys laboratory manuscripts (Gasiunas et al., 2012; Sapranauskas et al., 2011), there were six independent reports using the Cas9–guide RNA system to mediate programmable genome editing in vivo. These included four papers reporting Cas9 editing in mammalian cells (Cho et al., 2013; Cong et al., 2013; Jinek et al., 2013; Mali et al., 2013); one on zebrafish (Hwang et al., 2013); and one on bacteria (Jiang et al., 2013). Additionally, there was a seventh paper (Qi et al., 2013) showing that dCas9 could be used to inhibit transcription. Since that time there has been an explosion in the application and refinement of Cas9-mediated cleavage, as well as the discovery of novel CRISPR systems that can be adapted for genome editing. These include the discovery of a novel RNA-guided endonuclease, Cpf1 (Zetsche et al., 2015), and more recent work has shown that further CRISPR-targetable nucleases with the potential for differing capabilities are being discovered.

ACCURACY OF GENE EDITING

The potential impact of unintended changes to DNA is a key challenge for safe use of genome editing as a therapeutic strategy. Unintended changes to the genome could be caused by cleaving DNA at sites other than those that are being deliberately targeted.

The Challenge of Off-Target Toxicity

The site at which Cas9 cleaves DNA is determined by the complementarity of the DNA target with the RNA guide (typically 20 base pairs) adjacent to a protospacer adjacent motif (PAM) sequence (e.g., NGG for *Streptococcus pyogenes*, the most commonly used species of Cas9). In principle, this 22-base sequence would give enough diversity such that the cut site should be unique within even a 3 billion base-pair human genome. In practice, however, some base mismatches are tolerated leading to significant potential for off-target cutting. This has motivated efforts both to monitor the sites of off-target cutting as well as to enhance the specificity of the targeted nucleases. Initial efforts to define off-target cutting of Cas9 focused on specific searches for cutting at near-cognate sites. More recently these have been complemented by less biased genome-wide efforts. These can be divided into two broad classes: cell-based and cell-free (in vitro).

Genome-Wide Cell-Based Assays

Ostensibly, whole-genome sequencing (WGS), when conducted at a single-cell level, would seem to provide a definitive assessment of the accuracy of Cas9 genome editing. However, the depth of sequencing that would be required to certify the absence of off-target cutting is currently difficult to achieve for populations of cells. It should be possible, however, to estimate the sensitivity of the system for detecting off-target editing. Failure to detect editing with the assay would then indicate that the off-target editing rate was below the detection level.

Integrase-defective lentiviral vector (IDLV) capture (see Figure A-4a) is a genome-wide approach used to evaluate the specificity of genome-editing nucleases that was initially applied to engineered ZFNs and then later applied to TALENs and CRISPR/Cas9 (Gabriel et al., 2011; Wang et al., 2015). This method is based on the capture by NHEJ of IDLVs, which have linear double-stranded DNA genomes, into sites of nuclease-induced DSBs. Although the IDLV capture method directly identifies DSBs that occur in living cells, it is relatively insensitive and has a high background. To overcome these limitations, genome-wide unbiased identification of DSBs enabled by sequencing (GUIDE-seq) (see Figure A-4b) was developed (Tsai et al., 2015). GUIDE-seq exploits the efficient integration of a blunt, end-protected, double-stranded oligodeoxynucleotide (dsODN) tag, followed by tag-specific amplification and high-throughput sequencing. GUIDE-seq can detect off-target sites that are mutagenized by Cas9-sgRNAs with low frequencies (<0.1 percent) in a cell population, even with only a few million sequencing reads.

High-throughput genome-wide translocation sequencing (HTGTS) (see Figure A-4c) is another genome-wide method that identifies Cas9 off-target cleavage in live cells (Chiarle et al., 2011). HTGTS is based on the detection of translocations between a nuclease-induced "bait" DSB and off-target "prey" DSBs. A limitation of HTGTS is that nuclease-induced translocations represent rare events and thus require large numbers of input genomes for detection. A strategy for detecting genome-wide nuclease-induced DSBs in fixed cells, termed "BLESS" for breaks labeling, enrichment on streptavidin, and next-generation sequencing, captures a snapshot of transient DSBs that are present at a moment in time in a population of cells by direct in situ ligation of biotinylated hairpin adaptors in fixed and permeabilized cell nuclei (see Figure A-4d).

FIGURE A-4 Strategies for globally detecting off-target cutting events.
(a) Integrase-defective lentiviral vector (IDLV) capture. IDLVs (green) are integrated with a selectable marker into sites of nuclease-induced double-stranded breaks (DSBs) in living cells. Integration sites are recovered by linear amplification-mediated PCR (LAM-PCR), followed by high-throughput sequencing. (b) Genome-wide unbiased identification of DSBs enabled by sequencing (GUIDE-seq). An end-protected, short, double-stranded oligodeoxynucleotide (dsODN) is efficiently integrated into sites of nuclease-induced DSBs in living cells. This short sequence is used for tag-specific amplification followed by high-throughput sequencing to identify off-target cleavage sites. (c) High-throughput genome-wide translocation sequencing (HTGTS). Nuclease is expressed in a cell to generate a "prey" and "bait" DSB. Using a biotinylated primer designed against the targeted bait DSB junction, translocations between prey and bait are recovered by LAM-PCR and streptavidin-based enrichment for high-throughput sequencing. Off-target cleavage sites (prey) are identified by analysis of these translocation junctions. (d) Breaks labeling, enrichment on streptavidin, and next-generation sequencing (BLESS). Nuclease-treated cells are fixed, intact nuclei are isolated and permeabilized, and then sequencing adapters are ligated in situ to transient nuclease-induced DSBs. Adapter-ligated fragments are enriched and amplified for high-throughput sequencing. (e) Digested genome sequencing (Digenome-seq). Genomic DNA is isolated from cells and treated with Cas9 nuclease in vitro. Sequencing adapters are ligated and high-throughput sequencing is performed at standard whole-genome sequencing coverage. Absence of continuous sequence reads identifies cleavage sites.
SOURCE: Modified from Tsai and Joung, 2016.

Genome-Wide in In Vitro Assays

Digenome-seq (see Figure A-4e) is an in vitro method for detection of nuclease-induced DSBs in genomic DNA using whole-genome sequencing of Cas9-cleaved genomic DNA. Genomic DNA is isolated, and treated with high concentrations of Cas9–gRNA in vitro to maximize off-target cleavage and cleavage sites are identified by DNA sequencing. Because this assay is performed in vitro on purified DNA, it is not limited by cell-based factors such as chromatin context, epigenetic factors, subnuclear localization, or fitness effects. Digenome-seq thus may detect potential additional off-target cleavage at sites that would otherwise be obscured in cell-based methods. Thus, it could yield an overestimate of off-target events in vivo.

ENHANCING SPECIFICITY OF CRISPR/CAS9

Given its ease of use, flexibility, and versatility, the CRISPR/Cas9 system is rapidly becoming the tool of choice for gene editing. However, concerns about the potential risk of unwanted off-target effects have dominated many recent discussions. Most experiments that have detected significant off-targets have been performed in cancer cells (Fu et al., 2013; Hsu et al., 2013), which may have altered DNA repair pathways that could lead to elevated off-target events. In contrast, experiments in whole organisms such as mice (Yang et al., 2013), primates (Niu et al., 2014), zebrafish (Auer et al., 2014), or *Caenorhabditis elegans* (Dickinson et al., 2013) reported off-target frequencies that were low or not detectable, consistent with the high specificity of the CRISPR/Cas9-mediated gene targeting. It is possible that, in nontransformed cells, off-target cleavages are efficiently counter-selected by the endogenous DNA-damage response. Human pluripotent stem cells (hPSCs) are primary cells with genetically intact quality control mechanisms, and it seems possible that off-target events will accumulate less frequently in hPSCs or in normal somatic cells than has been observed in cancer cells. Nevertheless, it will be important to determine whether there are specific cell-types and conditions that predispose for the accumulation of off-target events. To address concerns about off-target events, diverse approaches to minimize mistargeting are being developed. Based on progress already made, it is anticipated that the risk of off-target events may be dramatically reduced, if not eliminated, in the near future for many genome-editing approaches. Below are three approaches and related progress.

Modification of Cas9 Structure

Protein engineering approaches can be deployed to develop better Cas9 variants that may be more accurate and efficient. Based on studies of

CRISPR/Cas9 structure, two recent papers report engineered substitutions such that the resulting Cas9 protein has a significantly reduced off-target rate (Kleinstiver et al., 2016; Slaymaker et al., 2016). The two studies focused on different DNA-binding domains of Cas9 but took the common strategy of reducing the relative affinity for nonspecific DNA binding. Remarkably this enhanced the specificity of Cas9 cutting without obviously impairing its overall efficiency. While these attempts are encouraging, other strategies will undoubtedly be forthcoming and should further improve the process, based on knowledge of CRISPR/Cas9 structure (Haurwitz et al., 2012; Jinek et al., 2014; Jore et al., 2011; Staals et al., 2013; Wiedenheft et al., 2009, 2011).

Engineered Combinations of Cas9 with Modified Cleavage Sites

This approach involves the use of two targeted DNA cuts, ensuring better fidelity than a single target cut. The basic rationale is that Cas9 protein has two active DNA-cleaving sites, involving aspartic acid, D10, and histidine, H840, each responsible for cutting a single strand of DNA thus generating the DSB (Jinek et al., 2014). Based on this feature, there are two ways of inactivating Cas9: single inactivation and double inactivation (Guilinger et al., 2014; Ran et al., 2013; Tsai et al., 2014). In one approach, Cas9 with a single inactivation, also named Cas9 nickase (Cas9n), in which only one of the active site residues (D10 or H840) is replaced with alanine (A), yields a Cas9 protein capable of cutting one strand of double-stranded DNA. Consequently, providing two guide RNAs that direct cutting on opposite strands in close proximity mediated by a dimer of Cas9n single cutters leads to an effective DSB and stimulation of both NHEJ and HDR to yield a DSB (see Figure A-3b). Remarkably these nicks can be effective even as far apart as ~100bp. In a second approach, both cleavage sites of Cas9 are inactivated, yielding nuclease-deficient dCas9, which is then fused to the FokI cleavage domain. As with ZFNs and TALENs, two Cas9 monomers provide recognition specificity for FokI dimerization and DNA cleavage (see Figure A-3c). In addition, these two strategies require appropriate length spacers between the targets: if the spacers are too short, there will be two competing Cas9 proteins, and if the spacers are too long, it is more difficult to execute effective cutting. Because of these stringent requirements, the off-target rate is greatly reduced, albeit with increased difficulty in target selection. These strategies have been shown to significantly reduce off-target rates (Guilinger et al., 2014; Ran et al., 2013; Tsai et al., 2014).

Cas9 Base-Editor:
Genome Editing Without Double-Stranded DNA Breaks

In an effort to increase the efficiency and precision of making point mutations in genomic DNA, the Liu group recently developed the so called "base editor" variant of Cas9 (see Figure A-5), which consists of a highly engineered fusion protein that recruits a cytosine deaminase domain, which converts cytosine to uracil, thereby effecting an irreversible C→T substitution (or G→A by targeting the complementary strand) without double-stranded cleavage of the DNA backbone (Komor et al., 2016).

Because cytosine deaminase acts only on single-stranded DNA, the C to U conversion activity is targeted to a small window of ~5 nucleotides near the 5′ end of the guide RNA-specified protospacer sequence on the displaced DNA strand. By avoiding DSBs, exogenous DNA templates, and stochastic DNA-repair processes, base editing introduces point mutations in unmodified mammalian cells with an efficiency as high as 75 percent and with a ratio of point mutation correction:indels exceeding 20:1. Moving forward it will be important to develop alternate base-editors capable

FIGURE A-5 Schematic of a CRISPR/Cas9 genome-editing system using a variant of the Cas9 nuclease. The "base editor" variant of Cas9 provides increased efficiency and precision when making changes to genomic DNA.
SOURCE: Modified from Komor et al., 2016.

of mediating a wider range of genetic changes ideally ultimately allowing conversion of any base to any other base within a user-defined window. Additionally, it will be important to robustly evaluate the propensity of the cytosine deaminase domain to introduce mutations outside of the DNA region targeted by the Cas9 guide RNA.

An alternative strategy for improving HDR, termed "CORRECT," (consecutive re-guide or re-Cas steps to erase CRISPR/Cas-blocked targets), exploits the observation that HDR accuracy is increased dramatically by incorporating silent CRISPR/Cas-blocking mutations along with the desired functional mutations (Paquet et al., 2016). This prevents recleavage and potential NHEJ repair that might disrupt successful HDR products. The authors show that by controlling the location of the introduced point mutation relative to the Cas9-mediated DSB they can alter the efficiency of mutagenesis, generating either heterozygous or homozygous alterations in human-induced pluripotent stem cells (hiPSCs).

QUALITY CONTROL AND QUALITY ASSURANCE FOR GENE EDITING

The specificity of genome editing is even more important in clinical applications than in laboratory research. As a medical product or medical practice, genome editing must be safe, efficacious, and cost-effective. Development of a regulatory framework for genome editing will need to address various issues associated with these requirements. As discussed above, although technical advances will likely make off-target events a manageable issue, this consideration will remain a concern that must be addressed by quality control (QC) and quality assurance (QA) procedures. In somatic genome editing, it may be relatively easy to set up assays or procedures to address off-target changes but it is probable that such rates will vary among cell types, necessitating measurement of off-target events in each cell type targeted. Although the specifics may vary from case to case, the general principle of monitoring to ensure safety and efficacy should be implemented. In contrast, it would be quite difficult to monitor embryos if they were to undergo editing. Functional equivalence assays need to be developed and agreed upon to serve as QC measures. Alternatives may be considered, such as editing performed on sperm progenitor cells.

USE OF dCAS9 TO REGULATE TRANSCRIPTION OR TO MAKE EPIGENETIC MODIFICATIONS

An alternate strategy for genome editing involves the use of catalytically dead variants of Cas9. This yields a programmable DNA-binding protein that is incapable of generating either single- or double-stranded breaks and thus does not typically lead to any changes in the DNA sequence of the genome. However, by fusing different effector domains to dCas9, it can be used either to turn on (CRISPRa) (Gilbert et al., 2014; Konermann et al., 2015; Perez-Pinera et al., 2013) or turn off (CRISPRi) transcription (Gilbert et al., 2013; Qi et al., 2013) or to make locus-specific changes to the epigenetic marks (modifications of the chromatin that regulate gene expression). It is likely that most if not all such epigenetic changes would fail to be passed to subsequent generations thus alleviating some of the concerns surrounding germline-editing approaches. By the same token, the transient nature of these changes limits their utility for correcting diseases caused by genetic mutations. Possible uses for such transient germline engineering, however, include the ability to expand germ cells, or the in vitro generation of desired stem cells or terminally differentiated cells. Additionally, the transient nature of the changes could expand the number of genes that could be safely targeted. For example, transient down-regulation of the HIV CCR5 coreceptor could protect against vertical passage of HIV, and this strategy could be expanded to other viral receptors. Additionally, it is possible to imagine that transient alterations to gene expression could lead to permanent developmental changes in an embryo, which could ameliorate the effects of disease-causing inherited mutations. Because no permanent, heritable changes are made to the individual, the use of dCas9 to alter gene expression does alleviate some ethical concerns. Nonetheless, at present the potential uses of dCas9 on embryos seem rather limited compared to approaches involving germline editing, and the more immediate therapeutic applications of dCas9 likely involve somatic alteration in gene expression.

GENOME TARGETING IN TRANSGENIC ANIMALS

Gene mutations can lead to abnormal development and to disease. Over the past several decades, a major advance in studying the consequence of mutations has been the development of the ability to experimentally introduce designed, targeted mutations into genes of organisms such as mice, fruit flies, and zebrafish, thus providing an important tool to understand the molecular-genetic basis of embryonic development and of disease. These methods can also be used to correct defective genes. Before describing the application of current precise genome-editing methods, we will summarize the major steps that were initially developed to genetically modify animals.

Random Insertion of Foreign DNA

The genetic manipulation of animals has been the basis for much of the research aimed at understanding embryonic development and human diseases. One powerful technology is based on manipulating mouse em-

FIGURE A-6 The generation of transgenic mice with randomly inserted transgenes. Embryos at the 4 to 8 cell stage are infected with retroviruses or DNA is injected into the male pronucleus of the zygote. The embryos can be transplanted into a foster mother. The exogenous DNA sequences are randomly integrated into the genome of the resulting transgenic mice directly or after incubation any time up until the blastocyst stage (~100 cells).

bryos in vitro and transferring the embryos to a foster mother to produce genetically altered animals (see Figure A-6).

Using these techniques, initially SV40 DNA (Jaenisch and Mintz, 1974) and later retroviruses (Jaenisch, 1976) were introduced into early mouse embryos leading to the generation of the first transgenic mice that transmitted the foreign DNA to the next generation according to Mendelian expectations. The most widely used method to generate genetically modified animals was microinjection of DNA into fertilized mouse or *Drosophila* eggs leading to the production of a large number of transgenic mice or flies that carried foreign DNA in their germline (Brinster et al., 1981; Costantini and Lacy, 1981; Gordon and Ruddle, 1981; Rubin and Spradling, 1982).

The random integration of foreign DNA into the genome of an animal can cause disruption of an endogenous gene leading to its inactivation. In this "insertional mutagenesis" approach the integrated DNA is used as a molecular tag for the isolation and identification of the mutated gene. The collagen I gene was the first endogenous gene inactivated by retroviral insertional mutagenesis resulting in mutant mice whose phenotype resembled brittle bone disease (Schnieke et al., 1983), a major disease of the skeletal system caused by mutations in a collagen gene. Similarly, injection of DNA into the zygote pronucleus produced mutant mice by insertional mutagenesis (Mahon et al., 1988). In addition to insertional mutagenesis, the integration of a gene into the genome can result in transcriptional activation of nearby genes, which has been widely used to study the consequences of ectopic transgene expression (Hammer et al., 1984).

While integration into the genome leading to insertional mutagenesis or ectopic transgene expression is efficient in generating transgenic animals, the approach suffers from unpredictability because the insertion of DNA into the genome is random and does not allow the targeting of predetermined genes or predictable transgene expression.

Gene Targeting in Embryonic Stem Cells

Embryonic stem (ES) cells, initially isolated from mouse blastocysts, are able to differentiate into all cell types of the body (Evans and Kaufman, 1981; Martin, 1981). Of great interest was that ES cells, when injected into a mouse carrier blastocyst, could integrate into the developing embryo and contribute to all somatic tissues and generate "chimeric mice." Of particular importance was the fact that the cells were able to contribute to the germline, thus allowing the derivation of animals from the cultured cells. Thus, the approach allowed the generation of mice carrying the alteration of an endogenous gene as a result of in vitro manipulation of the ES cells.

The first mouse strain derived from an ES cell carrying a mutation in a predetermined gene was a strain with inactivation of the HPRT gene, which is mutated in human patients with the severe mental disorder Lesch-Nyhan syndrome. The isolation of HPRT mutant ES cells was straightforward using a culture medium (HAT) that kills normal cells and selects for cells carrying an inactivated HPRT gene (Kuehn et al., 1987). This selective approach, while successful for HPRT, cannot be used for editing other genes.

Homologous Recombination

The discovery of homologous recombination represented a major breakthrough as it allowed the editing of any gene (Doetschman et al., 1987; Thomas and Capecchi, 1987). Targeting of genes requires the generation of a targeting vector containing DNA segments homologous to sequences of the endogenous gene flanking the desired modification (see Figure A-1). The vector is transfected into ES cells, and correctly targeted clones are selected (see Figure A-7a). Cells carrying the desired modification are injected into mouse blastocysts to generate chimeric mice (see Figure A-7b), which are bred with normal mice to obtain offspring carrying the mutant allele (see Figure A-7c). Homologous recombination in combination with ES cells has allowed scientists to efficiently create mice transmitting specific gene mutations to the next generation. Following the initial generation of mice carrying targeted mutations of the β_2-microglubulin and the c-Abl gene (Schwartzberg et al., 1989; Zijlstra et al., 1989), homologous recombination in ES cells has become a widely used tool for the study of mammalian development and the generation of animal models of human genetic diseases (Solter, 2006). Because chimera–competent ES cells were only available in the murine system, gene editing by homologous recombination was restricted to mice and could not readily be used in other species.

a.

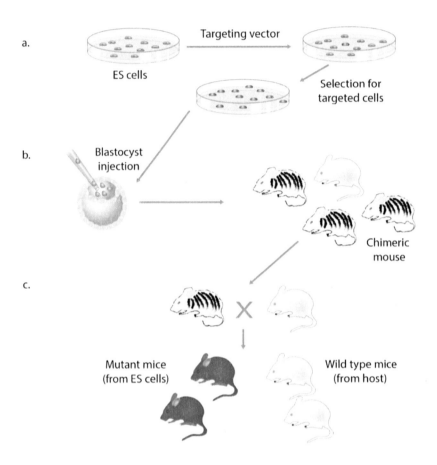

FIGURE A-7 The generation of defined genetically altered mice by homologous recombination (three-step process).

(a) In the first step a targeting vector with homology to the target gene is introduced into ES cells and correctly targeted clones are selected in culture. (b) The targeted ES cells are injected into an albino host blastocyst, which is transplanted into a foster mother to produce chimeric mice where the donor ES cells contribute to the tissues of the animal (as seen by coat color contribution derived from the ES cells). (c) Germline transmission of the ES cell clone is verified by mating of the chimeric mouse with the albino host strain. Pigmented offspring are derived from the donor ES cells.

Nuclear Cloning and the Generation of Mutant Animals

The transfer of a somatic nucleus into an enucleated egg resets the epigenetic state of the nucleus to an embryonic state and allows the generation of animals such as Dolly, the first cloned mammal (Wakayama et al., 1998; Wilmut et al., 1997). The production of animals from somatic cells by nuclear cloning allowed the generation of mutant animals in species where no ES cells were available. The first successful application of nuclear cloning in combination with homologous recombination to produce gene-altered farm animals used sheep fibroblasts. The human 1-antitrypsin gene was inserted into the 3' UTR of the COL1A1 gene, a convenient "safe harbor" locus giving predictable expression of the transgene. Transgenic sheep were derived from the targeted fibroblasts by nuclear-cloning, generating animals that expressed the therapeutically important human 1-antitrypsin protein (McCreath et al., 2000).

The strategies to produce animals carrying engineered gene alterations as summarized above relied on the manipulation of ES cells or on nuclear cloning, both of which are labor-intensive and require special skills. This changed dramatically when the new genome-editing methods based on ZFNs, TALENs, and CRISPR/Cas9 became available (Doudna and Charpentier, 2014). These approaches, described above, revolutionized the ability of researchers to edit genes in any species and to produce genetically altered animals with a fraction of the effort and time and much less sophistication and experimental skills needed than were required for the generation of gene-edited animals by strategies based on ES cells or nuclear transfer.

GENOME EDITING IN EMBRYOS

Homologous recombination in conventional gene targeting is an inefficient process and requires the selection of correctly targeted cell clones in cell culture. In a second step the targeted ES cell clone is injected into a host blastocyst to create a chimeric animal, which, in a third step, is mated to produce the desired mutant animal, a process that may take as much as 1 or 2 years (compare Figure A-7). In contrast, gene targeting by TALEN or by CRISPR/Cas9 is so efficient that no selection for correct targeting is required (Sakuma and Woltjen, 2014), making it possible to derive genetically modified animals in one step by direct genetic manipulation of the fertilized egg (see Figure A-8).

FIGURE A-8 The generation of gene-edited mice by CRISPR/Cas9 targeting in the zygote (one-step process). Cas9 RNA and guide RNA (gRNA) targeting a gene of interest are injected into the cytoplasm of the zygote. Mice carrying a mutation in both alleles of the targeted gene are derived in one step at a high frequency. If co-injected with a DNA vector, exogenous sequences will be inserted at some frequency at the double-strand break.

CRISPR/Cas9-Mediated Gene Editing in the Zygote

The injection of guide RNAs together with Cas9 RNA into the fertilized egg (zygote) was used to generate mice carrying mutations in several genes. The efficiency of Cas9-mediated DNA DSBs was high and resulted in 80 percent of pups carrying mutations in both alleles of two different genes (Wang et al., 2013). When the guide and Cas9 RNAs were co-injected with an oligonucleotide carrying a point mutation, the mutation was introduced into two target genes in 60 percent of the pups. In addition, the generation of conditional mutants requiring the insertion of two LoxP sites into the same allele was shown to be effective in the zygote. Thus, NHEJ-mediated mutation as well as insertion of DNA at the DSB site is extremely efficient, allowing the generation of mice carrying complex mutations within 3 weeks (the gestation time of the mouse) instead of 1 to 2 years when using ES cell–mediated gene targeting. The CRISPR/Cas9 gene-editing method was shown to work efficiently not only in mice but also in other species including rats (Li et al., 2013), zebrafish (Hwang et al., 2013), *C. elegans* (Friedland et al., 2013), and *Drosophila* (Zeng et al., 2015). Importantly, the approach allowed the generation of primates carrying mutations in specific genes (Niu et al., 2014). Most recently, two reports appeared that used genome editing in preimplantation human embryos that were defective and therefore could not be used to generate pregnancy (Kang et al., 2016; Liang et al., 2015).

The evidence summarized above indicates that animals carrying defined mutations in multiple genes can be generated in one step by manipulation of the fertilized egg. However, if intended for gene therapy (correction of mutant genes), several significant complications need to be considered. These include frequent mosaicism of manipulated embryos, the mutation of both alleles when the goal is to correct one mutant allele, and the impossibility of genotyping the one-cell embryo.

Mosaicism

The cleavage of the target gene and the insertion of DNA at the double-strand breakpoint may occur at a later stage than the zygote—such as the two-cell stage. The consequence of integration at a stage later than the one-cell zygote stage is that half (or less, depending on the time of DNA insertion) of the embryo's cells will carry the altered gene whereas the others will not. Animals with genetic alterations in only a subset of the cells are designated as "mosaics." The available evidence indicates that the incidence of mosaicism may be as high as 50 percent or higher (Wang et al., 2013). The high incidence of mosaicism has an important practical consequence: Preimplantation genetic diagnosis (PGD)—the biopsy of one or a few cells of the manipulated embryo—cannot be used to ascertain whether gene targeting resulted in the desired mutation because the biopsied cells may not reflect the genotype of the other cells of the embryo.

Mutation of the Wild-Type Allele by Cas9-Mediated Cleavage

Cleavage by Cas9 is significantly more efficient than insertion of a donor DNA at the cleavage site by homologous recombination. This poses a complication if the goal of gene editing in embryos is the correction of a mutant allele. To correct a given mutation, a guide RNA and a DNA target construct are injected into the embryo. While the DNA will integrate into the mutant allele at the DSB and correct the mutation, the other allele will often be cleaved, creating a new mutation by NHEJ. Given present technology, this poses a possibly serious problem for gene therapy as the mutant allele is corrected, but a new mutant allele is created. The inhibition of repair by end joining using a small molecule may help to mitigate this problem as this has been shown to favor the insertion of DNA by HDR over that by NHEJ (Maruyama et al., 2015). However, the unwanted mutation of the normal allele currently remains a complication of CRISPR/Cas9-mediated gene correction.

Genotyping of the One-Cell Embryo

Genome editing in embryos with the goal being to correct a mutant allele faces another problem: how to distinguish a wild type from a mutant embryo. If one parent carries a dominant mutant gene, 50 percent of the embryos will be affected and 50 percent will be wild type, and if both parents carry a recessive mutation, 75 percent of the embryos will be normal and 25 percent will be affected. Because it is not possible to use any current molecular test to distinguish mutant from normal embryos at the zygote stage, any gene-editing attempt will target (and modify) a large fraction of normal embryos. It is unlikely that a technological advance could resolve this dilemma in the foreseeable future.

GENE DRIVE: A MECHANISM TO SPREAD GENETIC ALTERATIONS THROUGH SEXUALLY REPRODUCING POPULATIONS

It has been proposed that naturally occurring "homing endonucleases" could cause mutant alleles to spread rapidly through sexually reproducing populations by a process designated as "gene drive" (Burt, 2003, 2014). The spreading of such a mutant allele through a population does not require a selective advantage for the carrier of the mutant gene but would rather propagate like a "selfish gene" (Esvelt et al., 2014; Oye et al., 2014).

Recently, a vector encoding both Cas9 and a guide RNA was introduced into a *Drosophila* genomic locus that governs cuticle color, creating a knock-out mutation. Cas9-mediated cleavage during development of the germline stimulated the copying of the insertion into the wild-type locus, such that all female gametes carried the insertion (see Figure A-9). Importantly, when these eggs were fertilized the mutation in the resulting heterozygous animals converted the wild-type allele into a mutant allele during meiosis by Cas9-mediated target gene cleavage, followed by HDR resulting in a homozygous mutation. Thus, the vector carrying the Cas9 gene and a guide RNA, when integrated into one allele, led to the conversion of the other allele during meiosis with an efficiency of 98 percent, causing the rapid spread of the mutant allele through the population (Gantz and Bier, 2015). This autocatalytic process was dubbed as a "mutagenic chain reaction."

If a vector carrying sequences correcting a given mutation in addition to the Cas9 and the guide RNA was inserted into one allele, these sequences could serve as a template during meiosis and convert the other allele by homologous recombination resulting in two repaired alleles (see Figure A-9a). Similarly, if a vector carrying sequences coding for another gene in addition to the Cas9 and the guide RNA were integrated into one allele, Cas9-mediated cleavage of the wild-type allele during meiosis would transfer the exogenous "cargo" gene into the other allele, leading to homozygous transgenic animals (Esvelt et al., 2014). Thus, gene-drive mechanisms can effectively propagate and spread mutant alleles or newly inserted genes through animal populations (see Figure A-9b).

So far gene-drive constructs have been demonstrated to spread through insect populations and have been proposed for use in mosquito popula-

FIGURE A-9 Gene drive. (a) Insertion of Cas9, guide RNA (g-DNA, targeting the gene) and "cargo" DNA sequences into a gene of interest. When expressed during meiosis, the guide RNA/Cas9 complex will introduce a double-strand break onto the other allele followed by homologous recombination driven repair, which will insert the Cas9/gRNA/transgene sequences into the wild-type allele. (b) The gene modification will rapidly spread through a sexually reproducing population
SOURCE: Information from Esvelt et al., 2014.

tion control. Gene drives have not as yet been shown to behave similarly in mammalian species. However, given the efficiency of genome editing in mammalian embryos it is possible, if not likely, that the underlying gene-drive mechanisms would also be effective in mammals and could in principle create gene modifications that could spread through the population. However, given the generation time and breeding patterns of humans, any such gene-drive application in the human species would require an inordinate numbers of years and seems inconceivable.

ALTERNATIVE ROUTES TO HERITABLE GERMLINE EDITING

The efficiency and precision of CRISPR/Cas9 gene-editing approaches have raised the potential that precise genome editing might be possible in cells that could contribute to the germline of the human species. For a genetic alteration to be passed on to the next generation, it has to be made in (1) *progenitor cells* that can give rise to the *gametes (eggs and sperm)*, (2) the eggs and sperm themselves, or (3) in the *fertilized zygote or early embryo*, when all cells can still contribute to the future germline.

As discussed in the preceding section, methods for germline editing have been most highly developed in the mouse and applied to a number of other mammalian species, particularly in relation to agricultural needs or the generation of preclinical disease models for human genetic diseases. Until the recent advent of advanced genome-editing tools, germline gene alterations in mice were primarily achieved via nontargeted introduction of transgenic DNA into the genome of the zygote or by targeted mutagenesis in ES cells. The latter approach involved the homologous recombination of targeting vectors into the host genome, the selection of the correctly targeted clones, and the generation of germline-transmitting chimeric animals (see details in the above section on germline genetic alteration). While this approach has proven to be extraordinarily powerful in producing knockout mice, conditional mutations, reporter lines, and a variety of human disease models, it is still relatively inefficient and has not been readily applicable to direct targeted genome alterations in zygotes. Thus, the idea of potential targeted gene alterations or corrections in human embryos was not under consideration.

However, more recently, the efficiency of CRISPR/Cas in targeting nuclease-enhanced editing to specific sites in the genome has raised new vistas including possible human germline editing. Soon after the demonstration that CRISPR/Cas could very efficiently target specific sites in the genome of mammalian cells, it was shown that this approach could be applied directly to the mouse zygote without the need for the intermediate ES cell step (see above section and Figure A-8). Thus, it became possible to consider genome editing directly in human embryos. The only publications to date on testing CRISPR on human zygotes demonstrated that targeted mutations could be generated, but also demonstrated that the resulting mutations were often complex and that only some embryos or embryonic cells carried the targeted event (Kang et al., 2016; Liang et al., 2015). As explained above, these intrinsic issues of CRISPR editing make the concept of using zygote genome editing to correct human genetic disease very challenging.

Editing the embryo genome, however, is not the only potential way to achieve modification of the genome in the germline. Approaches that directly modify the genome of the gametes—the eggs and sperm—before fertilization would overcome problems of mosaicism and would potentially allow preselection of the appropriately targeted gamete before in vitro fertilization.

Gamete Gene Editing: Current Status

There are a number of potential routes to gamete gene editing, some of which are already in use in the mouse and some of which remain to be fully developed.

Direct Introduction of Editing Factors into Oocytes

In the mouse it has been shown that maternally inherited Cas9 nuclease provides a very efficient means of generating targeted alterations in the resulting zygotes (Sakurai et al., 2016), presumably because of the immediate availability of the enzyme. While such an approach is, of course, not applicable to humans, it does suggest that preloading ovulated oocytes with the editing factors prior to in vitro fertilization might be a means of avoiding mosaic editing and enhancing efficiency. Whether this could actually promote gene targeting in the oocyte genome rather than after fertilization remains to be reported. Preselection of mutated or corrected oocytes would still be a challenge, but the reduction in mosaicism would allow PGD to be contemplated for identifying correctly targeted embryos.

Gene Editing in Sperm In Vitro

Sperm-mediated gene transfer is a fairly well established, although inefficient, route to transgenesis in a number of species, from fish to pigs (Lavitrano et al., 2013). Thus, it should be possible to introduce the components of genome-editing systems into sperm and have them carried into the zygote to promote genome editing there. More interesting is the possibility of direct genome editing in the sperm nuclei. Given that sperm are nondividing cells, currently only NHEJ-mediated gene editing would be possible, although the repair mechanism is presumably different from that in somatic cells (Ahmed et al., 2010). Homologous recombination-mediated gene correction or alteration has to date only been possible in dividing cells. However, there are indications that this block can be overcome (Orthwein et al., 2015). Izpisua Belmonte's group has recently developed an NHEJ-based gene knock-in method—homology-independent targeted gene integration (HITI). HITI allows the direct knock-in of DNA sequences at specific genomic loci in post-mitotic cells, for example, neurons (Suzuki et al., 2016b). HITI may open up new avenues to sperm (and even oocyte) gene editing. Insertion of a transient fluorescent reporter to identify sperm carrying the editing factors could help enrich for potentially gene-edited sperm. Final confirmation of the appropriately edited embryos after fertilization in vitro or intracytoplasmic sperm injection (ICSI) would require PGD.

Gene Editing in Germline Stem Cells

There is considerable biological and clinical interest in generating gametes from stem cell lines that can be propagated indefinitely in vitro. Spermatogonial stem cells (SSCs) have been isolated from mouse testes and have the capacity to regenerate fertilization-competent sperm when retransplanted to the germ cell–depleted adult testis (Kanatsu-Shinohara and Shinohara, 2013). Gene editing in SSCs would allow for the preselection of clonal lines with appropriate targeted mutations and the potential to prescreen for off-target effects or other unwanted genomic or epigenomic alterations before generating gametes. Proof of principle for such an approach has been published (Wu et al., 2015), in which the authors corrected a gene mutation that causes cataracts in mice by CRISPR/Cas9 editing in SSCs. SSCs were transferred back to the testis and round spermatids collected for ICSI. Offspring were correctly edited at 100 percent efficiency.

Translating this work into humans has many challenges. While SSC-like cells have been isolated from human testes (Wu et al., 2015), stable, self-renewing cell lines have not yet been achieved. If this challenge is overcome, there still remains the challenge of generating ICSI-competent gametes from the SSCs. In the mouse, this is achieved by transfer into the germ cell–depleted testis—not an easy solution in humans. Alternate approaches include generating a "reconstituted testis" with mixed SSCs and supporting cells of the testis and transplanting this under the testis capsule. This approach would also be ethically challenging in humans. The possible use of interspecies reconstitutions and transplants into immune-deficient mice would bring its own scientific and ethical challenges. The best solution would be to promote differentiation of the SSCs to mature haploid gametes in a fully defined culture system in vitro—a challenge not yet achieved in any system.

While the possibility of applying similar approaches to the female germline is attractive, the evidence for the existence of oogonial stem cells is controversial (Johnson et al., 2004). Most evidence suggests that there is a limited resource of oocytes in the adult mammalian ovary (Eggan et al., 2006) and no evidence for any endogenous stem cells.

Gene Editing in Pluripotent Stem Cells Followed by Germ Cell Differentiation

Pluripotent embryonic stem cells or induced pluripotent stem cells can be generated from both males and females, are readily amenable to CRISPR editing, and can be differentiated down the pathway toward meiotically competent germ cells. In the mouse, the most reliable reports of germ cell generation from ES cells have come from mimicking the known pathways that induce primordial germ cells from the pluripotent epiblast in the early embryo. Using this approach, Saitou's lab has generated primordial germ cell–like cells (PGC-LCs) from both male and female ES cells. When PGC-LCs were reconstituted with support cells from the testis or ovary respectively and transplanted back to the testis or ovary environment, investigators were able to recover spermatids or oocytes that could be used to generate viable offspring when combined with normal eggs and sperm (Hayashi et al., 2011, 2012). Recent advances have further extended this approach, either by coculture of the PGC-LCs with testis cells in culture to generate spermatid-like cells in vitro (Zhou et al., 2016), or by derivation of SSCs in cocultures of pluripotent embryonic stem cells with somatic testis cells and subsequent maturation to spermatids in adult testes (Ishikura et al., 2016). In both cases, spermatids were derived that were capable of fertilizing oocytes after ICSI and generating viable offspring. There are some concerns about whether epigenetic reprogramming would be complete in this culture system, but the overall results are quite remarkable. Another interesting development is from the Izpisua Belmonte, Okuda, and Matsui groups, who have shown that knockdown or knockout of *Max* in mouse embryonic stem cells (ESCs) strongly activates expression of germ cell–related genes and results in profound cytological changes to resemble cells undergoing meiotic division (Maeda et al., 2013; Suzuki et al., 2016a). Whether functional haploid cells can be generated using this approach remains to be seen.

These results in murine systems raise expectations that human haploid gametes could be generated from human pluripotent cells, with implications for understanding gametogenesis and causes of infertility and potentially offering new avenues for reproduction in infertile couples. It also would open up genetic modification of the stem cells to repair known genetic causes of infertility or to repair dominant gene mutations. However, to date, human gametes have not been generated successfully from pluripotent stem cells, although two recent papers report the generation of early PGC-LCs from human ES cells (Irie et al., 2015; Sasaki et al., 2015). Those studies revealed similarities and differences from the mouse germ cell differentiation pathway. This suggests that more knowledge of how germ cells actually develop in the human, or perhaps the nonhuman primate, embryo versus the mouse embryo is needed to move this research forward.

Gene Editing in Haploid ES Cells

Most animals are diploids, and natural haploid cells are typically limited to mature germ cells. Recently both androgenetic (male) and parthenogenetic (female) haploid ES cells (haESCs) have been derived in mice and rats (Leeb and Wutz, 2011; Li et al., 2012, 2014; Yang et al., 2012). haESCs contain only one copy of allelic genes of diploid cells and are amenable to genetic modification with traditional gene-targeting approaches and with new nuclease-based genome-editing strategies (Li et al., 2012, 2014). More interestingly, androgenetic haESCs, which contain a Y rather than an X chromosome, can produce viable and fertile offspring after intracytoplasmic injection into mature oocytes (Li et al., 2012, 2014). Haploid parthenogenetic mouse haESCs were also shown to be able to produce fertile mice when injected into oocytes in place of the maternal genome (Wan et al., 2013). Both strategies are possible to be used for introduction of genetic modifications to progeny. Most recently parthenogenetic human haESCs have also been successfully generated (Sagi et al., 2016). Human androgenetic haESCs have not yet been reported.

There are several limitations of haESCs. First, the haploid phenotype has been found to be unstable in culture. haESCs undergo spontaneous auto-diploidization and need several rounds of haploid purification by flow-activated cell sorting before becoming stable in culture. Also, there is a lack of androgenetic haESCs containing the Y chromosome (Li et al., 2012). This is due to the poor developmental potential of androgenetic embryos with YY chromosomes (Latham et al., 2000; Tarkowki, 1977). Therefore only female animals can currently be created. With further breeding, males can then be obtained. Another major drawback is that the efficiency for androgenetic haESCs to fertilize an egg is very low (less than 5 percent in mice and less than 2 percent in rats).

In summary, although the generation of human "artificial" gametes from stem cell lines is not currently achievable, work in the mouse suggests that this will likely be possible. Reconstituting the testis or ovary environment in vitro may be achieved by deriving both germ cells and supporting cells, such as Sertoli cells, and granulosa cells from in vitro differentiation of human ES cells. Further understanding of the endogenous signaling pathways that promote germ cell development and meiotic maturation will aid in the future derivation of human gametes in vitro. Such cells will be immediately useful for understanding gametogenesis and dissecting fertility problems, but safety concerns will need to be overcome before they could be used for human reproduction, with or without genome editing. The germline is generally considered to be somewhat protected from genetic damage, unlike that of somatic cells, and also undergoes extensive epigenetic remodeling before completion of gametogenesis. Both aspects would need to be replicated in the artificial gametes generated in vitro.

EDITING THE MITOCHONDRIAL GENOME

Mitochondrial diseases are a group of maladies caused by the dysfunction of mitochondria due to mutations in mitochondrial DNA (mtDNA). Mitochondrial diseases are associated with the degeneration of tissues and organs that have high energetic demands—including muscle, heart, and brain—that lead, among other pathologies, to myopathies, cardiomyopathies, neuropathies, encephalopathies, lactic acidosis, stroke-like syndrome, and blindness (Taylor and Turnbull, 2005). The percentage of mtDNA molecules that is mutated generally determines whether or not a patient is symptomatic. Currently, there are no cures for mitochondrial diseases, and for patients healthy enough to have children, genetic counseling and PGD represent the best options for preventing disease transmission. However, due to the non-Mendelian inheritance of mtDNA and the potentially different heteroplasmy levels among different blastomeres, PGD can only reduce, not eliminate, the risk of transmitting the disease. Recently developed mitochondrial replacement techniques involve a series of complex technical manipulations of nuclear genome between patient and donor oocytes that results in the generation of embryos carrying genetic material from three different origins (Paull et al., 2012; Tachibana et al., 2012). For these reasons, mitochondrial replacement techniques have raised biological, medical, and ethical concerns (Hayden, 2013; Reinhardt et al., 2013). Mitochondrial replacement techniques have low rates of success, and studies in lower organisms have reported potential issues arising from incompatibility between nuclear and mtDNA upon mitochondrial replacement (Reinhardt et al., 2013).

A novel alternative therapeutic approach was recently developed to eliminate the mutated mtDNA in the germline. Using mitochondria-targeted endonuclease, the targeted mtDNA in the mouse germline was successfully prevented from transmission to the next generation (Reddy et al., 2015). Due to the limited number of mtDNA mutations that can be targeted by restriction endonucleases, efforts have been made to target most of the mtDNA mutations using mitochondria-targeted transcription activator-like effector nucleases (mito-TALENs) and ZFNs (Bacman et al.,

2013; Gammage et al., 2014). The mito-TALENs were able to specifically eliminate the targeted mtDNA in the mouse germline (Reddy et al., 2015). Importantly, the technique of injection of nucleases (e.g., mito-TALENs) into oocytes or early embryos involves a simple microinjection of mRNA that encodes the nucleases. Moreover, the use of mitochondrial localization signal (e.g., Cox8 and ATP5b) restricts the translocation to mitochondria alone. A caveat of this technology is that elimination of high levels of mutated mtDNA in oocytes will lead to the generation of embryos with a low number of normal mtDNA that, if failing to replicate after implantation, could lead to pregnancy loss. PGD could be used for the selection and transfer of embryos containing higher levels of normal mtDNA. Importantly, unlike nuclear editing, mtDNA editing is not aimed to correct the mutations, but to eliminate mutated DNA, which is possible due to the presence of multiple copies of mtDNA in the oocytes. Moreover, due to the very low activity of repair mechanisms in mitochondria, the frequency of re-ligation of target mtDNA and introduction of new mutations would be very rare. In addition, similar mitochondrial editing tools in the future could also be used to eliminate mutated mtDNA in gametes derived from stem cells. Finally, a combination of mitochondrial gene-editing tools with mitochondrial replacement techniques may represent an alternative option, in the future, to prevent the germline transmission of mutations in the mtDNA responsible not only for mitochondrial specific diseases but also for situations where alterations in mitochondrial function contribute to pathologies such as cancer, diabetes, and aging-associated diseases.

THE CHALLENGE OF DELIVERY

In addition to the technical advances being made to genome-editing systems, an important challenge for in vivo use is effective delivery. Table A-1 highlights a number of strategies being explored for the delivery of genome-editing components, including a discussion of their advantages and disadvantages.

TABLE A-1 General Approaches to Delivering Genome-Editing Components

Method	Delivered Component	Explanation	Advantages	Disadvantages	Preferred Applications
		Nonviral			
Transfection	*Nuclease(s)* as plasmid DNA, RNA, or protein *guideRNA* as plasmid DNA or oligonucleotide is mixed with the nuclease RNA (can be complexed with nuclease as Ribonucleoprotein, RNP) *Template* as plasmid DNA or oligonucleotide (can be pre-complexed with RNP) (in some protocols nuclease(s) are delivered as mRNA, protein, or RNP by a nonviral method, most often electroporation, and template DNA is delivered separately by a viral vector, before or after delivery of the nuclease)	All components are assembled with a glyco/lipo-polymer vehicle that favors cell entry; the complex is applied to cells ex vivo or injected into a tissue or blood in vivo.	Relatively simple; can deliver all editing machinery together; transient expression limiting cytotoxicity and immunogenicity of editing machinery.	Cellular uptake and nuclear access can be rate-limiting; vehicle can cause cytotoxicity and inflammation in vivo; for in vivo delivery RNA needs to be modified for improved stability; cannot be targeted to specific tissues; formulation often proprietary.	Cell lines and some primary cells ex vivo

continued

TABLE A-1 Continued

Method	Delivered Component	Explanation	Advantages	Disadvantages	Preferred Applications
Nanoparticle		The complex, as above, is coupled to a nanoparticle (i.e., by gold, dextran) to enhance cellular uptake and delivery and biodistribution in vivo.	Cellular uptake can be enhanced; can be targeted to specific tissues; transient expression limiting cytotoxicity and potential immunogenicity of editing machinery.	Few	Tissues or systemic
Electroporation		A brief electric pulse is passed across a population of cells in a solution that contains the editing nuclease reagents with or without template.	Very effective method of delivery to a wide variety of cell types ex vivo; transient expression limiting cytotoxicity and potential immunogenicity of editing machinery.	Can cause cytotoxicity (increasingly from protein to mRNA to DNA; alleviated by using modified nucleic acids) but better tolerated than transfection; challenging to get delivery in vivo.	Cell lines and primary cells ex vivo
Squeeze Poration		A population of cells is passed through a small channel that is smaller than the diameter of the cells, creating small pores in the membrane to allow the nuclease and donor reagents to enter the cell.	New strategy that has not been widely validated.	Would not work for in vivo delivery.	

| Microinjection | Nuclease(s) as plasmid DNA, RNA, or protein; gRNA as plasmid DNA or RNA. The gRNA and nuclease can be pre-complexed as RNP. Template can be introduced as a plasmid, isolated DNA fragment, or oligonucleotide | The components can be introduced in a simple saline buffer, into the cytoplasm, or into the nucleus of cells or pronucleus of zygotes. | Efficiencies up to 100% | Technically more challenging than other methods, relatively few cells can be injected. | Zygotes and early embryos |

continued

TABLE A-1 Continued

Method	Delivered Component	Explanation	Advantages	Disadvantages	Preferred Applications
		Viral			
Lentiviral Vector (LV)	*Nuclease(s)* and *guideRNA* as gene expression cassettes delivered by the vector genome (can be driven by separate and tissue specific promoters) *Template DNA* (can be used for the delivery of template alone, in combination with electroporation of nuclease RNA, protein or RNP, or for the combined delivery of template and guideRNA and/or nuclease, on the same or separate vectors)	Replication-defective virus that can package ~8 kilobases of nucleic acid with an ability to enter almost all cell types; vector integrates quasi-randomly into cell genome, allowing for stable expression and transmission to the cell progeny; a modified version made with mutant integrase-defective lentiviral vector (IDLV), fails to integrate and is rapidly lost in proliferating cells.	Currently the most common tool for ex vivo gene transfer, also being explored for in vivo use; expression is stable for LV and transient for IDLV and can be made tissue-specific, regulated, or conditional; transduction of human cells well tolerated; IDLV provides for transient nuclease expression, thus limiting cytotoxicity and immunogenicity, and is well suited for template delivery.	Stable expression of nuclease by LV potentially leading to cytotoxicity and immunogenicity; potential risk of insertional mutagenesis by LV; vector manufacturing more complex and expensive than non-viral platform.	Cell lines and primary cells ex vivo

Adeno-Associated Virus (AAV) Vector	Replication-defective virus that can package ~4.7 kilobases of DNA with a broad number of variants (both natural and engineered serotypes) that can target different cell types.	Currently the most common tool for gene transfer in vivo; remains mostly episomal in the target cell nucleus; efficient delivery and robust expression in wide variety of cell types and tissues; transduction of human cells well tolerated; transient expression in dividing cells; well suited for nuclease and template delivery.	Limited capacity In non-proliferating cells and tissues, the vector can persist for years, leading to long-term expression of nuclease and potential cytotoxicity and immunogenicity; some people have pre-existing immunity to AAV, which can inhibit in vivo gene transfer or clear transduced cells.	Primary cells ex vivo and tissues or systemic in vivo
Adenoviral Vector	Replication-defective virus that can package >20 kilobases of DNA able to transduce a wide variety of cell types both ex vivo and in vivo.	Able to package large fragments of DNA; can be used for in vivo and ex vivo delivery; transient expression in dividing cells and tissues.	Has shown severe acute toxicity in some clinical trials; many people have pre-existing immunity; no longer commonly used gene therapy vector.	Primary cells ex vivo

NOTE: IDLV = integrase-defective lentiviral vector; RNP = ribonuclear protein complex; sgRNA = single guide RNA.

REFERENCES

Ahmed, E. A., P. de Boer, M. E. P. Philippens, H. B. Kal, and D. G. de Rooij. 2010. Parp1-XRCC1 and the repair of DNA double strand breaks in mouse round spermatids. *Mutation Research/Fundamental and Molecular Mechanisms of Mutagenesis* 683(1-2):84-90.

Auer, T. O., K. Duroure, A. De Cian, J. P. Concordet, and F. Del Bene. 2014. Highly efficient CRISPR/Cas9-mediated knock-in in zebrafish by homology-independent DNA repair. *Genome Research* 24(1):142-153.

Bacman, S. R., S. L. Williams, M. Pinto, S. Peralta, and C. T. Moraes. 2013. Specific elimination of mutant mitochondrial genomes in patient-derived cells by mitoTALENs. *Nature Medicine* 19(9):1111-1113.

Barrangou, R., C. Fremaux, H. Deveau, M. Richards, P. Boyaval, S. Moineau, D. A. Romero, and P. Horvath. 2007. CRISPR provides acquired resistance against viruses in prokaryotes. *Science* 315(5819):1709-1712.

Bibikova, M., D. Carroll, D. Segal, J. K. Trautman, J. Smith, Y. G. Kim, and S. Chandrasegaran. 2001. Stimulation of homologous recombination through targeted cleavage by chimeric nucleases. *Molecular and Cellular Biology* 21(1):289-297.

Bibikova, M., M. Golic, M., K. G. Golic, and D. Carroll. 2002. Targeted chromosomal cleavage and mutagenesis in *Drosophila* using zinc-finger nucleases. *Genetics* 161(3):1169-1175.

Bibikova, M., K. Beumer, J. K. Trautman, and D. Carroll. 2003. Enhancing gene targeting with designed zinc finger nucleases. *Science* 300(5620):764.

Brinster, R. L., H. Y. Chen, M. Trumbauer, A. W. Senear, R. Warren, and R. D. Palmiter. 1981. Somatic expression of herpes thymidine kinase in mice following injection of a fusion gene into eggs. *Cell* 27(1 Pt. 2):223-231.

Burt, A. 2003. Site-specific selfish genes as tools for the control and genetic engineering of natural populations. *Proceedings of The Royal Society B: Biological Sciences* 270(1518):921-928.

Burt, A. 2014. Heritable strategies for controlling insect vectors of disease. *Philosophical Transactions of the Royal Society B: Biological Sciences* 369(1645):20130432.

Carroll, D. 2014. Genome engineering with targetable nucleases. *Annual Review of Biochemistry* 83:409-439.

Chevalier, B. S., T. Kortemme, M. S. Chadsey, D. Baker, R. J. Monnat, and B. L. Stoddard. 2002. Design, activity, and structure of a highly specific artificial endonuclease. *Molecular Cell* 10(4): 895-905.

Chiarle, R., Y. Zhang, R. L. Frock, S. M. Lewis, B. Molinie, Y. J. Ho, D. R. Myers, V. W. Choi, M. Compagno, D. J. Malkin, D. Neuberg, S. Monti, C. C. Giallourakis, M. Gostissa, and F. W. Alt. 2011. Genome-wide translocation sequencing reveals mechanisms of chromosome breaks and rearrangements in B cells. *Cell* 147(1):107-119.

Cho, S. W., S. Kim, J. M. Kim, and J. S. Kim. 2013. Targeted genome engineering in human cells with the Cas9 RNA-guided endonuclease. *Nature Biotechnology* 31(3):230-232.

Cong, L., F. A. Ran, D. Cox, S. Lin, R. Barretto, N. Habib, P. D. Hsu, X. Wu, W. Jiang, L. A. Marraffini, and F. Zhang. 2013. Multiplex genome engineering using CRISPR/Cas systems. *Science* 339(6121):819-823.

Costantini, F., and E. Lacy. 1981. Introduction of a rabbit beta-globin gene into the mouse germ line. *Nature* 294(5836):92-94.

Cox, D. B. T., R. J. Platt, and F. Zhang. 2015. Therapeutic genome editing: Prospects and challenges. *Nature Medicine* 21(2):121-131.

Deltcheva, E., K. Chylinski, C. M. Sharma, K. Gonzales, Y. Chao, Z. A. Pirzada, M. R. Eckert, J. Vogel, and E. Charpentier. 2011. CRISPR RNA maturation by trans-encoded small RNA and host factor RNase III. *Nature* 471(7340):602-607.

Desjarlais, J. R., and J. M. Berg. 1992. Toward rules relating zinc finger protein sequences and DNA binding site preferences. *Proceedings of the National Academy of Sciences of the United States of America* 89(16):7345-7349.

Dickinson, D. J., J. D. Ward, D. J. Reiner, and B. Goldstein. 2013. Engineering the *Caenorhabditis elegans* genome using Cas9-triggered homologous recombination. *Nature Methods* 10(10):1028-1034.

Doetschman, T., R. G. Gregg, N. Maeda, M. L. Hooper, D. W. Melton, S. Thompson, and O. Smithies. 1987. Targeted correction of a mutant HPRT gene in mouse embryonic stem cells. *Nature* 330:576-578.

Doudna, J. A., and E. Charpentier. 2014. Genome editing: The new frontier of genome engineering with CRISPR-Cas9. *Science* 346(6213):1258096.

Eggan, K., S. Jurga, R. Gosden, I. M. Min, and A. J. Wagers. 2006. Ovulated oocytes in adult mice derive from non-circulating germ cells. *Nature* 441(7097):1109-1114.

Esvelt, K. M., A. L. Smidler, F. Catteruccia, and G. M. Church. 2014. Concerning RNA-guided gene drives for the alteration of wild populations. *eLife* e03401.

Evans, M. J., and M. H. Kaufman. 1981. Establishment in culture of pluripotential cells from mouse embryos. *Nature* 292(5819):154-156.

Friedland, A. E., Y. B. Tzur, K. M. Esvelt, M. P. Colaiacovo, G. M. Church, and J. Calarco. 2013. Heritable genome editing in *C. elegans* via a CRISPR-Cas9 system. *Nature Methods* 10(8):741-743.

Fu, Y., J. A. Foden, C. Khayter, M. L. Maeder, D. Reyon, J. K. Joung, and J. D. Sander. 2013. High-frequency off-target mutagenesis induced by CRISPR-Cas nucleases in human cells. *Nature Biotechnology* 31(9):822-826.

Gabriel, R., A. Lombardo, A. Arenas, J. C. Miller, P. Genovese, C. Kaeppel, A. Nowrouzi, C. C. Bartholomae, J. Wang, G. Friedman, M. C. Holmes, P. D. Gregory, H. Glimm, M. Schmidt, L. Naldini, and C. von Kalle. 2011. An unbiased genome-wide analysis of zinc-finger nuclease specificity. *Nature Biotechnology* 29(9):816-823.

Gammage, P. A., J. Rorbach, A. I. Vincent, E. J. Rebar, and M. Minczuk. 2014. Mitochondrially targeted ZFNs for selective degradation of pathogenic mitochondrial genomes bearing large-scale deletions or point mutations. *EMBO Molecular Medicine* 6(4):458-466.

Gantz, V., and E. Bier. 2015. The mutagenic chain reaction: A method for converting heterozygous to homozygous mutations. *Science* 348(6233):442-444.

Garneau, J. E., M. E. Dupuis, M. Villion, D. A. Romero, R. Barrangou, P. Boyaval, C. Fremaux, P. Horvath, A. H. Magadan, and S. Moineau. 2010. The CRISPR/Cas bacterial immune system cleaves bacteriophage and plasmid DNA. *Nature* 468(7320):67-71.

Gasiunas, G., R. Barrangou, P. Horvath, and V. Siksnys. 2012. Cas9-crRNA ribonucleoprotein complex mediates specific DNA cleavage for adaptive immunity in bacteria. *Proceedings of the National Academy of Sciences of the United States of America* 109(39):E2579-E2586.

Gilbert, L. A., M. H. Larson, L. Morsut, Z. Liu, G. A Brar, S. E. Torres, N. Stern-Ginossar, O. Brandman, E. H. Whitehead, J. A. Doudna, W. A. Lim, J. S. Weissman, and L. S. Qi. 2013. CRISPR-mediated modular RNA-guided regulation of transcription in eukaryotes. *Cell* 154(2):442-451.

Gilbert, L. A., M. A. Horlbeck, B. Adamson, J. E. Villalta, Y. Chen, E. H. Whitehead, C. Guimaraes, B. Panning, H. L. Ploegh, M. C. Bassik, L.S. Qi, M. Kampmann, and J. S. Weissman. 2014. Genome-scale CRISPR-mediated control of gene repression and activation. *Cell* 159(3):647-661.

Gordon, J. W., and F. H. Ruddle. 1981. Integration and stable germ line transmission of genes injected into mouse pronuclei. *Science* 214(4526):1244-1246.

Guilinger, J. P., D. B. Thompson, and D. R. Liu. 2014. Fusion of catalytically inactive Cas9 to FokI nuclease improves the specificity of genome modification. *Nature Biotechnology* 32(6):577-582.

Hammer, R. E., R. D. Palmiter, and R. L. Brinster. 1984. Partial correction of murine hereditary growth disorder by germ-line incorporation of a new gene. *Nature* 311(5981):65-67.

Haurwitz, R. E., S. H. Sternberg, and J. A. Doudna. 2012. Csy4 relies on an unusual catalytic dyad to position and cleave CRISPR RNA. *The EMBO Journal* 31(12):2824-2832.

Hayashi, K., H. Ohta, K. Kurimoto, S. Aramaki, and M. Saitou. 2011. Reconstitution of the mouse germ cell specification pathway in culture by pluripotent stem cells. *Cell* 146(4):519-532.

Hayashi, K., S. Ogushi, K. Kurimoto, S. Shimamoto, H. Ohta, and M. Saitou. 2012. Offspring from oocytes derived from in vitro primordial germ cell-like cells in mice. *Science* 338(6109):971-975.

Hayden, E. C. 2013. Regulators weigh benefits of "three-parent" fertilization. *Nature* 502(7471):284-285.

Hsu, P. D., D. A. Scott, J. A. Weinstein, F. A. Ran, S. Konermann, V. Agarwala, Y. Li, E. J. Fine, X. Wu, O. Shalem, T. J. Cradick, L. A. Marraffini, G. Bao, and F. Zhang. 2013. DNA targeting specificity of RNA-guided Cas9 nucleases. *Nature Biotechnology* 31(9):827-832.

Hwang, W. Y., Y. Fu, D. Reyon, M. L. Maeder, S. Q. Tsai, J. D. Sander, R. T. Peterson, J. R. Yeh, and J. K. Joung. 2013. Efficient genome editing in zebrafish using a CRISPR-Cas system. *Nature Biotechnology* 31(3):227-229.

Irie, N., L. Weinberger, W. W. Tang, T. Kobayashi, S. Viukov, Y. S. Manor, S. Dietmann, J. H. Hanna, and M. A. Surani. 2015. SOX17 is a critical specifier of human primordial germ cell fate. *Cell* 160(1-2):253-268.

Ishikura, Y., Y. Yabuta, H. Ohta, K. Hayashi, T. Nakamura, I. Okamoto, T. Yamamoto, K. Kurimoto, K. Shirane, H. Sasaki, and M. Saitou. 2016. *In Vitro Derivation and Propagation of Spermatogonial Stem Cell Activity from Mouse Pluripotent Stem Cells.* Cell Reports 17(10):2789-2804.

Jaenisch, R. 1976. Germ line integration and Mendelian transmission of the exogenous Moloney leukemia virus. *Proceedings of the National Academy of Sciences of the United States of America* 73(4):1260-1264.

Jaenisch, R., and B. Mintz. 1974. Simian virus 40 DNA sequences in DNA of healthy adult mice derived from preimplantation blastocysts injected with viral DNA. *Proceedings of the National Academy of Sciences of the United States of America* 71(4):1250-1254.

Jamieson, A. C., S. H. Kim, and J. A. Wells. 1994. In vitro selection of zinc fingers with altered DNA-binding specificity. *Biochemistry* 33(19):5689-5695.

Jiang, W., D. Bikard, D. Cox, F. Zhang, and L. A. Marraffini. 2013. RNA-guided editing of bacterial genomes using CRISPR-Cas systems. *Nature Biotechnology* 31(3):233-239.

Jinek, M., K. Chylinski, I. Fonfara, M. Hauer, J.A. Doudna, and E. Charpentier. 2012. A programmable dual-RNA-guided DNA endonuclease in adaptive bacterial immunity. *Science* 337(6096):816-821.

Jinek, M., A. East, A. Cheng, S. Lin, E. Ma, and J. Doudna. 2013. RNA-programmed genome editing in human cells. *eLife* 2:e00471.

Jinek, M., F. Jiang, D. W. Taylor, S. H. Sternberg, E. Kaya, E. Ma, C. Anders, M. Hauer, K. Zhou, S. Lin, M. Kaplan, A. T. Iavarone, E. Charpentier, E. Nogales, and J. A. Doudna. 2014. Structures of Cas9 endonucleases reveal RNA-mediated conformational activation. *Science* 343(6176):1247997.

Johnson, J., J. Canning, T. Kaneko, J. K. Pru, and J. L. Tilly. 2004. Germline stem cells and follicular renewal in the postnatal mammalian ovary. *Nature* 428(6979):145-150.

Jore, M. M., M. Lundgren, E. van Duijn, J. B. Bultema, E. R. Westra, S. P. Waghmare, B. Wiedenheft, Ü. Pul, R. Wurm, R. Wagner, M. R. Beijer, A. Barendregt, K. Zhou, A. P. L. Snijders, M. J. Dickman, J. A. Doudna, E. J. Boekema, A. J. R. Heck, J. van der Oost, and S. J. J. Brouns. 2011. Structural basis for CRISPR RNA-guided DNA recognition by Cascade. *Nature Structural & Molecular Biology* 18(5):529-536.

Joung, J. K., and J. D. Sander. 2013. TALENs: A widely applicable technology for targeted genome editing. *Nature Reviews Molecular Cell Biology* 14(1):49-55.

Kanatsu-Shinohara, M., and T. Shinohara. 2013. Spermatogonial stem cell self-renewal and development. *Annual Reviews Cell and Developmental Biology* 29:163-187.

Kang, X., W. He, Y. Huang, Q. Yu, Y. Chen, X. Gao, X. Sun, and Y. Fan. 2016. Introducing precise genetic modifications into human 3PN embryos by CRISPR/Cas-mediated genome editing. *Journal of Assisted Reproduction and Genetics* 33(5):581-588.

Kim, Y. G., J. Cha, and S. Chandrasegaran. 1996. Hybrid restriction enzymes: Zinc finger fusions to Fok I cleavage domain. *Proceedings of the National Academy of Sciences of the United States of America* 93(3):1156-1160.

Kleinstiver, B. P., V. Pattanayak, M. S. Prew, S. Q. Tsai, N. T. Nguyen, Z. Zheng, and J. K. Joung. 2016. High-fidelity CRISPR-Cas9 nucleases with no detectable genome-wide off-target effects. *Nature* 529(7587):490-495.

Komor, A. C., Y. B. Kim, M. S. Packer, J. A. Zuris, and D. R. Liu. 2016. Programmable editing of a target base in genomic DNA without double-stranded DNA cleavage. *Nature* 533(7603):420-424.

Konermann, S., M. D. Brigham, A. E. Trevino, J. Joung, O. O. Abudayyeh, C. Barcena, P. D. Hsu, N. Habib, J. S. Gootenberg, H. Nishimasu, O. Nureki, and F. Zhang. 2015. Genome-scale transcriptional activation by an engineered CRISPR-Cas9 complex. *Nature* 517(7536):583-588.

Kuehn, M., A. Bradley, E. Robertson, and M. Evans. 1987. A potential animal model for Lesch-Nyhan syndrome through introduction of HPRT mutations into mice. *Nature* 326(6110):295-298.

Latham, K. E., B. Patel, F. D. Bautista, and S. M. Hawes. 2000. Effects of X chromosome number and parental origin on X-linked gene expression in preimplantation mouse embryos. *Biology of Reproduction* 63(1):64-73.

Lavitrano, M., R. Giovannoni, and M. G. Cerrito. 2013. Methods for sperm-mediated gene transfer. In *Spermatogenesis: Methods and protocols*, Vol. 927, edited by D. Carrell and K. I. Aston. New York: Humana Press. Pp. 519-529.

Leeb, M., and A. Wutz. 2011. Derivation of haploid embryonic stem cells from mouse embryos. *Nature* 479(7371):131-134.

Li, W., L. Shuai, H. Wan, M. Dong, M. Wang, L. Sang, C. Feng, G.Z. Luo, T. Li, X. Li, L. Wang, Q. Y. Zheng, C. Sheng, H. J. Wu, Z. Liu, L. Liu, L. Wang, X. J. Wang, X. Y. Zhao, and Q. Zhou. 2012. Androgenetic haploid embryonic stem cells produce live transgenic mice. *Nature* 490(7420):407-411.

Li, W., F. Teng, T. Li, and Q. Zhou. 2013. Simultaneous generation and germline transmission of multiple gene mutations in rat using CRISPR-Cas systems. *Nature Biotechnology* 31(8):684-686.

Li, W., X. Li, T. Li, M. G. Jiang, H. Wan, G. Z. Luo, C. Feng, X. Cui, F. Teng, Y. Yuan, Q. Zhou, Q. Gu, L. Shuai, J. Sha, Y. Xiao, L. Wang, Z. Liu, X. J. Wang, X. Y. Zhao, and Q. Zhou. 2014. Genetic modification and screening in rat using haploid embryonic stem cells. *Cell Stem Cell* 14(3):404-414.

Liang, P., Y. Xu, X. Zhang, C. Ding, R. Huang, Z. Zhang, J. Lv, X. Xie, Y. Chen, Y. Li, Y. Sun, Y. Bai, Z. Songyang, W. Ma, C. Zhou, and J. Huang. 2015. CRISPR/Cas9-mediated gene editing in human tripronuclear zygotes. *Protein & Cell* 6(5):363-372.

Maeda, I., D. Okamura, Y. Tokitake, M. Ikeda, H. Kawaguchi, N. Mise, K. Abe, T. Noce, A. Okuda, and Y. Matsui. 2013. Max is a repressor of germ cell-related gene expression in mouse embryonic stem cells. *Nature Communications* 4:1754.

Mahon, K. A., P. A. Overbeek, and H. Westphal. 1988. Prenatal lethality in a transgenic mouse line is the result of a chromosomal translocation. *Proceedings of the National Academy of Sciences of the United States of America* 85(4):1165-1168.

Makarova, K. S., N. V Grishin, S. A Shabalina, Y. I. Wolf, and E. V. Koonin. 2006. A putative RNA-interference-based immune system in prokaryotes: Computational analysis of the predicted enzymatic machinery, functional analogies with eukaryotic RNAi, and hypothetical mechanisms of action. *Biology Direct* 1(1):7.

Mali, P., L. Yang, K. M. Esvelt, J. Aach, M. Guell, J. E. DiCarlo, J. E. Norville, and G. M. Church. 2013. RNA-guided human genome engineering via Cas9. *Science* 339(6121): 823-826.

Martin, G. R. 1981. Isolation of a pluripotent cell line from early mouse embryos cultured in medium conditioned by teratocarcinoma stem cells. *Proceedings of the National Academy of Sciences of the United States of America* 78(12):7634-7638.

Maruyama, T., S. K. Dougan, M. C. Truttmann, A. M. Bilate, J. R. Ingram, and H. L. Ploegh. 2015. Increasing the efficiency of precise genome editing with CRISPR-Cas9 by inhibition of nonhomologous end joining. *Nature Biotechnology* 33(5):538-542.

McCreath, K. J., J. Howcroft, K. H. Campbell, A. Colman, A. E. Schnieke, and A. J. Kind. 2000. Production of gene-targeted sheep by nuclear transfer from cultured somatic cells. *Nature* 405(6790):1066-1069.

Mojica, F. J. M., C. Diez-Villasenor, J. Garcia-Martinez, and E. Soria. 2005. Intervening sequences of regularly spaced prokaryotic repeats derive from foreign genetic elements. *Journal of Molecular Evolution* 60(2):174-182.

Naldini, L. 2015. Gene therapy returns to centre stage. *Nature* 526(7573):351-360.

Niu, Y., B. Shen, Y. Cui, Y. Chen, J. Wang, L. Wang, Y. Kang, X. Zhao, W. Si, W. Li, A. P. Xiang, J. Zhou, X. Guo, Y. Bi, C. Si, B. Hu, G. Dong, H. Wang, Z. Zhou, T. Li, T. Tan, X. Pu, F. Wang, S. Ji, Q. Zhou, X. Huang, W. Ji, and J. Sha. 2014. Generation of gene-modified cynomolgus monkey via Cas9/RNA-mediated gene targeting in one-cell embryos. *Cell* 156(4):836-843.

Orthwein, A., S. M. Noordermeer, M. D. Wilson, S. Landry, R. I. Enchev, A. Sherker, M. Munro, J. Pinder, J. Salsman, G. Dellaire, B. Xia, M. Peter, and D. Durocher. 2015. A mechanism for the suppression of homologous recombination in G1 cells. *Nature* 528(7582):422-426.

Oye, K. A., K. Esvelt, E. Appleton, F. Catteruccia, G. Church, T. Kuiken, S. B. Lightfoot, J. McNamara, A. Smidler, and J. P. Collins. 2014. Biotechnology: Regulating gene drives. *Science* 345(6197):626-628.

Paquet, D., D. Kwart, A. Chen, A. Sproul, S. Jacob, S. Teo, K. M. Olsen, A. Gregg, S. Noggle, and M. Tessier-Lavigne. 2016. Efficient introduction of specific homozygous and heterozygous mutations using CRISPR/Cas9. *Nature* 533(7601):125-129.

Paull, D., V. Emmanuele, K.A. Weiss, N. Treff, L. Stewart, H. Hua, M. Zimmer, D. J. Kahler, R. S. Goland, S. A. Noggle, R. Prosser, M. Hirano, M. V. Sauer, and D. Egli. 2012. Nuclear genome transfer in human oocytes eliminates mitochondrial DNA variants. *Nature* 493(7434):632-637.

Perez-Pinera, P., D. D. Kocak, C. M. Vockley, A. F. Adler, A. M. Kabadi, L. R. Polstein, P. T. Thakore, K. A. Glass, D. G. Ousterout, K. W. Leong, F. Guilak, G. E. Crawford, T. E. Reddy, and C. A. Gersbach. 2013. RNA-guided gene activation by CRISPR-Cas9-based transcription factors. *Nature Methods* 10(10):973-976.

Pourcel, C., G. Salvignol, and G. Vergnaud. 2005. CRISPR elements in *Yersinia pestis* acquire new repeats by preferential uptake of bacteriophage DNA, and provide additional tools for evolutionary studies. *Microbiology* 151(Pt. 3):653-663.

Qasim, W., H. Zhan, S. Samarasinghe, S. Adams, P. Amrolia, S. Stafford, K. Butler, C. Rivat, G. Wright, and K. Somana. 2017. Molecular remission of infant B-ALL after infusion of universal TALEN gene-edited CAR T cells. *Science Translational Medicine* 9(374):eaaj2013

Qi, L. S., M. H. Larson, L. A. Gilbert, J. A. Doudna, J. S. Weissman, A. P. Arkin, and W. A. Lim. 2013. Repurposing CRISPR as an RNA-guided platform for sequence-specific control of gene expression. *Cell* 152(5):1173-1183.

Ran, F. A., P. D. Hsu, C. Y. Lin, J. S. Gootenberg, S. Konermann, A. E. Trevino, D. A. Scott, A. Inoue, S. Matoba, Y. Zhang, and F. Zhang. 2013. Double nicking by RNA-guided CRISPR Cas9 for enhanced genome editing specificity. *Cell* 154(6):1380-1389.

Rebar, E. J., and C. O. Pabo. 1994. Zinc finger phage: Affinity selection of fingers with new DNA-binding specificities. *Science* 263(5147):671-673.

Reddy, P., A. Ocampo, K. Suzuki, J. Luo, S. R. Bacman, S. L. Williams, A. Sugawara, D. Okamura, Y. Tsunekawa, J. Wu, D. Lam, X. Xiong, N. Montserrat, C. R. Esteban, G. H. Liu, I. Sancho-Martinez, D. Manau, S. Civico, F. Cardellach, M. del Mar O'Callaghan, J. Campistol, H. Zhao, J. M. Campistol, C. T. Moraes, and J. C. I. Belmonte. 2015. Selective elimination of mitochondrial mutations in the germline by genome editing. *Cell* 161(3):459-469.

Reinhardt, K., D. K. Dowling, and E. H. Morrow. 2013. Medicine: Mitochondrial replacement, evolution, and the clinic. *Science* 341(6152):1345-1346.

Rouet, P., F. Smih, and M. Jasin. 1994. Introduction of double-strand breaks into the genome of mouse cells by expression of a rare-cutting endonuclease. *Molecular and Cellular Biology* 14(12):8096-8106.

Rubin, G. M., and A. C. Spradling. 1982. Genetic transformation of *Drosophila* with transposable element vectors. *Science* 218(4570):348-353.

Sagi, I., G. Chia, T. Golan-Lev, M. Peretz, U. Weissbein, L. Sui, M. V. Sauer, O. Yanuka, D. Egli, and N. Benvenisty. 2016. Derivation and differentiation of haploid human embryonic stem cells. *Nature* 532(7597):107-111.

Sakuma, T., and K. Woltjen. 2014. Nuclease-mediated genome editing: At the front-line of functional genomics technology. *Development, Growth & Differentiation* 56(1):2-13.

Sakurai, T., A. Kamiyoshi, H. Kawate, C. Mori, S. Watanabe, M. Tanaka, R. Uetake, M. Sato, and T. Shindo. 2016. A non-inheritable maternal Cas9-based multiple-gene editing system in mice. *Scientific Reports* 6:20011.

Sapranauskas, R., G. Gasiunas, C. Fremaux, R. Barrangou, P. Horvath, and V. Siksnys. 2011. The *Streptococcus thermophilus* CRISPR/Cas system provides immunity in *Escherichia coli*. *Nucleic Acids Research* 39(21):9275-9282.

Sander, J. D., and J. K. Joung. 2014. CRISPR-Cas systems for editing, regulating and targeting genomes. *Nature Biotechnology* 32(4):347-350.

Sasaki, K., S. Yokobayashi, T. Nakamura, I. Okamoto, Y. Yabuta, K. Kurimoto, H. Ohta, Y. Moritoki, C. Iwatani, H. Tsuchiya, S. Nakamura, K. Sekiguchi, T. Sakuma, T. Yamamoto, T. Mori, K. Woltjen, M. Nakagawa, T. Yamamoto, K. Takahashi, S. Yamanaka, and M. Saitou. 2015. Robust in vitro induction of human germ cell fate from pluripotent stem cells. *Cell Stem Cell* 17(2):178-194.

Schnieke, A., K. Harbers, and R. Jaenisch. 1983. Embryonic lethal mutation in mice induced by retrovirus insertion into the a1(I) collagen gene. *Nature* 304(5924):315-320.

Schwartzberg, P., S. Goff, and E. Robertson. 1989. Germ-line transmission of a c-Abl mutation produced by targeted gene disruption in ES cells. *Science* 246(4931):799-803.

Silva, G., L. Poirot, R. Galetto, J. Smith, G. Montoya, P. Duchateau, and F. Paques. 2011. Meganucleases and other tools for targeted genome engineering: Perspectives and challenges for gene therapy. *Current Gene Therapy* 11(1):11-27.

Slaymaker, I. M., L. Gao, B. Zetsche, D. A. Scott, W. X. Yan, and F. Zhang. 2016. Rationally engineered Cas9 nucleases with improved specificity. *Science* 351(6268):84-88.

Solter, D. 2006. From teratocarcinomas to embryonic stem cells and beyond: A history of embryonic stem cell research. *Nature Reviews Genetics* 7:319-327.

Staals, R. H., J. Y. Agari, S. Maki-Yonekura, Y. Zhu, D. W. Taylor, E. van Duijn, A. Barendregt, M. Vlot, J. J. Koehorst, K. Sakamoto, A. Masuda, N. Dohmae, P. J. Schaap, J. A. Doudna, A. J. R. Heck, K. Yonekura, J. van der Oost, and A. Shinkai. 2013. Structure and activity of the RNA-targeting Type III-B CRISPR-Cas complex of *Thermus thermophilus*. *Molecular Cell* 52(1):135-145.

Suzuki, A., M. Hirasaki, T. Hishida, J. Wu, D. Okamura, A. Ueda, M. Nishimoto, Y. Nakachi, Y. Mizuno, Y. Okazaki, Y. Matsui, J. C. I. Belmonte, and A. Okuda. 2016a. Loss of MAX results in meiotic entry in mouse embryonic and germline stem cells. *Nature Communications* 7:11056.

Suzuki, K., Y. Tsunekawa, R. Hernandez-Benitez, J. Wu, J. Zhu, E. J. Kim, F. Hatanaka, M. Yamamoto, T. Araoka, Z. Li, M. Kurita, T Hishida, M. Li, E. Aizawa, S. Guo, S. Chen, A. Goebl, R. D. Soligalla, J. Qu, T. Jiang, X. Fu, M. Jafari, C. R. Esteban, W. T. Berggren, J. Lajara, E. Nuñez-Delicado, P. Guillen, J. M. Campistol, F. Matsuzaki, G. H. Liu, P. Magistretti, K. Zhang, E. M. Callaway, K. Zhang, and J. C. Belmonte. 2016b. In vivo genome editing via CRISPR/Cas9 mediated homology-independent targeted integration. *Nature* 540:144-149.

Tachibana, M., P. Amato, M. Sparman, J. Woodward, D. M. Sanchis, H. Ma, N. M. Gutierrez, R. Tippner-Hedges, E. Kang, H. S. Lee, C. Ramsey, K. Masterson, D. Battaglia, D. Lee, D. Wu, J. Jensen, P. Patton, S. Gokhale, R. Stouffer, and S. Mitalipov. 2012. Towards germline gene therapy of inherited mitochondrial diseases. *Nature* 493(7434):627-631.

Tarkowki, A. K. 1977. In vitro development of haploid mouse embryos produced by bisection of one-cell fertilized eggs. *Journal of Embryology and Experimental Morphology* 38:187-202.

Taylor, R. W., and D. M. Turnbull. 2005. Mitochondrial DNA mutations in human disease. *Nature Reviews Genetics* 6(5):389-402.

Thomas, K., and M. Capecchi. 1987. Site directed mutagenesis by gene targeting in mouse embryo-derived stem cells. *Cell* 51(3):503-512.

Tsai, S. Q., and J. K. Joung. 2016. Defining and improving the genome-wide specificities of CRISPR-Cas9 nuclease. *Nature Reviews Genetics* 17(5):300-312.

Tsai, S. Q., N. Wyvekens, C. Khayter, J.A. Foden, V. Thapar, D. Reyon, M. J. Goodwin, M. J. Aryee, and J. K. Joung. 2014. Dimeric CRISPR RNA-guided FokI nucleases for highly specific genome editing. *Nature Biotechnology* 32(6):569-576.

Tsai, S. Q., Z. Zheng, N. T. Nguyen, M. Liebers, V. V. Topkar, V. Thapar, N. Wyvekens, C. Khayter, A. J. Iafrate, L. P. Le, M. J. Aryee, and J. K. Joung. 2015. GUIDE-seq enables genome-wide profiling of off-target cleavage by CRISPR-Cas nucleases. *Nature Biotechnology* 33(2):187-197.

Wakayama, T., A. C. Perry, M. Zuccotti, K. R. Johnson, and R. Yanagimachi. 1998. Full-term development of mice from enucleated oocytes injected with cumulus cell nuclei. *Nature* 394(6691):369-374.

Wan, H., Z. He, M. Dong, T. Gu, G. Z. Luo, F. Teng, B. Xia, W. Li, C. Feng, X. Li, T. Li, L. Shuai, R. Fu, L. Wang, X. J. Wang, X. Y. Zhao, and Q. Zhou. 2013. Parthenogenetic haploid embryonic stem cells produce fertile mice. *Cell Research* 23(11):1330-1333.

Wang, H., H. Yang, C. S. Shivalila, M. M. Dawlaty, A. W. Cheng, F. Zhang, and R. Jaenisch. 2013. One-step generation of mice carrying mutations in multiple genes by CRISPR/Cas-mediated genome engineering. *Cell* 153(4):910-918.

Wang, X., Y. Wang, X. Wu, J. Wang, Y. Wang, Z. Qiu, T. Chang, H. Huang, R. J. Lin, and J. K. Yee. 2015. Unbiased detection of off-target cleavage by CRISPR-Cas9 and TALENs using integrase-defective lentiviral vectors. *Nature Biotechnology* 33(2):175-178.

Wiedenheft, B., K. Zhou, M. Jinek, S. M. Coyle, W. Ma, and J. A. Doudna. 2009. Structural basis for DNase activity of a conserved protein implicated in CRISPR-mediated genome defense. *Structure* 17(6):904-912.

Wiedenheft, B., G. C. Lander, K. Zhou, M. M. Jore, S. J. J. Brouns, J. van der Oost, J. A. Doudna, and E. Nogales. 2011. Structures of the RNA-guided surveillance complex from a bacterial immune system. *Nature* 477(7365):486-489.

Wilmut, I., A. E. Schnieke, J. McWhir, A. J. Kind, and K. H. Campbell. 1997. Viable offspring derived from fetal and adult mammalian cells. *Nature* 385(6619):810-813.

Wu, Y., H. Zhou, X. Fan, Y. Zhang, M. Zhang, Y. Wang, Z. Xie, M. Bai, Q. Yin, D. Liang, W. Tang, J. Liao, C. Zhou, W. Liu, P. Zhu, H. Guo, H. Pan, C. Wu, H. Shi, L.Wu, F. Tang, and J. Li. 2015. Correction of a genetic disease by CRISPR-Cas9-mediated gene editing in mouse spermatogonial stem cells. *Cell Research* 25(1):67-79.

Yang, H., L. Shi, B. A. Wang, D. Liang, C. Zhong, W. Liu, Y. Nie, J. Liu, J. Zhao, X. Gao, D. Li, G. L. Xu, and J. Li. 2012. Generation of genetically modified mice by oocyte injection of androgenetic haploid embryonic stem cells. *Cell* 149(3):605-617.

Yang, H., H. Wang, C. S. Shivalila, A. W. Cheng, L. Shi, and R. Jaenisch. 2013. One-step generation of mice carrying reporter and conditional alleles by CRISPR/Cas-mediated genome engineering. *Cell* 154(6):1370-1379.

Zeng, H., S. Wen, W. Xu, Z. He, G. Zhai, Y. Liu, Z. Deng, and Y. Sun. 2015. Highly efficient editing of the actinorhodin polyketide chain length factor gene in Streptomyces coelicolor M145 using CRISPR/Cas9-CodA(sm) combined system. *Applied Microbiology and Biotechnology* 99(24):10575-10585.

Zetsche, B., J. S. Gootenberg, O. O. Abudayyeh, I. M. Slaymaker, K. S. Makarova, P. Essletzbichler, S. E. Volz, J. Joung, J. Van der Oost, A. Regev, E. V. Koonin, and F. Zhang. 2015. Cpf1 is a single RNA-guided endonuclease of a class 2 CRISPR-Cas system. *Cell* 163(3):759-771.

Zhou, Q., M. Wang, Y. Yuan, X. Wang, R. Fu, H. Wan, M. Xie, M. Liu, X. Guo, Y. Zheng, G. Feng, Q. Shi, X.Y. Zhao, J. Sha, and Q. Zhou. 2016. Complete meiosis from embryonic stem cell-derived germ cells in vitro. *Cell Stem Cell* 18(3):330-340.

Zijlstra, J., E. Li, F. Sajjadi, S. Subramani, and R. Jaenisch. 1989. Germ line transmission of a disrupted b2-microglobulin gene produced by homologous recombination in embryonic stem cells. *Nature* 342(6248):435-438.

B

International Research
Oversight and Regulations

T he governance of research and clinical trials using human genome editing is expected to draw on the foundation of international and national regulations, policies, and guidance that apply to other areas of clinical research and development, including other types of genetic technologies, stem cells, reproductive medicine, and research involving human embryos. This appendix provides further information on some of these systems. It is not meant to be comprehensive, but rather to provide perspectives on how issues are addressed in countries other than the United States.

PUBLIC CONSULTATION CAN FORM PART
OF A GOVERNANCE STRATEGY

There are numerous examples around the world of the use of public consultation on a wide range of biomedical and environmental policies (see Box B-1 for two examples described in greater detail). In the United States, the National Environmental Policy Act is unusual among environmental laws, because rather than directly regulating action, it simply provides that when the government makes a major decision, it must be subjected to a higher than usual degree of public scrutiny. By incorporating public comment, such public scrutiny creates political pressure that can drive decisions in one way or another, and it allows for some interplay between government expertise/authority and public consultation. Canada, when it looked at assisted reproduction across many different forms, formed a royal commission on new reproductive technologies that traveled the country from east to west, holding public hearings on the topic. In the European Union

BOX B-1
Two Examples of Public Consultation

This box discusses examples from France and the United Kingdom in which public consultations have been undertaken on human application of emerging technologies. The consultative approaches have similarities and differences that may be informative as other countries consider how to address scientific and ethical issues associated with human genome editing.

In France, a General Public Discussion ("Les états généraux de la bioéthique") was organized prior to the 2009 revision of French Bioethics Laws. In addition to institutional reports and an interactive website, the consultation included three "Consensus Conferences" on bioethical issues, including embryo research and access to new reproductive technologies. A representative sample of 25 citizens was chosen using an opinion-poll method to participate in each conference. These participants attended weekend seminars and received instruction on the issues by a multidisciplinary team of experts. The citizens were also invited to a public debate where topical experts answered their questions. At the end of the process, each group of citizens drafted recommendations that were synthesized in the consultation's final report. Criticisms raised after the consultation included an impression that few citizen recommendations were incorporated in subsequent legal revisions and that the revisions did not address some of the social concerns raised by citizen panels. On the other hand, the consultative process provided an opportunity to broaden participation in the revision of the bioethics law, which was first implemented in 1994, based largely on recommendations of a national bioethics committee that consisted of experts such as doctors, biomedical researchers,

(EU), genetically engineered foods are of special interest, and an EU directive requires public access to information whenever a product potentially affects biodiversity or other environmental elements. Public consultation is considered an alternative to a directive centralized form of governance, in which the public can, through its own decentralized processes, exert pressure on government or on industry and alter the direction or the speed of biotechnology innovation (Charo, 2016b).

VOLUNTARY REGULATION THROUGH GUIDELINES IS ANOTHER COMPONENT OF GOVERNANCE

Beyond consultation are voluntary self-regulation and nonbinding agreements. These are self-imposed rules that are seriously constraining with respect to donation of tissues, recruitment of donors, and experimentation that raises concerns, such as the use of chimeras. Examples include the guidelines adopted by the International Society for Stem Cell Research, philosophers, and representatives of religious denominations. Social values raised by consulted citizens, such as the desire for children to know their history or for a committed couple to access reproductive technologies regardless of sexual orientation, also had the opportunity to be expressed in an official forum, covered by the media, and to contribute to subsequent public discussions.

More recently, the United Kingdom undertook consultations on mitochondrial replacement therapy, following a 2008 revision of the Human Fertilisation and Embryology Act. Public workshops and debates and interactive websites focused on ethical issues the use of mitochondrial techniques might raise and whether such techniques should be permitted for use in clinical practice in the United Kingdom. The balance of views from this exercise, reported in 2013, was that such treatment techniques should be allowed but that their use should be carefully controlled. Further consultation was undertaken in 2014 on draft regulations. To ensure a large audience, a range of organizations was solicited, including patient groups, professional bodies, research bodies, genetic interest groups, and faith and community organizations, as well as individuals. A number of responses (1,857) were received from interested parties as well as from a number of individuals giving their views on the draft regulations. In comparison to the French process, the HFEA process included multisite public forums and a larger number of citizens providing input, as well as more focused recommendations due to the single-issue consultation. On the other hand, criticisms levied included that the processes and modalities were rule-guided rather than based on dialogue and deliberation, and that there was a lack of identifiable links between the consultation and the ultimate legislative outcome.

which have been amended to cover all forms of embryo research, from basic science to clinical trials with stem cells (ISSCR, 2016). Guidance also comes in the form of persuasive, albeit unenforceable, international instruments, such as those issued by the Council for International Organizations of Medical Sciences (CIOMS) for global standards for human subjects research (Gallagher et al., 2000).

At the far end of the spectrum, of course, there is regulation and legislation. Specifically with respect to gene therapy and germline manipulation, there are a number of international instruments of varying degrees of enforceability. For example, the Council of Europe's Oviedo Convention says that predictive genetic tests should be used only for medical purposes. It specifically calls for a prohibition on the use of genetic engineering of the germline or changing the makeup of the following generations. It builds on earlier European conventions, but like many international instruments, it is not ratified by every member country and, even when ratified, does not necessarily get implemented with domestic legislation. It has great normative value, but its enforcement-level value is uneven.

REGULATORY APPROACHES VARY BY COUNTRY

According to one recent review of gene-transfer trial information from regulatory and other sources, as of June 2012 more than 1,800 trials have been approved, initiated, or completed in 31 countries (Ginn et al., 2013; IOM, 2014). By mid-2016 that number had grown to more than 2,400, with trials primarily located in the Americas and Europe but nonetheless ongoing on every populated continent, and the number of studies generally growing every year.[1] The 2013 review reported that 65.1 percent of the trials were based in the Americas, 28.3 percent in Europe, and 3.4 percent in Asia. Data from 2015 and 2016 show a similar pattern. Because more than half of all trials (63.7 percent, or 1,174) are associated with U.S. investigators or institutions (Ginn et al., 2013), U.S. regulations that govern research funded by the National Institutes of Health (NIH) or subject to the NIH rules due to a federal-wide assurance will have some effect on how the work proceeds outside the United States. The U.S. Food and Drug Administration (FDA) rules will also apply for products for which FDA approval is sought so that sale can proceed in the United States, regardless of funding source or whether the trial site is in the United States or abroad.

Countries approach the structure of their regulatory pathways in different ways. Japan has a regulatory pathway that tries to identify prospectively those things that are going to be high, medium, or low risk, and regulate them accordingly. The United States follows a similar process in its regulation of medical devices. But for drug regulation, the United States treats everything ab initio as equally dangerous and runs every proposed drug through the same rules for testing safety and efficacy. By contrast, in Japan there is an initial determination about the level of risk that is likely to be present for each proposed drug and the degree of stringency that the regulatory process must apply as a result. Japan has also added a conditional approval pathway specifically for regenerative medicine and gene therapy products, but it is too new for evaluation (Charo, 2016b).

Singapore also has a risk-based approach similar to Japan's, and for cell therapy it uses variables that include whether the manipulation is substantial or minimal, whether or not the intended use is homologous or nonhomologous, and whether or not this is going to be combined with some drug, device, or other biologic.

---

[1]Gene Therapy Clinical Trials Worldwide, provided by the *Journal of Gene Medicine*. http://www.abedia.com/wiley/years.php (accessed January 30, 2017).

Brazil provides an example of regulation and governance by accretion. It has approved laws related specifically to genetically engineered foods and stem cell research and cell therapy, but they are layered on top of earlier, more general rules, including constitutional prohibitions on the sale of any kind of human tissue and 1996 laws on the patenting of human biological materials, creating a situation of confusion. The result has been a degree of paralysis while the interplay among the laws is being managed.

More generally, discourse in Latin America on human somatic cell genome editing has been informed by concerns about genetically modified plants and animals, biopiracy, biosecurity, and use of stem cells for clinical care. Mexico addresses genetic engineering in the context of GMOs and biosecurity in its general health law and in its research regulations.[2] Brazil addresses gene editing in its Biosafety Law, implicitly permitting at least some somatic gene-editing research in humans, although its primary focus is clearly on GMOs.[3] Similarly, Ecuador's Constitution has provisions addressing genomic heritage in the setting of GMOs and biopiracy, and in its guarantee of personal integrity it prohibits the use of genetic material for scientific research in violation of human rights.[4]

A few jurisdictions in Latin America have explicitly addressed somatic genome editing, typically imposing restrictions aimed at prohibiting uses that might be perceived as "enhancement" rather than treatment or prevention of disease and injury. Chile states that gene editing "in somatic cells will be authorized only for the treatment of diseases or to prevent their occurrence" in a far-reaching law that also addresses intellectual property, discrimination, and protection of genetic identity, as well as prohibiting "eugenic practices" (with an exception for genetic counseling).[5] In Panama and Mexico City, use of genetic manipulation except for the elimination or treatment of a serious defect or disease is punishable by a prison sentence of 2 to 6 years.[6] Colombia's penal code similarly permits genetic modification

---

[2]Ley General de Salud, Titulo Decimo Segundo. Capitulo XII, Artículo 282. And Reglamento de la Ley General de Salud en Materia de Investigacíon para la Salud, Titulo Cuarto, Capitulo II, Articulos 85-88 (recombinant DNA research).

[3]Public Law No. 11.105, Chapter 1, Article 6, as translated by WIPO.

[4]Constitución de la Republica del Ecuador 2008, Titulo II, Articulo 66, 1.3(d). Interestingly, Ecuador promulgated an extensive set of regulations governing the use of biological samples and genomic data, specifically citing, inter alia, the biopiracy of DNA from an indigenous population in that country. Ministero de Salud Pública (MSP), Reglamento para uso del material genético humano en Ecuador. Ministereo de Salud Pública, Dirección Nacional de Noamrtización y Programa Nacional de Genética, 2013.

[5]Public Law No. 20.120 On the Scientific Investigation of the Human Genome, Its Genoma, & Prohibition of Human Cloning, Articles 1, 3, 4, 7, 8, 12, and 13, 2006 (English translation).

[6]Ley Penal en General. Capítulo II, Artículo 145. (2010); Código Penal para el Distrito Federal. Capítulo II, Artículo 154 (also bars employment and other benefits this period).

for treatment, diagnosis, and research to alleviate suffering or improve human health, while imposing a prison sentence of 1 to 5 years for other uses.[7]

In the European Union, the European Medicines Agency (EMA) has the responsibility to evaluate and supervise human and veterinary medicines to protect public and animal health (EMA, 2013). In 2007, the EMA established the Committee for Advanced Therapies as the unit responsible for assessing the quality, safety, and efficacy of medicines made from genes and cells—medicines that are termed "advanced therapy medicinal products." This committee provides a centralized procedure for the assessment and approval of medicines for marketing in the European Union. The process is mandatory for biologics, including gene and cell therapy products, and a number of other product categories, including medicines for the treatment of HIV/AIDS and cancer (Cichutek, 2008).

The EMA, however, does not have authority to review and approve protocols for clinical research, including gene-transfer research (Pignatti, 2013). That authority resides with national regulatory agencies, but every EU state has adopted the EU Directive on Clinical Trials (Kong, 2004). It requires member states to adopt a system for the review of clinical research consistent with internationally recognized standards for good clinical practice for the ethical and scientifically valid design, conduct, and report of trials (Kong, 2004). The FDA, which participated in the international process for developing these standards, also recognizes these standards and publishes them as guidance documents (FDA, 2012).[8]

As with Europe, China has a regulatory framework for the development and use of human medical products. Although it is not yet amended to address genome editing specifically, frameworks governing gene and cell therapies have been implemented and the State Food and Drug Administration (the predecessor of the current China Food and Drug Administration [CFDA]) approved a gene therapy product for marketing. In addition, regulatory guidelines for human embryo research and in vitro fertilization (IVF) practices have been published by Chinese agencies (China Ministry of Health, 2001, 2003). Within the current regulatory framework, human somatic cell genome editing may be considered a third category therapeutic technology rather than a drug. If so, it would be regulated by CFDA, and procedures would include evaluations for safety and efficacy through preclinical testing and clinical trials, similar to processes used by the FDA and EMA. In addition to CFDA, the Health and Family Planning Commission

---

[7]Código Penal Colombiano, Capítulo Octavo, Artículo 132 (2015).

[8]Information on the national regulatory frameworks likely to apply to somatic and germline human genome editing in a number of European countries is described in a background document produced for a 2016 workshop on human genome editing in the EU. http://acmedsci. ac.uk/file-download/41517-573f212e2b52a.pdf (accessed January 30, 2017).

(HFPC), which regulates IVF clinics, is likely to be involved in oversight of human genome editing. Consultations would likely occur with agencies such as the Ministry of Science and Technology, Chinese Academy of Sciences, Chinese Academy of Medical Sciences, and Chinese Academy of Engineering to enable their positions to be incorporated into regulations.

HERITABLE GENETIC MODIFICATIONS
RAISE ADDITIONAL ISSUES

A number of special regulatory and governance issues may arise around use of human embryos and the potential for genetic changes to be made to the human germline. Discussions of such issues have been informed by debates about topics such as embryonic stem cells, cloning assisted reproductive technologies, and the beginning of life.

As noted above, the Convention for the protection of Human Rights and Dignity of the Human Being with regard to the Application of Biology and Medicine: Convention on Human Rights and Biomedicine ("Oviedo Convention") develops principles concerning a number of medical topics that raise bioethics issues. For countries that have signed and ratified the treaty, the genetic constitution of the individual is to be protected against unlawful interventions seeking to modify the germline. A number of countries have also enacted national laws, regulations, or guidelines that restrict human germline modifications (see Figure B-1).

INTERNATIONAL COOPERATION ON THE GOVERNANCE
OF HUMAN GENOME EDITING IS DESIRABLE ALTHOUGH
FORMAL REGULATORY HARMONIZATION SEEMS INFEASIBLE

Given the global nature of scientific and medical advances and the diversity and complexity of approaches to regulating human genetic technologies, there have been calls for international collaboration, cooperation, and even harmonization of regulations governing human genome editing. Arguments can be made both for and against an international convergence of national regulation of genomic technologies (Breggin et al., 2009; Marchant et al., 2012). A compelling argument for creating uniform or consistent regulations of gene editing is to avoid "regulatory havens" that circumvent restrictions if providers or consumers travel to jurisdictions with more lenient or non-existent regulations in order to undertake the restricted procedures (Charo, 2016a). The potential for lucrative medical tourism may create a "race to the bottom" that encourages laxer standards in nations seeking revenues from medical tourism (Abbott et al., 2010). Consistent standards may also promote equal health protection for citizens of all nations and provide consistent requirements for companies and sci-

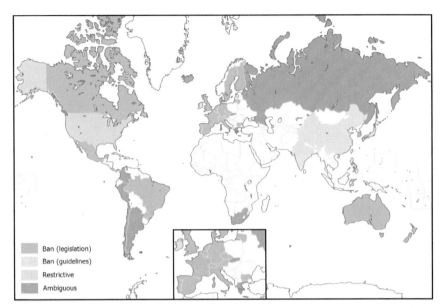

FIGURE B-1 Countries take varying approaches to the regulation of human heritable germline modifications. The countries in red have enacted legal prohibitions on germline modification, while those in pink prohibit such modification through recommendations or guidelines. Countries in grey have varying levels of regulation, with light grey representing restrictive and dark grey representing ambiguous regulations.
SOURCE: Araki and Ishii, 2014.

entists in the field, reducing transaction costs and increasing economies of scale (Vogel, 1998). Harmonized standards also provide economies of scale for regulators, reduce administrative costs in adopting and administering national laws, and increase opportunities to share regulatory resources and workload. Finally, the process of harmonization can promote the exchange of good practices and build regulatory capacity (OECD, 2013).

On the other hand, nations have different historical, economic, social, and cultural systems and values, which may translate into different approaches to the regulation of a powerful technology such as human genome editing. Uniform national regulations may also subject every nation to the lowest common regulatory denominator, depending on how harmonization is achieved. As a practical matter, reaching consensus among 100 or more nations on regulatory requirements for any technology is a laborious and resource-intensive undertaking that in the end may not be successful. Diversity in regulatory approaches also provides a natural experiment to evaluate

TABLE B-1 Three General Approaches to International Regulatory Convergence

Convergence Process	Definition	Example
Transnational Regulatory Dialogue and Networking	Informal process of communication and policy learning between regulators	International Dialogue on Responsible Nanotechnology
International Coordination/Cooperation	Nonbinding international instruments such as guidelines, principles, and standards	ISSCR Guidelines for Embryonic Stem Cell Research
Treaty-Based Harmonization	Formal negotiation of binding treaties	United Nations Convention on Cloning (failed)

SOURCE: Adapted from Breggin et al. (2009). We are grateful to Chatham House, the Royal Institute of International Affairs, for permission to reproduce a figure from the work titled: *Securing the Promise of Nanotechnologies: Towards Transatlantic Regulatory Cooperation,* authored by Linda Breggin, Robert Falkner, Nico Jaspers, John Pendergrass, and Read Porter, 2009.

the effects of different regulatory frameworks, providing a "laboratory of nations" that "fosters innovation and rapid learning about the impact of striking different balances between innovation and precaution" (Evans, 2015). However, realizing this benefit requires procedures that facilitate the exchange of information and promote learning.

As summarized in Table B-1, there is a continuum of approaches to aligning national regulatory requirements (Breggin et al., 2009). Harmonization usually involves the enforcement of identical or equivalent regulatory requirements under the national laws of participating countries. Harmonization is usually accomplished through an international treaty or other formal and binding legal instrument, implemented through the amendment of national laws to conform to treaty requirements (OECD, 2013). International treaties and other formal agreements are difficult and time consuming to negotiate, and often present difficult enforcement issues.[9] Given these obstacles, there has been a trend away from treaties in the international governance of technologies and products in favor of mechanisms of international cooperation and coordination (Falkner, 2013; Susskind, 2008).

Informal mechanisms of international coordination and cooperation do not create legal requirements to implement specific provisions, but

---

[9]An example of the challenges associated with negotiating and enforcing treaties was the unsuccessful attempt through the United Nations system in the early 2000s to create a binding international treaty banning human cloning (Cameron and Henderson, 2008).

rather provide general agreement between governments in the form of non-binding guidelines, recommendations, consensus documents, statements of principles, or voluntary standards. Such normative guidelines may be agreed upon in free-standing negotiations, but are often negotiated within an appropriate international organization (Abbott, 2014). International cooperation and coordination approaches can also be achieved through nongovernmental organizations, such as scientific societies, for example through the International Society for Stem Cell Research (ISSCR) Guidelines for Embryonic Stem Cell Research (Daley et al., 2007).

The least formal mechanism of international convergence is policy diffusion through transnational regulatory dialogue and networking. This approach usually does not involve the creation of instruments that set forth specific substantive or procedural recommendations for nations to follow. Rather, it provides a forum for regulators from different nations to share information, approaches, challenges, and ideas. An example is the International Dialogue on Responsible Nanotechnology, in which experts from 25 national governments convened in a series of meetings every 2 years to report on their regulatory activities and challenges (Meridian Institute, 2004). Regulators who have been involved in international coordination activities state that such person-to-person contacts and communications provide one of the most effective mechanisms for promoting international cooperation and understanding (Saner and Marchant, 2015).

A convergence of regulatory approaches for human genome editing would have some beneficial effects as described above, but countries have already adopted diverse laws relevant to human genome editing and a formal or complete harmonization does not seem feasible—and may not even be entirely desirable—at this time. Moreover, national responses to human genome editing reflect unique historical, cultural, economic, and social factors. Notwithstanding these important differences that prevent uniform international standards, there are important benefits for providing for robust communication and coordination between regulators in different countries, and potential opportunities for identifying common ground on specific substantive or technical aspects as well as opportunities to produce learning benefits (e.g., Zhai et al., 2016).

REFERENCES

Abbott, K. W. A. 2014. International organisations and international regulatory co-operation: Exploring the links. In *International regulatory co-operation and international organisations: The Cases of the OECD and the IMO*. Paris: OECD Publishing. Pp. 17-44.

Abbott, K. W. A., D. J. Sylvester, and G. E. Marchant. 2010. Transnational regulation: Reality or romanticism? In *International handbook on regulating nanotechnologies*, edited by G. Hodge, D. Bowman, and A. Maynard. Cheltenham, UK: Edward Elgar Publishing. Pp. 525-544.

Araki, M., and T. Ishii. 2014. International regulatory landscape and integration of corrective genome editing into in vitro fertilization. *Reproductive Biology and Endocrinology* 12:108. http://www.rbej.com/content/12/1/108 (accessed January 25, 2017).

Breggin, L., R. Falkner, N. Jaspers, J. Pendergrass, and R. Porter. 2009. *Securing the promise of nanotechnologies: Towards transatlantic regulatory cooperation.* London, UK: Chatham House. https://www.chathamhouse.org/sites/files/chathamhouse/public/Research/Energy,%20Environment%20and%20Development/r0909_nanotechnologies.pdf (accessed November 7, 2016).

Cameron, N. M. de S., and A.V. Henderson. 2008. Brave new world at the General Assembly: The United Nations Declaration on Human Cloning. *Minnesota Journal of Law, Science and Technology* 9(1):145-238.

Charo, R. A. 2016a. On the road (to a cure?): Stem-cell tourism and lessons for gene editing. *New England Journal of Medicine* 374(10):901-903.

Charo, R. A. 2016b. The legal and regulatory context for human gene editing. *Issues in Science and Technology* 32(3). http://issues.org/32-3/the-legal-and-regulatory-context-for-human-gene-editing (accessed November 7, 2016).

China Ministry of Health (People's Republic of China Ministry of Health). 2001. *Guidelines on human assisted reproductive technologies* [in Chinese]. http://go.nature.com/1ztc8qb (accessed November 7, 2016).

China Ministry of Health (People's Republic of China Ministry of Health). 2003. *Guidelines on human embryonic stem cell research.* http://www.cncbd.org.cn/News/Detail/3376 (accessed November 7, 2016).

Cichutek, K. 2008. Gene and cell therapy in Germany and the EU. *Journal fur Verbraucherschutz und Lebensmittelsicherheit* 3(Suppl. 1):73-76.

Daley, G. Q., L. Ahrlund-Richter, J. M. Auerbach, N. Benvenisty, R. A. Charo, G. Chen, H. K. Deng, L. S. Goldstein, K. L. Hudson, I. Hyun, S. C. Junn, J. Love, E. H. Lee, A. McLaren, C. L. Mummery, N. Nakatsuji, C. Racowsky, H. Rooke, J. Rossant, H. R. Scholer, J. H. Solbakk, P. Taylor, A. O. Trounson, I. L. Weissman, I. Wilmut, J. Wu, and L. Zoloth. 2007. The ISSCR guidelines for human embryonic stem cell research. *Science* 315:603-604.

EMA (European Medicines Agency). 2013. *Legal foundation.* http://www.ema.europa.eu/ema/index.jsp?curl=pages/about_us/general/general_content_000127.jsp&mid=WC0b01ac0580029320 (accessed January 25, 2017).

Evans, B. J. 2015. *Panel: Governance at the institutional and national levels: National regulatory frameworks.* Presentation at International Summit on Gene Editing, Washington, DC, December 2.

Falkner, R. 2013. The crisis of environmental multilateralism: A liberal response. In *The green book: New Directions for liberals in government*, edited by D. Brack, P. Burall, N. Stockley, and M. Tuffrey. London, UK: Biteback Publishing. Pp. 347-358.

FDA (U.S. Food and Drug Administration). 2012. *Vaccine, blood, and biologics: SOPP 8101.1: Scheduling and conduct of regulatory review meetings with sponsors and applicants.* Rockville, MD: FDA. http://www.fda.gov/BiologicsBloodVaccines/GuidanceComplianceRegulatoryInformation/ProceduresSOPPs/ucm079448.htm (accessed January 25, 2017).

Gallagher, J., S. Gorovitz, and R. J. Levine. 2000. *Biomedical research ethics: Updating international guidelines: A consultation.* Geneva, Switzerland: Council for International Organizations of Medical Sciences (CIOMS). http://www.cioms.ch/index.php/publications/available-publications/540/view_bl/61/bioethics-and-health-policy/3/biomedical-research-ethics-updating-international-guidelines-a-consultation?tab=getmybooksTab&is_show_data=1 (accessed November 7, 2016).

Ginn, S. L., I. E. Alexander, M. L. Edelstein, M. R. Abedi, and J. Wixon. 2013. Gene therapy clinical trials worldwide to 2012—An update. *Journal of Gene Medicine* 15(2):65-77.

IOM (Institute of Medicine). 2014. *Oversight and review of clinical gene transfer protocols: Assessing the role of the Recombinant DNA Advisory Committee.* Washington, DC: The National Academies Press.

ISSCR (International Society for Stem Cell Research). 2016. *Guidelines for stem cell research and clinical translation.* http://www.isscr.org/docs/default-source/guidelines/isscr-guidelines-for-stem-cell-research-and-clinical-translation.pdf?sfvrsn=2 (accessed November 7, 2016).

Kong, W. M. 2004. The regulation of gene therapy research in competent adult patients, today and tomorrow: Implications of EU directive 2001/20/EC. *Medical Law Review* 12(2):164-180.

Marchant, G. E., K. W. Abbott, D. J. Sylvester, and L. M. Gaudet. 2012. Transnational new governance and the international coordination of nanotechnology oversight. In *The nanotechnology challenge: Creating law and legal institutions for uncertain risks,* edited by D. A. Dana. Cambridge, UK: Cambridge University Press. Pp. 179-202.

Meridian Institute. 2004. *International dialogue on responsible research and development of nanotechnology.* Washington, DC: Meridian Institute. http://www.temas.ch/nano/nano_homepage.nsf/vwRes/SafetyAlexandria/$FILE/Final_Report_Responsible_Nanotech_RD_040812.pdf (accessed November 7, 2016).

OECD (Organisation for Economic Co-operation and Development). 2013. *International regulatory co-operation: Addressing global challenges.* Paris: OECD Publishing.

Pignatti, F. 2013. *Harmonizing across regions.* Presentation at Implementing a National Cancer Clinical Trials System for the 21st Century, Washington, DC, February 12.

Saner, M. A., and G. E. Marchant. 2015. Proactive international regulatory cooperation for governance of emerging technologies. *Jurimetrics* 55(2):147-178.

Susskind, L. 2008. Strengthening the global environmental treaty system. *Issues in Science and Technology* 25(1):60-68.

Vogel, D. 1998. Globalization of pharmaceutical regulation. *Governance* 11(1):1-22.

Zhai, X., V. Ng, and R. Lie. 2016. No ethical divide between China and the West in human embryo research. *Developing World Bioethics* 16(2):116-120.

C

Data Sources and Methods

The National Academy of Sciences and the National Academy of Medicine Committee on Human Gene Editing: Scientific, Medical, and Ethical Considerations was tasked with studying the scientific underpinnings of human gene-editing technologies—including human germline editing—and the clinical, ethical, legal, and social implications of their use. The committee also explored fundamental, underlying principles that could be adapted by any nation considering the development of guidelines for human gene editing. To respond comprehensively to its charge, the committee examined data from a variety of sources, including a review of the literature, open-session meetings and conference calls, public testimony and input, and other publicly available resources.

COMMITTEE COMPOSITION

The National Academies of Sciences, Engineering, and Medicine (the National Academies) appointed a committee of 22 experts to undertake the statement of task. The committee was composed of members with expertise in basic science, clinical research and medicine, law and regulation, ethics and religion, patient advocacy, science communication, public engagement, and the biomedical industry. Appendix D provides the biographical information for each committee member.

MEETINGS AND INFORMATION-GATHERING ACTIVITIES

The committee deliberated from December 2015 to January 2017 to conduct its assessment, and gathered information and data relevant to its statement of task by conducting a review of available literature, inviting stakeholders to share perspectives at public meetings, and soliciting public comments both online and in person.

Literature Review

Several strategies were used to identify literature relevant to the committee's charge. A search of bibliographic databases, including PubMed, Scopus, Web of Science, ProQuest Research Library, Medline, Embase, and LexisNexis, was conducted to obtain articles from peer-reviewed journals that discussed basic research, clinical applications, patient safety, scientific standards, ethics, oversight, and social issues associated with human gene editing. Staff reviewed recent news and literature to identify articles relevant to the committee's charge and created a database of references. In addition, committee members, speakers, sponsors, and other interested parties submitted articles, reports, and policy statements on these topics. The committee's database included several hundred relevant articles and reports, and was updated continuously throughout the study process.

Public Meetings

Four of the five meetings held over the course of the study included sessions in which committee members obtained input from a range of stakeholders and members of the public. Three meetings were held in Washington, DC (December 2015, February 2016, and July 2016), and one meeting was held in Paris, France, hosted by the French National Academy of Medicine (April 2016).

The committee's first meeting in December 2015 was held in association with the 3-day International Summit on Human Gene Editing: A Global Discussion, co-hosted by the U.S. National Academy of Sciences, U.S. National Academy of Medicine, Chinese Academy of Sciences, and The Royal Society of the United Kingdom. Although a separate ad hoc committee planned the summit, it provided a critical opportunity for the study committee to gather information. The summit convened experts from around the world to discuss scientific, ethical, and governance issues associated with human gene-editing research.[1]

---

[1]The list of speakers at the International Summit included Peter Braude, Annelien Bredenoord, Philip Campbell, Alta Charo, George Church, Ralph Cicerone, Chad Cowan, George Daley,

The committee's second meeting in February 2016 included perspectives from potentially affected stakeholder communities such as patient groups and representatives from companies developing gene editing–based therapeutics. It also featured presentations from experts on models for public engagement as well as federal and institutional oversight bodies.

The study's third meeting in April 2016, hosted by the French National Academy of Medicine in Paris, France, explored the principles underlying governance of gene editing. Speakers during the meeting provided international perspectives spanning permissive, neutral, precautionary, and preventive governance approaches. Meeting discussions also addressed potential therapeutic clinical applications for human germline gene editing. This meeting was held the day following a gene-editing workshop convened by the Federation of European Academies of Medicine, the U.K. Academy of Medical Sciences, and the French Academy of Medicine (FEAM, UKAMS, and ANM, 2017). A number of committee members were able to participate in the preceding FEAM workshop, which provided an important opportunity to learn further about gene-editing regulatory and governance concerns and strategies across the European community.[2]

Finally, the study's fourth meeting in July 2016 provided input on several of the social issues associated with human gene editing, including race and genetics in U.S. history and the intersection of moral views and public policy. The list of speakers who provided input to the committee in these meeting sessions is below.

Public Comments

The committee's data-gathering meetings also provided opportunities for the committee to engage and interact with a variety of stakeholders. Each public meeting included a public comment period, in which the committee invited input from any interested party. The committee also worked to make its activities as transparent and accessible as possible and to ac-

---

Marcy Darnovsky, Victor Dzau, Fola Esan, Barbara Evans, William Foster, Bärbel Friedrich, Hille Haker, John Harris, John Holdren, Rudolf Jaenisch, Weizhi Ji, Pierre Jouannet, J. Keith Joung, Daniel Kevles, Jonathan Kimmelman, Eric Lander, Ephrat Levy Lahad, Jinsong Li, Robin Lovell-Badge, Gary Marchant, Jennifer Merchant, Keymanthri Moodley, Indira Nath, Staffan Normark, Kyle Orwig, Pilar Ossorio, Duanquing Pei, Matthew Porteus, K. Vijay Raghavan, Klaus Rajewsky, Thomas Reiss, Janet Rossant, Ismail Serageldin, Bill Skarnes, John Skehel, Azim Surani, Sharon Terry, Adrian Thrasher, Fyodor Urnov, Marco Weinberg, Ernst-Ludwig Winnacker, Zhihong Xu, and Feng Zhang. Presentations and other materials from the Summit are available at http://nationalacademies.org/gene-editing/Gene-Edit-Summit/index.htm (accessed January 7, 2017).

[2]The formal report of the FEAM workshop is available at http://www.feam-site.eu/cms/docs/activities/humangenomeeditingworkshop2016report.pdf.

commodate those with special needs or those who may not have been able to attend in person.

The study website was updated regularly to reflect the recent and planned activities of the committee. Study outreach also included a study-specific email address for comments and questions and social media feeds and tags. A subscription to regular email updates was available to share further information and solicit additional comments and input to the committee.

Live video streams with closed captioning and links to an online public comment tool were provided throughout the course of the study to allow the opportunity for input from those unable to attend meetings in person. All online comments and submissions were catalogued in the study's public access file. Any information provided to the committee from outside sources or through the online comment tool is available by request through the National Academies' Public Access Records Office.

Speakers

The following individuals were invited speakers at data-gathering sessions of the committee:

Roberto Andorno, University of Zurich
Mónica López Barahona, Centro de Estudios Biosanitarios
Pierre Bégué, Académie Nationale de Médecine, France
Nick Bostrom, University of Oxford
Abby Bronson, Parent Project Muscular Dystrophy
Dominique Brossard, University of Wisconsin–Madison
Jacqueline Chin, National University of Singapore
Hans Clevers, Hubrecht Institute
Ronald Cole-Turner, Pittsburgh Theological Seminary
Francis Collins, National Institutes of Health
George William Foster, Congressman, IL-11
Søren Holm, University of Manchester
Rahman Jamal, National University of Malaysia
Bartha Knoppers, McGill University
Fredrik Lanner, Karolinska Institute
James Lawford-Davies, Hempsons Law Firm, United Kingdom
John Leonard, Intellia Therapeutics
Bruce Lewenstein, Cornell University
Andrew May, Caribou Biosciences
Vic Myer, Editas Medicine
Alondra Nelson, Columbia University
Erik Parens, Hastings Center

Guido Pennings, Ghent University, Belgium
Pearl O'Rourke, Partners HealthCare
Jackie Leach Scully, Newcastle University
Oliver Semler, University of Cologne
Trevor Thompson, Sickle Cell Foundation of Tennessee
Anna Veiga, Center of Regenerative Medicine, Barcelona, Spain
Thomas Voit, University College London
Elizabeth Vroom, United Parent Projects Muscular Dystrophy
Keith Wailoo, Princeton University
Michael Werner, Alliance for Regenerative Medicine
Nancy Wexler, Hereditary Disease Foundation
Bethan Wolfenden, Bento Bioworks
Carrie Wolinetz, National Institutes of Health
Philip Yeske, United Mitochondrial Disease Foundation
Xiaomei Zhai, Peking Union Medical College, China

D

Committee Member Biographies

R. Alta Charo, J.D. (*Co-Chair*), is a member of the National Academy of Medicine, and is the Warren P. Knowles Professor of Law and Bioethics and the Sheldon B. Lubar Distinguished Research Chair in Law at the University of Wisconsin–Madison, where she is on the faculties of the law and medical schools and teaches public health law, biotechnology regulation, and bioethics. She received her B.A. in biology from Harvard University and J.D. from Columbia University. Professor Charo was a member of President Obama's transition team, focusing on science policy, and from 2009 to 2011 was a senior policy advisor on emerging technology issues in the Office of the Commissioner at the U.S. Food and Drug Administration. Her other federal service includes the congressional Office of Technology Assessment, the U.S. Agency for International Development, the National Institutes of Health Human Embryo Research Panel, and President Clinton's National Bioethics Advisory Commission. At the National Academies of Sciences, Engineering, and Medicine she co-chaired (with Richard Hynes) the Committee on Guidelines for Embryonic Stem Cell Research and has been a member of the Board on Life Sciences; Board on Population Health and Public Health Practice; Committee on Science, Technology, and Law; and Board on Health Sciences Policy.

Richard O. Hynes, Ph.D. (*Co-Chair*), is Daniel K. Ludwig Professor for Cancer Research at the Massachusetts Institute of Technology (MIT) and an investigator at the Howard Hughes Medical Institute. He received his B.A. in biochemistry from the University of Cambridge, United Kingdom,

279

and his Ph.D. in biology from MIT in 1971. After postdoctoral work at the Imperial Cancer Research Fund in London, where he initiated his work on cell adhesion, he returned to MIT as a faculty member. Dr. Hynes is a fellow of The Royal Society of London, the American Academy of Arts and Sciences, and the American Association for the Advancement of Science, and is a member of the National Academy of Sciences and the National Academy of Medicine. He has received the Gairdner Foundation International Award for achievement in medical science and the Pasarow Award for Cardiovascular Research. He was previously associate head and then head of the Biology Department and served for 10 years as director of the MIT Center for Cancer Research. He was a governor of the Wellcome Trust U.K. from 2007 to 2016. At the National Academies he has previously co-chaired (with Jonathan Moreno and R. Alta Charo) committees on guidelines for human embryonic stem cell research.

David W. Beier, J.D., is a managing director of Bay City Capital and has been with the firm since 2013. He is a globally recognized leader in health care policy, pricing, intellectual property, government affairs, regulatory affairs, health care economics, and product commercialization. In addition, having spent two decades as part of the senior management teams for Amgen and Genentech, the two largest biotechnology companies in the world, he contributes invaluable perspective regarding strategy for entrepreneurial biotechs, the needs of potential acquirers, and the global health care industry in general. Mr. Beier served in the White House as the Chief Domestic Policy Advisor to Vice President Al Gore during the Clinton Administration. He has served as an appointee of President Clinton on his Advisory Committee for Trade Policy and Negotiations, on the Institute of Medicine panel on the Future of Health and Human Services, and as an advisor to the President's Council of Advisors on Science and Technology. Mr. Beier was also formerly a partner in the international law firm Hogan and Hartson and was formerly Counsel to the U.S. House of Representatives Committee on the Judiciary. He has testified before Congress and the Federal Trade Commission, has written numerous law review articles and technical legal works, is regularly invited to author expert op-eds on health care, and has contributed to books on topics ranging from intellectual property, trade, privacy, and justice issues. He currently serves as an appointee of Governor Brown on the California State Government Organization and the Economy Commission, as a fellow of the Center for Global Enterprise, and teaches as an adjunct lecturer at the Haas School of Business at the University of California, Berkeley. Mr. Beier received his J.D. from Albany Law School at Union University and his undergraduate degree at Colgate University. He is admitted to practice law in New York and the District of Columbia.

Ellen Wright Clayton, M.D., J.D., is an internationally respected leader in the field of law and genetics who holds appointments in both the law and medical schools at Vanderbilt University, where she also co-founded and directed the Center for Biomedical Ethics and Society. She has published 2 books and more than 150 scholarly articles and chapters in medical journals, interdisciplinary journals, and law journals on the intersection of law, medicine, and public health. In addition, she has collaborated with faculty and students throughout Vanderbilt and in many institutions around the country and the world on interdisciplinary research projects, and helped to develop policy statements for numerous national and international organizations. She currently chairs the Paediatric Platform of the international Public Population Program in Genomics. An active participant in policy debates, she has advised the National Institutes of Health as well as other federal and international bodies on an array of topics ranging from children's health to the ethical conduct of research involving human subjects. Professor Clayton has worked on a number of projects for the National Academy of Medicine, of which she is a member of the Executive Committee of its National Advisory Council, chair of the National Academies of Sciences, Engineering, and Medicine's Board on Population Health and Public Health Practice, and was chair of its committee to define myalgic encephalomyelitis/chronic fatigue syndrome. She is also a member of the National Academies' Report Review Committee. She is an elected fellow of the American Academy for the Advancement of Science.

Barry S. Coller, M.D., is the Physician in Chief, Vice President for Medical Affairs, David Rockefeller Professor of Medicine, and Head, Allen and Frances Adler Laboratory of Blood and Vascular Biology at The Rockefeller University. He is a leader in investigating platelet physiology, vascular biology, and adhesion phenomena in sickle-cell disease. He produced monoclonal antibodies that inhibit platelet aggregation and adhesion of sickle red blood cells to the blood vessel walls. He produced one of the earliest monoclonal antibodies to platelets and played a leading role in its development into a drug used to prevent thrombosis after coronary artery angioplasty and stent placement in humans. He has also identified mutations in genes that cause human bleeding disorders. Dr. Coller received the Pasarow Award in 2005, the Warren Alpert Foundation Award in 2001, and a National Research Achievement Award from the American Heart Association in 1998. He is a member of the National Academy of Medicine, the National Academy of Sciences, and the American Academy of Arts and Sciences. Dr. Coller is a past president of the American Society of Hematology and was founding president of the Society for Clinical and Translational Science. He currently serves on the National Academies of Sciences, Engineering, and Medicine's Board on Health Sciences Policy. Dr.

Coller received his B.A. from Columbia University in 1966 and his M.D. from the New York University School of Medicine in 1970. He completed his residency in internal medicine at Bellevue Hospital in New York City and received advanced training in hematology and clinical pathology at the National Institutes of Health. He was at Stony Brook University from 1976 to 1993, and from 1993 to 2001 he served as a professor of medicine and chairman of the Department of Medicine at Mount Sinai School of Medicine. Dr. Coller joined The Rockefeller University in 2001 and currently serves as principal investigator of the university's Clinical and Translational Science Award and director of The Rockefeller University Center for Clinical and Translational Science.

John H. Evans, Ph.D., is a professor of sociology at the University of California, San Diego. Dr. Evans earned his B.A. from Macalester College and his Ph.D. from Princeton University. He has been a postdoctoral fellow at Yale University and a visiting member of the Institute for Advanced Study in Princeton, New Jersey, and has held visiting professorial fellowships at the University of Edinburgh and the University of Muenster. His research concerns religion, culture, politics, and science. He has published a book about the ethical debates about human genetic engineering in the second half of the 20th century. Another book examines what religious people in the United States think about reproductive genetic technologies. A recent book concerns how societal views can be included in public bioethical debates about issues such as genetic modification. A forthcoming book examines what Americans think a human is, and how that relates to how we should treat each other. He is writing a book about what the relationship is between religion and science for American citizens. In addition to these books, Dr. Evans has written more than 40 articles and book chapters on topics in religion, culture, politics, and science.

Juan Carlos Izpisua Belmonte, Ph.D., is a professor in the Gene Expression Laboratory at the Salk Institute for Biological Studies in La Jolla, California since 1993. From 2005 to 2013 he was also director of the Center for Regenerative Medicine in Barcelona. Dr. Izpisua Belmonte's research interests are focused on the understanding of stem cell biology, organogenesis, regeneration, and aging. He has published more than 400 articles in internationally peer-reviewed journals and book chapters in these areas. The ultimate goal of his research is to translate it toward the development of cell- and gene-based therapies as well as new molecules for the treatment of human disease. Dr. Izpisua Belmonte graduated from the University of Valencia, Spain, with a bachelor's degree in pharmacy and science and a master's degree in pharmacology, and he received his Ph.D. from the University of Bologna, Italy, and the University of Valencia, Spain, in 1987. He completed his postdoctoral work at the European Molecular Biology Lab in Heidelberg, Germany, and at the University of California, Los Angeles.

Rudolf Jaenisch, M.D., is a founding member of the Whitehead Institute for Biomedical Research and professor of biology at the Massachusetts Institute of Technology. Dr. Jaenisch studies the epigenetic regulation of gene expression with the goal of efficiently changing one differentiated cell type into another. This has led to groundbreaking work with mammalian embryonic stem cells and adult cells that have been reprogrammed to an embryonic stem cell–like state, called induced pluripotent stem (iPS) cells. Dr. Jaenisch continues to push iPS cell methodology forward and has demonstrated iPS cells' therapeutic potential in models of sickle-cell anemia and Parkinson's disease. For his work, Dr. Jaenisch has been honored with the first Peter Gruber Foundation Award in Genetics, Brupracher Foundation Cancer Award, Cozzarelli Prize from the *Proceedings of the National Academy of Sciences of the United States of America*, Robert Koch Prize for Excellence in Scientific Achievement, Meira and Shaul G. Massry Prize, Ernst Schering Prize, Vilcek Prize, and Wolf Prize in Medicine, and is a recipient of the United States National Medal of Science. Dr. Jaenisch is a member of the National Academy of Sciences, a member of the National Academy of Medicine, and a fellow of the American Academy of Arts and Sciences.

Jeffrey Kahn, Ph.D., M.P.H., is the Andreas C. Dracopoulos Director of the Johns Hopkins Berman Institute of Bioethics. He is also Robert Henry Levi and Ryda Hecht Levi Professor of Bioethics and Public Policy, and Professor in the Department of Health Policy and Management in the Johns Hopkins Bloomberg School of Public Health. His research interests include the ethics of research, ethics and public health, and ethics and emerging biomedical technologies. He speaks widely both in the United States and abroad and has published 4 books and more than 125 articles in the bioethics and medical literature. He is an elected member of the National Academy of Medicine and a fellow of the Hastings Center, and he has chaired or served on committees and panels for the National Institutes of Health, the Centers for Disease Control and Prevention, and the Institute of Medicine/National Academy of Medicine. He is currently chair of the National Academies of Sciences, Engineering, and Medicine's Board on Health Sciences Policy. His education includes a B.A. from the University of California, Los Angeles, a Ph.D. from Georgetown University, and an M.P.H. from the Johns Hopkins Bloomberg School of Public Health.

Ephrat Levy-Lahad, M.D., is a professor of internal medicine and medical genetics at the Hebrew University of Jerusalem and director of the Medical Genetics Institute at Shaare Zedek Medical Center in Jerusalem, Israel. She

received her medical degree from the Hebrew University-Hadassah Medical
School in Jerusalem, and is board certified in internal medicine (Israel) and
in clinical genetics and clinical molecular genetics (Israel and the United
States). Dr. Levy-Lahad's clinical laboratory includes cancer genetics diagnostics and a large preimplantation diagnosis service. Her research laboratory focuses on the genetics of breast cancer, in particular the BRCA1 and
BRCA2 genes, and on genetic and environmental factors that affect the risk
associated with these mutations. She also studies the application of genetic
testing to population screening and large-scale prevention efforts. Another
focus of her research is elucidating the genetic basis of rare diseases, including discoveries of novel genes for neurological phenotypes and for defects
in ovarian development. Dr. Levy-Lahad is highly involved in bioethical
aspects of genetic research, and is currently co-chair of the Israel National
Bioethics Council. She is a member of Israel's National Council for Gynecology, Perinatal Medicine, and Genetics and the National Council for
Digital Health Innovation. Internationally, she was a member of the United
Nations Educational, Scientific and Cultural Organization's International
Bioethics Committee (2006-2009) and the International Society for Stem
Cell Research's Task Force on the Clinical Translation of Stem Cells.

Robin Lovell-Badge, Ph.D., is a senior group leader at The Francis Crick
Institute. Dr. Lovell-Badge has had longstanding interests in the biology of
stem cells, how genes work in the context of embryo development, and how
decisions of cell fate are made. Major themes of his current work include
sex determination, development of the nervous system and pituitary, and
the biology of stem cells within the early embryo. He is also very active in
both public engagement and policy work, notably around stem cells, genetics, human embryo and animal research, and in ways science is regulated
and disseminated. He is a co-opted member of the Human Fertilisation and
Embryology Authority's Scientific and Clinical Advances Advisory Committee and a member of its panel looking at the science and safety of ways to
avoid mitochondrial diseases. He was a member of the U.K. Academy of
Medical Sciences' committees on Interspecies-Embryos, Animals Containing Human Material, and a joint U.K. academies committee on Human
Enhancement and the Future of Work. He is also a member of the steering
committee of the Hinxton Group, the Royal Society's Public Engagement
Committee, and the U.K. Science Media Centre's Advisory Board. He was
elected a member of EMBO in 1993, a fellow of the Academy of Medical Sciences in 1999, and a fellow of The Royal Society in 2001. He has
received the Louis Jeantet Prize for Medicine in 1995, the Amory Prize,
awarded by the American Academy of Arts and Sciences, in 1996, the Feld-
berg Foundation Prize in 2008, and the Waddington Medal of the British
Society for Developmental Biology in 2010. He was also a distinguished

visiting professor at the University of Hong Kong from 2009 to 2015 and the president of the Institute of Animal Technologists. Dr. Lovell-Badge obtained his B.Sc. in zoology at the University College London in 1975 and his Ph.D. in embryology at the University College London in 1978.

Gary Marchant, J.D., Ph.D., is Regents' Professor and Lincoln Professor of Emerging Technologies, Law and Ethics at the Sandra Day O'Connor College of Law at Arizona State University (ASU). He is also a professor of life sciences at ASU and executive director of the ASU Center for the Study of Law, Science and Technology. Professor Marchant has a Ph.D. in genetics from the University of British Columbia, a masters of public policy degree from the Kennedy School of Government, and a law degree from Harvard University. Prior to joining the ASU faculty in 1999, he was a partner in a Washington, DC, law firm where his practice focused on environmental and administrative law. Professor Marchant teaches and researches in the subject areas of environmental law, risk assessment and risk management, genetics and the law, biotechnology law, food and drug law, legal aspects of nanotechnology, and law, science, and technology.

Jennifer Merchant, Ph.D., is a professor of Anglo-American legal and political institutions at the Université de Paris II (Panthéon-Assas). She is a leading researcher in bioethical issues of comparative public policy with expertise in comparative North American and European policy, politics, and regulation of medical technologies involving human reproduction. She is also an expert in French law and politics on embryo research and assisted reproductive technology. Her academic interests include comparative public policy, reproduction, bioethics, civil society, science, and government. Dr. Merchant is a member of the French National University Institute, the Centre for the Study and Research of Administrative and Political Sciences, the Ethics Committee of the French National Institute of Health and Medical Research, and the International Network on Feminist Approaches to Bioethics (FAB) Association as well as FAB Country Representative for France. She has been the co-editor-in-chief of the *Revue Tocqueville/Tocqueville Review* since 2001 and a member of the Global Ethics Observatory and the United Nations Educational, Scientific and Cultural Organization since 2005.

Luigi Naldini, M.D., Ph.D., is professor of cell and tissue biology and of gene and cell therapy at the San Raffaele University School of Medicine and scientific director of the San Raffaele Telethon Institute for Gene Therapy, Milan, Italy. Dr. Naldini has pioneered the development and applications of lentiviral vectors for gene transfer, which have become one of the most widely used tool in biomedical research and, upon recently entering clinical testing, are providing a long sought hope of cure for several currently untreatable and otherwise deadly human diseases. Since then he has continued to investigate new strategies to overcome the major hurdles to safe and effective gene transfer, translate them into new therapeutic strategies for genetic disease and cancer, and allowed novel insights into hematopoietic stem cell function, induction of immunological tolerance, and tumor angiogenesis. His recent work also contributed to advancing the use of engineered nucleases for targeted genome editing in cell and gene therapy. Dr. Naldini is a member of the European Molecular Biology Organization, has been president of the European Society of Gene and Cell Therapy (ESGCT), and was awarded an European Research Council Advanced Investigator Grant in 2009, the Outstanding Achievement Award from the American Society of Gene and Cell Therapy in 2014 and from ESGCT in 2015, an Honorary doctorate from the Vrije University, Brussel, in 2015, and the Jimenez Diaz Prize in 2016. He received his M.D. from the University of Torino and his Ph.D. in cell and tissue biology from the University of Rome La Sapienza.

Duanqing Pei, Ph.D., is professor and director general of Guangzhou Institutes of Biomedicine and Health, Chinese Academy of Sciences. Dr. Pei joined the medical faculty at Tsinghua University in Beijing, China, in 2002 and moved to the newly formed Guangzhou Institutes of Biomedicine and Health in 2004. Prior to this appointment, he served as a faculty member at the University of Minnesota School of Medicine. Dr. Pei studied the transcription regulation of hepatitis B virus (HBV) for his Ph.D. thesis and worked on extracellular matrix remodeling as a postdoctoral fellow and faculty member. Upon returning to China, he first started to work on stem cell pluripotency and then on reprogramming. The Pei lab in Tsinghua has published on the structure and function of Oct4, Sox2, FoxD3, Essrb, and Nanog, and their interdependent relationship toward pluripotency. The Pei lab was the first in China to create mouse induced pluripotent stem (iPS) cells using a nonselective system, and then improved the iPS process systematically. The Pei lab subsequently disseminated the iPS technology in China by providing resources and training workshops. Recent publications from the Pei lab includes the discovery of vitamin C as a potent booster for iPS cell generation and that a mesenchymal to epithelial transition initiates the reprogramming process of mouse fibroblasts. Dr. Pei's lab continues to explore new ways to improve iPS technology, dissect the reprogramming mechanisms driven by Oct4/Sox2/Klf4 or fewer factors, develop alternative reprogramming methods, employ iPS cells to model human diseases in vitro, and use gene-editing tools to correct mutations in stem cells for regenerative medicine. Dr. Pei obtained his Ph.D. from the University of Pennsylvania in 1991 and trained as a postdoctoral fellow at the University of Michigan.

Matthew Porteus, M.D., Ph.D., is associate professor of pediatrics, Divisions of Stem Cell Transplantation and Regenerative Medicine, Hematology/Oncology, and Human Gene Therapy at Stanford School of Medicine. He completed his combined M.D.-Ph.D. at Stanford Medical School, with his Ph.D. focusing on understanding the molecular basis of mammalian forebrain development with his Ph.D. thesis titled "Isolation and Characterization of TES-1/DLX-2: A Novel Homeobox Gene Expressed During Mammalian Forebrain Development." After completion of his dual-degree program, he was an intern and resident in pediatrics at Boston Children's Hospital and then completed his pediatric hematology/oncology fellowship in the combined Boston Children's Hospital/Dana Farber Cancer Institute program. For his fellowship and postdoctoral research he worked with Dr. David Baltimore at the Massachusetts Institute of Technology and the California Institute of Technology where he began his studies in developing homologous recombination as a strategy to correct disease-causing mutations in stem cells as definitive and curative therapy for children with genetic diseases of the blood, particularly sickle-cell disease. Following his training with Dr. Baltimore, he took an independent faculty position at University of Texas Southwestern in the Departments of Pediatrics and Biochemistry before again returning to Stanford University in 2010 as an associate professor. During this time his work has been the first to demonstrate that gene correction could be achieved in human cells at frequencies that were high enough to potentially cure patients and is considered one of the pioneers and founders of the field of genome editing—a field that now encompasses thousands of labs and several new companies throughout the world. He has extensive experience with the major engineered nuclease platforms including zinc finger nucleases, transcription activator-like effector nucleases, and CRISPR/Cas9 nucleases. He has used genome-editing strategies in a variety of different stem cells including hematopoietic stem and progenitor cells, neural stem cells, spermatogonial stem cells, human embryonic stem cells, and induced pluripotent cells. His research program continues to focus on developing genome editing by homologous recombination as curative therapy for patients with both genetic and nongenetic diseases. Clinically, Dr. Porteus attends at the Lucille Packard Children's Hospital where he takes care of pediatric patients undergoing hematopoietic stem cell transplantation. Administratively, Dr. Porteus is the associate director of the Stanford Medical Scientist-Training Program where he oversees the admission and progress of students obtaining both M.D. and Ph.D. degrees at Stanford University.

Janet Rossant, Ph.D., is a senior scientist in the Developmental and Stem Cell Biology Program at The Hospital for Sick Children and is a professor in the Department of Molecular Genetics, and the Department of Obstetrics and Gynaecology at the University of Toronto. Her research focuses on understanding the genetic control of normal and abnormal development in the early mouse embryo using both cellular and genetic manipulation techniques. Her interests in the early embryo have led to the discovery of a novel placental stem cell type, the trophoblast stem cell. Dr. Rossant is also the president and scientific director of the Gairdner Foundation. She is actively involved in the international developmental and stem cell biology communities and has contributed to the scientific and ethical discussion on public issues related to stem cell research. She chaired the working group of the Canadian Institutes of Health Research (CIHR) on stem cell research, which came up with guidelines for CIHR-funded research in this area. Dr. Rossant trained at Oxford University and Cambridge University in the United Kingdom and has been in Canada since 1977, first at Brock University and then at the Samuel Lunenfeld Research Institute, Mount Sinai Hospital, Toronto, from 1985 to 2005.

Dietram A. Scheufele, Ph.D., is the John E. Ross Professor in Science Communication and Vilas Distinguished Achievement Professor at the University of Wisconsin–Madison and in the Morgridge Institute for Research. He is also an Honorary Professor of Communication at the Technische Universität Dresden, Germany. Dr. Scheufele has co-chaired the National Academies of Sciences, Engineering, and Medicine's Roundtable on Public Interfaces of the Life Sciences and the National Conference of Lawyers and Scientists, a joint committee of the American Association for the Advancement of Science and the American Bar Association. He is a fellow of the American Association for the Advancement of Science, the International Communication Association, and the Wisconsin Academy of Sciences, Arts, and Letters, and a member of the German National Academy of Science and Engineering. He currently serves on the National Academies of Sciences, Engineering, and Medicine's Division on Earth and Life Studies Advisory Committee. In the past, Dr. Scheufele has been a tenured faculty member at Cornell University, a Shorenstein fellow at Harvard University, and a visiting scholar at the Annenberg Public Policy Center of the University of Pennsylvania. His consulting experience includes work for the Public Broadcasting System, World Health Organization, and World Bank.

Ismail Serageldin, Ph.D., is the founding director of the Bibliotheca Alexandrina (BA), the new Library of Alexandria, inaugurated in 2002. He also chairs the Boards of Directors for each of the BA's affiliated research institutes and museums. He is advisor to the Egyptian Prime Minister in matters concerning culture, science and museums. He serves as chair or member of a number of advisory committees for academic, research, scientific, and international institutions and civil society efforts, including the

Advisory Committee of the World Social Science Report for 2013, as well as the United Nations Educational, Scientific and Cultural Organization–supported World Water Scenarios (2013), and chairs the Executive Council of the World Digital Library (2010), the Executive Council of the Encyclopedia of Life (2010), and the Internet Corporation for Assigned Names and Numbers Panel for the Review of the Internet Future (2013). He also co-chaired the African Union's High-Level Panel on Modern Biotechnology (2006) and again on Science, Technology and Innovation in 2012-2013. He has previously held positions including vice president of the World Bank (1992-2000), chairman of the Consultative Group on International Agricultural Research (1994-2000), and founder and former chairman of the Global Water Partnership (1996-2000) and the Consultative Group to Assist the Poorest, a microfinance program (1995-2000). He was chair of Savoirs Contre Pauvreté (Knowledge Against Poverty), at Collège de France, Paris, and distinguished professor at Wageningen University in the Netherlands. He is a member of many academies, including the U.S. National Academy of Sciences (Public Welfare Medalist), the American Philosophical Society, the American Academy of Arts and Sciences, the World Academy of Sciences, the World Academy of Arts and Sciences, the European Academy of Sciences and Arts, the African Academy of Sciences, Institut d'Egypte (Egyptian Academy of Science), the Royal Belgian Academy, the Bangladesh Academy of Sciences, and the Indian National Academy of Agricultural Sciences. Dr. Serageldin has published more than 100 books and more than 500 papers on a variety of topics, including biotechnology, rural development, sustainability, and the value of science to society. He has hosted a cultural program on television in Egypt (more than 130 episodes) and developed a television Science Series in Arabic and English. He holds a bachelor of science degree in engineering from Cairo University, a master's degree and a Ph.D. from Harvard University, and has received 34 honorary doctorates.

Sharon Terry, M.A., is president and CEO of Genetic Alliance, a network of more than 10,000 organizations, of which 1,200 are disease advocacy organizations. Genetic Alliance engages individuals, families, and communities to transform health. Ms. Terry is also the founding CEO of PXE International, a research advocacy organization for the genetic condition pseudoxanthoma elasticum (PXE), which affects Ms. Terry's two adult children. As co-discoverer of the gene associated with PXE, she holds the patent for ABCC6 to act as its steward and has assigned her rights to the foundation. She developed a diagnostic test and conducts clinical trials. She is the author of 140 peer-reviewed papers, of which 30 are PXE clinical studies. Ms. Terry is also a co-founder of the Genetic Alliance Registry and Biobank. In her focus at the forefront of consumer participation in genetics research, services, and policy, she serves in a leadership role on many of the major international and national organizations, including the Accelerating Medicines Partnership, the National Academies of Sciences, Engineering, and Medicine's Science and Policy Board, the National Academies' Roundtable on Translating Genomic-Based Research for Health, the PubMed Central National Advisory Committee, the PhenX scientific advisory board, the Global Alliance for Genomics and Health, the International Rare Disease Research Consortium Executive Committee, and as Founding President of EspeRare Foundation of Geneva, Switzerland. She is on the editorial boards of several journals and is an editor of *Genome*. She led the coalition that was instrumental in the passage of the Genetic Information Nondiscrimination Act. She received an honorary doctorate from Iona College for her work in community engagement in 2006; the first Patient Service Award from the University of North Carolina Institute for Pharmacogenomics and Individualized Therapy in 2007; the Research!America Distinguished Organization Advocacy Award in 2009; and the Clinical Research Forum and Foundation's Annual Award for Leadership in Public Advocacy in 2011. In 2012, she became an honorary professor of Hebei United University in Tangshan, China, and also received the Facing Our Risk of Cancer Empowered (FORCE) Spirit of Empowerment Advocacy Award. She was named one of the U.S. Food and Drug Administration's "30 Heroes for the Thirtieth Anniversary of the Orphan Drug Act" in 2013. In 2012 and 2013, Ms. Terry won $400,000 in first prizes in three large competitions for the Platform for Engaging Everyone Responsibly (PEER). PEER was awarded a $1 million contract from the Patient-Centered Outcomes Research Institute in 2014.

Jonathan Weissman, Ph.D., is a professor of cellular and molecular pharmacology at the University of California, San Francisco, and a Howard Hughes Medical Institute investigator. His research explores how cells ensure that proteins fold into their correct shape, as well as the role of protein misfolding in disease and normal physiology. He is also developing experimental and analytical approaches for exploring the organizational principles of biological systems and globally monitoring protein translation through ribosome profiling. A broad goal of his work is to bridge large-scale approaches and in-depth mechanistic investigations to reveal the information encoded within genomes.

Keith Yamamoto, Ph.D., is University of California, San Francisco, vice chancellor for science policy and strategy. He also serves as vice dean for research for the School of Medicine, and professor of cellular and molecular pharmacology. Dr. Yamamoto's research focuses on signaling and transcriptional regulation by nuclear receptors, which mediate the actions of essential hormones and cellular signals; he uses mechanistic and systems approaches to pursue these problems in pure molecules, cells, and whole organisms. He has led or served on numerous national committees focused on public and scientific policy, public understanding and support of biological research, and science education; he chairs the Coalition for the Life Sciences, and sits on the National Academy of Medicine Council and the National Academies of Sciences, Engineering, and Medicine's Division on Earth and Life Studies Advisory Committee. He has chaired or served on many committees that oversee training and the biomedical workforce, research funding, and the process of peer review and the policies that govern it at the National Institutes of Health. He is a member of the advisory board for Lawrence Berkeley National Laboratory and the board of directors of Research!America. He was elected to the National Academy of Sciences, the National Academy of Medicine, the American Academy of Arts and Sciences, and the American Academy of Microbiology, and is a fellow of the American Association for the Advancement of Science.

E

Glossary

Adult stem cell—An undifferentiated cell found in a differentiated tissue in an adult organism that can renew itself and can differentiate to yield specialized cell types of the tissue in which it is found (NRC, 2002, p. 259).

Allele—A variant form of a gene at a particular locus on a chromosome. Different alleles produce variations in inherited characteristics (NASEM, 2016a, p. 180).

Aneuploidy—The presence of an abnormal number of chromosomes in a cell.

Assisted reproductive technology (ART)—A fertility treatment or procedure that involves laboratory handling of gametes (eggs and sperm) or embryos. Examples of ART include in vitro fertilization (IVF) and intracytoplasmic sperm injection (ICSI) (NRC, 2002, p. 260).

Autologous transplant—Transplanted tissue derived from the intended recipient of the transplant. Such a transplant helps to avoid complications of immune rejection (IOM, 2005, p. 115).

Blastocyst—A preimplantation embryo in placental mammals (about 5 days after fertilization in humans) of 50-150 cells. The blastocyst consists of a sphere made up of an outer layer of cells (the trophectoderm), a fluid-filled cavity (the blastocoel or blastocyst cavity), and a cluster of cells in the in-

293

terior (the inner cell mass) (IOM, 2005, p. 115). Cells from the inner cell mass, if grown in culture, can give rise to embryonic stem cell lines.

Cas9 (CRISPR Associated Protein 9)—A specialized enzyme known as a nuclease that has the ability to cut DNA sequences. Cas9 makes up part of the "toolkit" for the CRISPR/Cas9 method of genome editing.

Chimera—An organism composed of cells derived from at least two genetically different individuals (NRC, 2002, p. 261).

Choriocarcinoma—A type of tumor that originates from the trophoblast, the precursor of the placenta, and invades the uterine wall.

Chromatin—The complex of DNA and proteins that forms chromosomes. Some of the proteins are structural, helping to organize and protect the DNA, while others are regulatory, acting to control whether genes are active or not, and to promote DNA replication or repair.

Chromosome—A thread-like structure that contains a single length of DNA, usually carrying many hundreds of genes. This is packaged with proteins to form chromatin. The DNA within the complete cellular set of chromosomes (23 pairs in humans) comprises two copies of the genome, one from each parent. The chromosomes usually reside in the nucleus of a cell, except during cell division when the nuclear membrane breaks down and the chromosomes become condensed and can be visualized as discrete entities.

Cleavage—The process of cell division in the very early embryo before it becomes a blastocyst (NRC, 2002, p. 261). Also used to describe breaking or cutting DNA.

Clinical application—The use of a biomedical reagent, procedure, or device to treat a clinical condition.

Clinical trial—A supervised and monitored experimental test in patients of a newly developed clinical application to ensure minimization of risk and optimization of efficacy. Clinical trials are required before a treatment is approved for general use.

CRISPR (Clustered Regularly-Interspaced Short Palindromic Repeats)—A naturally occurring mechanism found in bacteria that involves the retention of fragments of foreign DNA, providing the bacteria with some immunity to viruses. The system is sometimes referred to as CRISPR/Cas9 to denote the entire gene-editing platform in which RNA homologous with the targeted gene is combined with Cas9 (CRISPR Associated Protein 9), which is a DNA-cutting enzyme (nuclease) to form the "toolkit" for the CRISPR/Cas9 method of genome editing.

CRISPRa—CRISPR activation, using a guide RNA and nuclease-deficient or nuclease-dead Cas9 (dCas9) linked to one or more activation domains to increase transcription of a target gene.

CRISPRr/CRISPRi—CRISPR repression, or CRISPR interference, using a dCas9 or dCas9-repressor with a guide RNA to decrease transcription of a target gene.

Cultured cell—A cell maintained in a tissue culture allowing expansion of its numbers.

dCas9 (Nuclease-deficient Cas9 or nuclease-dead Cas9)—This can still bind DNA, together with a guide RNA, but not cut it. It is often linked to a transcription factor, chromatin-modifying enzyme, or fluorescent protein to mediate alterations to gene expression or to mark specific sites.

Deontology ethics—A normative theory regarding which choices are morally required, forbidden, or permitted.

Deoxyribonucleic acid (DNA)—A two-stranded molecule, arranged as a double helix, that contains the genetic instructions used in the development, functioning, and reproduction of all known living organisms.

Differentiation—The process whereby an unspecialized early embryonic cell acquires the features of a specialized cell, such as a heart, liver, or muscle cell (IOM, 2005, p. 116).

Diploid—Cells that contain a full set of DNA—half from each parent. In humans, diploid cells contain 46 chromosomes (in 23 pairs).

Divergence (evolutionary)—During evolution, variations occur in the sequences of genes; if these variations confer some advantage natural selection increases their prevalence. Different selective pressures select for different variations so that the prevalence of different gene variants diverges in different populations.

Dominant—A pattern of inheritance of a gene or trait in which a single copy of a particular allele (gene variant) confers a function independent of the nature of the second copy of the gene in a diploid cell of an organism.

Double-strand break (DSB)—A break in the DNA double helix in which both strands are cut, as distinct from a single-strand break or "nick."

Ectoderm—The outermost of the three primitive germ layers of the embryo; it gives rise to skin, nerves, and brain (IOM, 2005, p. 116).

Ectopic—Found in an unusual location, such as an ectopic pregnancy outside the uterus.

Embryo—An animal in the early stages of growth and differentiation that are characterized by cleavage (cell division of the fertilized egg), differentiation of fundamental cell types and tissues, and the formation of primitive organs and organ systems; the developing human individual from the time of implantation to the end of the eighth week after conception, after which stage it becomes known as a fetus (adapted from IOM, 2005, p. 116).

Embryonic germ (EG) cell—A pluripotent stem cell that migrates during early development to the future gonads to form the progenitors of egg or sperm cells. The properties of EG cells are similar to those of embryonic stem cells, but may differ in the DNA methylation of some imprinted regions (NRC, 2002, p. 263).

Embryonic stem (ES) cell—A primitive (undifferentiated) cell from the embryo that has the potential to become a wide variety of specialized cell types (i.e., is pluripotent). It is derived from the inner cell mass of the blastocyst. An embryonic stem cell is not an embryo; by itself, it cannot produce the necessary cell types, such as trophectoderm cells, so as to give rise to a complete organism (NAS, 2002, p. 263). Embryonic stem cells can be maintained as pluripotent cells in culture and induced to differentiate into many different cell types .

Endoderm—Innermost of the three primitive germ layers of the embryo; it later gives rise to the lungs, liver, and digestive organs (IOM, 2005, p. 116).

Endogenous—Originating from within a cell or an organism.

Endometrium—The inner epithelial lining of the uterus into which embryos implant.

Endonuclease—An enzyme that breaks down a nucleotide chain into two or more shorter chains by cleaving at internal phosphodiester bonds.

Enhancement—Improving a condition or trait beyond a typical or normal level.

Enucleated cell—A cell whose nucleus has been removed (IOM, 2005, p. 116).

Enucleation—A process whereby the nuclear material of a cell is removed, leaving only the cytoplasm. When applied to an egg, can involve the removal of the maternal chromosomes, when they are not surrounded by a nuclear membrane (adapted from NRC, 2002, p. 263).

Enzyme—A protein that acts as a biological catalyst, speeding up chemical reactions.

Epiblast—A specific layer of cells in an early vertebrate embryo that gives rise to the entire embryo other than yolk sac and placenta. Epiblast cells are pluripotent and can give rise to embryonic stem cells.

Epigenetic effects—Changes in gene expression that occur without changing the DNA sequence of a gene; for example, in the epigenetic effect called genomic imprinting, chemical molecules called methyl groups attach to DNA and alter the gene's expression (NRC, 2002, p. 263).

Epigenome—A set of chemical modifications to the DNA of the genome and to proteins that bind to DNA in the chromosomes to affect whether and how genes are expressed.

Ex vivo—Latin: "out of the living"; outside an organism.

Exogenous—Introduced or originating from outside a cell or an organism.

Fertilization—The process whereby male and female gametes (sperm and egg) unite (NRC, 2002, p. 264).

FokI—The nuclease from which the cleavage domain has been abstracted and joined to zinc finger (ZF) or transcription activator-like effector (TALE) DNA-binding domains. The FokI cleavage domain cuts only one strand of the DNA (a nick), so a pair of ZFNs or TALENs is required to create double-strand breaks. The FokI cleavage domain has also been linked to nuclease-deficient Cas9 (dCas9), and this fusion must also dimerize to cut DNA.

Gain of function—A type of mutation that results in an altered gene product that possesses a new molecular function or a new pattern of gene expression (NRC and IOM, 2015, p. 1).

Gamete—A reproductive cell (egg or sperm). Gametes are haploid (having only half the number of chromosomes found in somatic cells—23 in humans), so that when two gametes unite at fertilization, the resulting one-cell embryo (zygote) has the full number of chromosomes (46 in humans) (NRC, 2002, p. 264).

Gastrulation—The procedure by which an animal embryo at an early stage of development produces the three primary germ layers—ectoderm, mesoderm, and endoderm (IOM, 2005, p. 117).

Gene—A functional unit of heredity that is a segment of DNA in a specific site on a chromosome. A gene typically directs the formation of a protein or RNA molecule (NRC, 2002, p. 264).

Gene drive—A system of biased inheritance in which the ability of a particular genetic sequence to pass from a parent to its offspring through sexual reproduction is enhanced (NASEM, 2016a, p. 182). Gene drive technology actively copies a sequence on one chromosome to its partner chromosome, so that the organism carries two copies of the intentionally modified gene. This process ensures that all of an organism's offspring and subsequent generations will inherit the edited genome and related trait(s). Thus, the result of a gene drive is the preferential increase of a specific genotype from one generation to the next, and potentially throughout a population (NASEM, 2016a, p. 182).

Gene editing—A technique that allows researchers to alter the DNA of cells or organisms to insert, delete, or modify a gene or gene sequences to silence, enhance, or otherwise change the gene's characteristics (NASEM, 2016a, p. 182).

Gene expression—The process by which RNA and proteins are made from the instructions encoded in genes. Gene expression is controlled by proteins and RNA molecules that bind to the genome or to the RNA copy and regulate their levels of production and those of their products. Alterations in gene expression change the functions of cells, tissues, organs, or whole organisms and sometimes result in observable characteristics associated with a particular gene (adapted from NRC, 2002, p. 264).

Gene targeting—A procedure used to produce an alteration in a specific gene (IOM, 2005, p. 117).

Gene therapy—Introduction of exogenous genes into cells with the goal of ameliorating a disease condition.

Gene transfer—Any process often used to describe the transfer of genes into cells—as used in gene therapy.

Genetic element—A segment of the DNA in a genome that has some particular property conferred by its sequence, such as a gene encoding a protein or RNA—more often used to refer to sequences that are not such genes but may control gene expression or genome organization.

Genome—The complete set of DNA that makes up an organism (NASEM, 2016a, p. 182). In humans, the genome is organized into 23 pairs of homologous chromosomes.

Genome editing—The process by which the genome sequence is changed through the intervention of a DNA break or other DNA modification.

Genotype—Genetic constitution of an individual (IOM, 2005, p. 117).

Germ cell (or germline cell)—A cell at any point in the lineage of cells that will give rise to sperm or eggs. The germline is this lineage of cells. Eggs and sperm fuse during sexual reproduction to create an embryo. In so doing, the germline continues into the next generation.

Germ layer—In early development, the embryo differentiates into three distinct germ layers (ectoderm, endoderm, and mesoderm), each of which gives rise to different parts of the developing organism (IOM, 2005, p. 117).

Gestation—The period of development of an organism from fertilization of the egg until birth (NRC, 202, p. 265).

Governance The process of exercising oversight through traditions (standards of practice) or regulations by which individuals and communities are held accountable. Governance often involves such policy tools as professional standards of practice and codes of conduct; formal guidelines, agreements, and treaties; and legislation or other governmental regulation (NASEM, 2016a, p. 183).

Guide molecule—A protein or short section of RNA used to guide the genome-editing machinery to the desired location in the DNA sequence.

Guide RNA (gRNA)—Short segments of RNA used to direct the DNA-cutting enzyme to the target location in the genome. gRNA segments contain the region of homology to the target sequence (usually 20 bases), and a sequence that interacts with the nuclease (e.g., Cas9). gRNAs used in genome editing are synthetic and do not occur in nature.

Haploid—Refers to a cell (usually a gamete or its immediate precursor) having only one set of chromosomes (23 in humans). In contrast, body cells (somatic cells) are diploid, having two sets of chromosomes (46 in humans) (adapted from NRC, 2002, p. 265).

Heritable genetic change—Modifications to genes that could be passed down through generations.

Heterozygous—Having two different variants (alleles) of a specific gene on the two homologous chromosomes of a cell or an organism.

Homologous recombination—Recombining of two like DNA molecules, including a process by which gene targeting produces an alteration in a specific gene (adapted from IOM, 2005, p. 118).

Homology-directed repair (HDR)—A natural repair process used to repair broken DNA, which relies on a DNA "template" with homology to the broken stretch of DNA. This usually occurs during or after DNA synthesis, which provides this template. In genome editing via HDR, the DNA template is synthesised or made by recombinant DNA techniques, and usually contains regions of exact homology to the target locus at each end, with the desired alteration contained within the middle.

Homozygous—Having the same variant (allele) of a specific gene on both homologous chromosomes of a cell or an organism.

Human Fertilisation and Embryology Authority (HFEA)—The United Kingdom's independent regulator overseeing the use of germ cells and embryos in fertility treatment and research (HFEA, 2013). It also stands for the Human Fertilisation and Embryology Act, the law under which the Authority operates and which it upholds.

Implantation—The process by which an embryo becomes attached to the inside of the uterus (7-14 days in humans) (NRC, 2002, p. 265).

In utero—Latin: "in the uterus."

In vitro—Latin: "in glass"; in a laboratory dish or test tube; in an artificial environment (NRC, 2002, p. 265).

In vitro fertilization (IVF)—An assisted reproduction technique in which fertilization is accomplished outside the body (NRC, 2002, p. 265).

In vivo—Latin: "in the living"; in a natural environment, usually in the body of the subject. This term is often also used to refer to events in "living" cells in culture (adapted from NRC, 2002, p. 265).

Indel—An insertion or deletion of DNA sequence. Small indels (e.g., one to four base pairs) are often associated with nonhomologous end joining. These often result in the disruption of a gene by shifting the open reading frame and/or creating premature stop codons.

Induced pluripotent stem (iPS) cell—A cell induced by the introduction or activation of genes conferring pluripotency and stem celllike properties. Thus, cells already committed to a particular fate (e.g., skin) can be induced to become pluripotent. This is useful in regenerative medicine because the iPS cells can be introduced back into the donor of the original cells with much less risk of transplant rejection.

Insertional mutagenesis—The alteration of the sequence of a gene by the insertion of exogenous sequence such as by integration of viral sequences.

Institutional review board (IRB)—An administrative body in an institution (such as a hospital or a university) established to protect the rights and welfare of human research subjects recruited to participate in research activities conducted under the auspices of that institution. The IRB has the authority to approve, require modifications in, or disapprove research activities in its jurisdiction, as specified by both federal regulations and local institutional policy (NRC, 2002, p. 266).

Lentivirus—A subclass of retroviruses, viruses whose genome are made of RNA but during viral replication becomes copied into a DNA form that can integrate into the DNA genome of a cell. Often used as carriers of genes (vectors) to introduce genes into cells.

Ligase—An enzyme that catalyzes joining of two pieces of DNA.

Loss of function—A type of mutation in which the altered gene product lacks the molecular function of the wild-type gene (MGI, 2017).

Meganuclease—A special type of enzyme that binds to and cuts DNA at specific DNA sequences of a length that occurs at few sites in the genome. These are natural enzymes (and their synthetic derivatives) that catalyze DNA rearrangement events via DNA cleavage.. They can be used in genome editing for both nonhomologous end joining and homology directed repair–mediated alterations. It was the study of these that first revealed the basic mechanisms of DNA cleavage and the DNA repair processes on which genome editing depends.

Mesoderm—The middle layer of the embryo, which consists of a group of cells derived from the inner cell mass of the blastocyst; it is formed at gastrulation and is the precursor to blood, bone, muscle, and connective tissue.

Mitochondrial transfer (or mitochondrial replacement)—Novel procedures designed to prevent the maternal transmission of mitochondrial DNA (mtDNA) diseases (NASEM, 2016b, p. 1).

Mitochondrion (plural, Mitochondria)—A cellular structure in the cytoplasm that provides energy to the cell. Each cell contains many mitochondria. In humans, a single mitochondrion contains 37 genes on a circular mitochondrial DNA, compared with about 35,000 genes contained in the nuclear DNA (NRC, 2002, p. 267).

Mosaicism—Variation among cells, such that the cells are not all the same—for example, in an embryo when not all the cells are edited.

Multipotent stem cells—Stem cells from the embryo, fetus, or adult, whose progeny are of multiple differentiated cell types and usually, but not necessarily, all of a particular tissue, organ, or physiological system (NRC, 2002, p. 267).

Murine—Derived from mice.

Mutation—A change in a DNA sequence. Mutations can occur spontaneously during cell division or can be triggered by environmental stresses, such as sunlight, radiation, and chemicals (NRC, 2002, p. 267).

Nickase—A nuclease that cuts only one strand of the DNA double helix.

Nonhomologous end joining (NHEJ)—A natural repair process used to join the two ends of a broken DNA strand back together. This is prone to errors where short indels (usually of two to four base pairs of DNA) are introduced.

Normative theory—A theory of how people should make decisions, as opposed to how they actually do or will make decisions.

Nuclease—An enzyme that can cut through DNA or RNA strands.

Off-target effect—A direct or indirect, unintended, short- or long-term consequence of an intervention on an organism other than the intended effect on that organism (NASEM, 2016, p. 184).

Off-target event (or off-target cleavage)—when a genome-editing nuclease cuts DNA at a location other than the one for which it was targeted. This can occur because the off-target sequence is similar to but not identical with the intended target sequence.

Oocyte—Developing egg; usually a large and immobile cell.

Phenotype—Observable properties of an organism that are influenced by both its genotype and its environment.

Plasmid—A self-replicating circular DNA molecule. A plasmid can be engineered to carry and express genes of interest in target cells.

Pluripotent stem cell (PSC)—A stem cell that includes in its progeny all cell types that can be found in a postimplantation embryo, fetus, or developed organism (NRC, 2002, p. 268).

Population—All of the individuals of a given species within a defined ecological area (NASEM, 2016a, p. 184).

Preclinical research—Research conducted to investigate potential clinical applications but not involving humans. For example, research on molecules, cells, tissues, or animals.

Precursor cell or Progenitor cell—In fetal or adult tissues, it is a partially committed but not fully differentiated cell that divides and gives rise to differentiated cells (adapted from NRC, 2002, p. 269).

Preimplantation genetic diagnosis (PGD)—Before an in vitro–fertilized embryo is implanted in a woman's uterus, it can be screened for specific genetic mutations that are known to cause particular genetic diseases or for chromosomal abnormalities. One or more cells are removed from the preimplantation embryo for testing (NRC, 2002, p. 269) and the surviving embryo that is implanted is one that is not carrying the genetic abnormality.

Prenatal diagnosis—Detection of abnormalities and disease conditions while a fetus is developing in the uterus. Many techniques for prenatal diagnosis, such as chorionic villus sampling and amniocentesis, require sampling placental tissue or fetal cells found in the amniotic fluid or feto-maternal circulation. Others, such as ultrasonography, can be performed without cell or tissue samples (NRC, 2002, p. 269).

Primitive streak—An elongated band of cells that forms along the axis of an embryo early in gastrulation by the movement of lateral cells toward the axis and that develops a groove along its midline through which cells move to the interior of the embryo to form the mesoderm (adapted from Grossinger, 2000, p. 815).

Pronucleus—The haploid nucleus of an oocyte or sperm, either prior to fertilization or immediately after fertilization, before the sperm and egg nuclei have fused into a single diploid nucleus.

Protein—A large complex molecule made up of one or more chains of amino acids. Proteins perform a wide variety of activities in the cell (NRC, 2002, p. 269).

Recessive—A recessive allele of a gene is one whose effects are masked by the second allele present in a diploid cell or organism, which is referred to as dominant.

Recombinant DNA—A recombinant DNA molecule is made up of DNA sequences that have been artificially modified or joined together so that the new genetic sequence differs from naturally occurring genetic material (IOM, 2014, p. 23).

Recombinant DNA Advisory Committee (RAC)—Oversees and reviews proposals for research funded by the National Institutes of Health (NIH) or similar projects conducted at institutions funded by NIH that involve recombinant or synthetic DNA, such as gene therapy (adapted from NASEM, 2016b, p. 62).

Recombination—The process, natural or engineered, in which two pieces of DNA undergo breakage and reunion to generate a new combination of DNA segments.

Regenerative medicine—Medical treatments that seek to replace defective, damaged, or missing tissue by engineered cells, tissues, or implants, often involving stem cells.

Restriction enzyme—An enzyme from bacteria that is used to cut DNA at defined sequences, used in DNA analysis and in joining DNA fragments through the cut ends.

Retrovirus—A virus whose genome is made of RNA but during viral replication becomes copied into a DNA form that can integrate into the DNA genome of a cell. Often used as carriers of genes (vectors) to introduce genes into cells. A subset of retroviruses is called lentiviruses.

Risk—The probability of an effect on a specific endpoint or a set of endpoints due to a specific set of a stressor or stressors. An effect can be beneficial or harmful (NASEM, 2016a, p. 185).

Risk assessment—The process by which all available evidence on the probability of effects is collected, evaluated, and interpreted to estimate the probability of the sum total of effects (NASEM, 2016a, p. 185).

RNA (ribonucleic acid)—A chemical that is similar in structure to DNA. One of its main functions is to translate the genetic code of DNA into structural proteins.

RNP (ribonuclear protein complex)—Many types exist within cells, and this is a general term encompassing all of these, but in the context of genome editing it is often used to refer to a guide RNA molecule combined with a DNA-cutting enzyme such as Cas9.

Selective advantage—Some variants of genes provide a trait that confers a survival or a reproductive advantage that can be selected by natural selection and therefore increases in prevalence in a population.

Single guide RNA (sgRNA)—A short piece of RNA that binds to a nuclease such as Cas9 and also to a specific DNA sequence to guide the nuclease to a specific location in the genome. This term is synonymous with guide RNA (vide infra) in most usages.

Somatic cell—Any cell of a plant or animal other than a reproductive cell or reproductive cell precursor. Latin: soma = body (NRC, 2002, p. 270).

Somatic cell nuclear transfer (SCNT)—The transfer of a cell nucleus from a somatic cell into an egg (oocyte) whose nucleus has been removed (IOM, 2005, p. 119).

Spermatogonial stem cells—The self-replicating precursors of sperm cells.

Stem cell—A nonspecialized cell that has the capacity to divide indefinitely in culture and to differentiate into more mature cells with specialized functions.

Stem cell therapy—The use of stem cells in regenerative medicine to replace defective, damaged, or missing tissue.

Syncytiotrophoblast cell—A cell derived from trophectodermal cells from the early mammalian embryo that fuse (into multinucleate syncitia) and contribute to the structure and function of the placentae.

Synthetic biology—The development of living cells from separate genetic components, using engineering principles to build desired functions into living organisms.

Synthetic DNA—DNA molecules that are chemically or by other means synthesized or amplified; they may be chemically or otherwise modified but can base pair, or be recombined with, naturally occurring DNA molecules.

T cells—Types of white blood cells that are of crucial importance in the immune system. They cooperate with other immune cells in killing infected or cancerous cells but can also participate in inflammation or in autoimmunity when they become activated against an organism's own cells or tissues.

Target sequence—Specific sequence of DNA bases within the genome that is the target of genome-editing tools. For CRISPR/Cas9 methods this will be a 20 nucleotide sequence that the gRNAs are designed to recognize (i.e., they will contain a complementary sequence of the same length).

Therapy (or therapeutic intervention)—The treatment or prevention of disease or disability.

Tissue culture—The growth of cells or tissue segments in vitro in an artificial medium for experimental research (IOM, 2005, p. 120).

Totipotent cell—A stem cell that has unlimited developmental capability. The totipotent cells of the very early embryo (an embryo prior to the blastocyst stage) have the capacity to differentiate into extraembryonic tissues, membranes, the embryo, and all postembryonic tissues and organs (NRC, 2002, p. 271).

Transcription—Making an RNA copy from a gene or other DNA sequence. Transcription is the first step in gene expression (NRC, 2002, p. 271).

Transcription Activator-Like Effector Nuclease (TALEN)—A class of engineered restriction enzymes generated by the fusion of a transcription activator-like effector DNA-binding domain (that binds to a specific DNA sequence) to a DNA-cleavage domain (nuclease) to be used as a genome-editing tool (adapted from NASEM, 2016a, p. 186). TALENs followed zinc finger nucleases and preceded CRISPR/Cas9 as genome-editing tools.

Transcription factor—A protein that binds to control regions (enhancers and promoters) of genes to activate or repress their transcription (or expression).

Transfection—A method by which experimental DNA may be introduced into a cell (adapted from IOM, 2005, p. 120).

Transgene—A gene or genetic material that has been introduced into a cell or organism. Transgenes can be integrated at random, or targeted to a specific site by homologous recombination or by genome editing using methods of homology-directed repair.

Transgenic organism—An organism into which one or more genes from another species (transgenes) have been transferred or otherwise artificially introduced.

Transhumanism—A class of philosophies of life that seek the continuation and acceleration of the evolution of intelligent life beyond its currently human form and human limitations by means of science and technology, guided by life promoting principles and values (More, 1990).

Translation—The process of forming a protein molecule from information contained in a messenger RNA (NRC, 2002, p. 271)—a step in gene expression following transcription (copying of RNA from DNA).

Trophectoderm—The outer layer of the developing blastocyst that will ultimately form the embryonic side of the placenta (NRC, 2002, p. 271).

Undifferentiated—Not having developed into a specialized cell or tissue type (NRC, 2002, p. 271).

Unipotent stem cell—A stem cell that both divides and gives rise to a single mature cell type, such as a spermatogenic stem cell, which only gives rise to sperm (NRC, 2002, p. 271). Alternatively called a progenitor.

Utilitarianism—The morally right action as the action that produces the most "good."

Variant—Genes have many variants in a population that can differ somewhat in function, some being advantageous and some being deleterious or nonfunctional.

Vector—A vehicle that transfers a gene into a new site (analogous to insect vectors that transfer a virus or parasite into a new animal host). Vectors used in molecular cell biology and genetic engineering include plasmids and modified viruses engineered to carry and express genes of interest in target cells. The most clinically relevant viral vectors for gene transfer include retroviral, lentiviral, adenoviral, and adeno-associated viral vectors.

Virtue ethics—A focus on moral character as opposed to duties (deontology) or consequences (consequentialism).

Wild type (noun); Wild-type (adjective)—The "normal" type of an organism or a gene.

X-inactivation—The process in which one X chromosome of the two present in a female mammalian cell is inactivated so that only the genes of one X chromosome are expressed.

Zinc finger—A small protein structure based on naturally occurring transcription factors that bind to defined DNA sequences to control the activity of nearby genes. Zinc fingers can be custom engineered to target a specific section of the DNA sequence for use in genome engineering.

Zinc finger nuclease (ZFN)—A class of engineered enzymes generated by the fusion of zinc finger DNA-binding domains to a DNA-cleavage enzyme (usually FokI) that can be used as a genome-editing tool (adapted from

NASEM, 2016a, p. 186). One of the first and a reliable method of genome editing.

Zygote—The one-cell embryo formed by the union of sperm and egg at fertilization (NRC, 2002, p. 272).

REFERENCES

Grossinger, R. 2000. *Embryogenesis: Species, gender, and identity.* Berkeley, CA: North Atlantic Books.

HFEA (Human Fertilisation and Embryology Authority). 2013. *What we do.* http://www.hfea.gov.uk/133.html (accessed May 10, 2017).

IOM (Institute of Medicine). 2005. *Guidelines for human embryonic stem cell research*, Vol. 23. Washington, DC: The National Academies Press.

IOM. 2014. *Oversight and review of clinical gene transfer protocols: Assessing the role of the recombinant DNA advisory committee.* Washington, DC: The National Academies Press.

MGI (Mouse Genome Informatics). 2017. *MGI glossary*, s.v. "loss of function." http://www.informatics.jax.org/glossary/loss-of-function (accessed May 10, 2017).

More, M. 1990. "Religion, Eupraxophy, and Transhumanism" in *Transhumanism: Towards a futurist philosophy.* https://www.scribd.com/doc/257580713/Transhumanism-Toward-a-Futurist-Philosophy (accessed January 25, 2017).

NASEM (National Academies of Sciences, Engineering, and Medicine). 2016a. *Gene drives on the horizon: Advancing science, navigating uncertainty, and aligning research with public values.* Washington, DC: The National Academies Press.

NASEM. 2016b. *Mitochondrial replacement techniques: Ethical, social, and policy considerations.* Washington, DC: The National Academies Press.

NRC (National Research Council). 2002. *Scientific and medical aspects of human reproductive cloning.* Washington, DC: National Academy Press.

NRC and IOM (Institute of Medicine). 2015. *Potential risks and benefits of gain-of-function research: Summary of a workshop.* Washington, DC: The National Academies Press.